SOAP

for

The Rotations

SOAP

for
The Rotations

SECOND EDITION

PETER S. UZELAC, MD, FACOG, HCLD (ABB)
Founder and CEO
Marin Fertility Center
Lab Director
MFC Lab, Inc.
Greenbrae, California

Special Contributor
DANIEL C. MALDONADO, MD
Attending Physician of Family Medicine
Assistant Director of Inpatient Medicine
White Memorial Medical Center (WMMC)
WMMC Family Practice Residency Program
Los Angeles, California
Assistant Clinical Professor
Department of Family Medicine
University of Southern California, Keck School of Medicine
Los Angeles, California

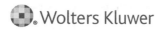
. Wolters Kluwer

Philadelphia · Baltimore · New York · London
Buenos Aires · Hong Kong · Sydney · Tokyo

Acquisitions Editor: Matt Hauber
Development Editor: Andrea Vosburgh
Editorial Coordinator: Julie Kostelnik
Marketing Manager: Phyllis Hitner
Senior Production Project Manager: Alicia Jackson
Design Coordinator: Elaine Kasmer
Manufacturing Coordinator: Margie Orzech
Prepress Vendor: TNQ Technologies

9 8 7 6 5 4 3 2 1

Printed in China

Library of Congress Cataloging-in-Publication Data

ISBN-13: 978-1-975107-65-9

Cataloging in Publication data available on request from publisher.

For Alina, Pierce, Alain, and Elle

CONTENTS

ACKNOWLEDGMENTS

I would like to thank all of the SOAP authors for their hard work and commitment to making this series a success. I would also like to express special appreciation to Matt Hauber, Julie Kostelnik, and Andrea Vosburgh at Wolters Kluwer for their patience and persistence in keeping this project on track.

CONTRIBUTORS

Jennifer Agard, MD, FACOG
Marin Fertility Center
Greenbrae, California
Section 3: Obstetrics and Gynecology

Terako Amison, MD
Assistant Professor, Department of Psychiatry
Psychiatry Clerkship Director, Vanderbilt School of Medicine
Nashville, Tennessee
Section 5: Psychiatry

Spencer Degerstedt
Interventional Radiology Resident
Oregon Health & Science University
Portland, Oregon
Section 4: Surgery and Emergency Medicine

Zaiba Jetpuri, DO
Assistant Professor
Department of Family and Community Medicine
University of Texas, Southwestern Medical Center
Dallas, Texas
Section 2: Pediatrics

Daniel C. Maldonado, MD
Attending Physician of Family Medicine
Assistant Director of Inpatient Medicine
White Memorial Medical Center (WMMC)
WMMC Family Practice Residency Program
Los Angeles, California
Assistant Clinical Professor
Department of Family Medicine
University of Southern California, Keck School of Medicine
Los Angeles, California
Section 1: Internal Medicine

Nida Zahra, MD
Assistant Professor and Medical Director
Department of Family and Community Medicine
University of Texas, Southwestern Medical Center
Dallas, Texas
Section 2: Pediatrics

Like most medical students, I started my ward experience head down and running, eager to finally make contact with real patients. What I found was a confusing world, completely different from anything I had known during the first 2 years of medical school. New language, foreign abbreviations, and residents too busy to set my bearings straight: Where would I begin?

Pocket textbooks, offering medical knowledge in a convenient and portable package, seemed to be the logical solution. Unfortunately, I found myself spending valuable time sifting through large amounts of text, often not finding the answer to my question, and in the process missing out on teaching points during rounds!

I designed the SOAP series to provide medical students and house staff with pocket manuals that truly serve their intended purpose: quick accessibility to the most practical clinical information in a user-friendly format. At the inception of this project, I envisioned all of the benefits the SOAP format would bring to the reader:

- Learning through this model reinforces a thought process that is already familiar to students and residents, facilitating easier long-term retention.
- SOAP promotes good communication between physicians and facilitates the teaching/learning process.
- SOAP puts the emphasis back on the patient's clinical problem and not the diagnosis.
- In the age of managed care, SOAP meets the challenge of providing efficiency while maintaining quality.
- As sound medical-legal practice gains attention in physician training, SOAP emphasizes adherence to a documentation style that leaves little room for potential misinterpretation.

Rather than attempting to summarize the contents of a 1,000-page textbook into a miniature form, the SOAP series focuses exclusively on guidance through patient encounters. In a typical use, "finding out where to start" or "refreshing your memory" with SOAP books should be possible in less than a minute. Subjects are always confined to 2 pages, and the most important points have been highlighted. Topics have been limited to those problems you will most commonly encounter repeatedly during your training, and contents are grouped according to the hospital or clinic setting. Facts and figures that are not particularly helpful to surviving life on the wards, such as demographics, pathophysiology, and busy tables and graphs, have purposely been omitted (such details are much better studied in a quiet environment using large and comprehensive texts).

Congratulations on your achievements thus far, and I wish you a highly successful medical career!

Peter S. Uzelac, MD, FACOG, HCLD (ABB)

ABBREVIATIONS

17OHP4	17-alpha hydroxy-progesterone
A1c	hemoglobin A1c
A-a gradient	alveolar-to-arterial gradient
AAA	abdominal aortic aneurysm
AAP	American Academy of Pediatrics
ABC	airway, breathing, circulation
Abd	abdomen
ABG	arterial blood gas
AC	abdominal circumference
ACE	angiotensin-converting enzyme
ACLS	advanced cardiac life support
ACS	acute coronary syndrome
ADA	American Diabetic Association
ADH	antidiuretic hormone
ADHD	attention deficit hyperactivity disorder
AFB	acid-fast bacilli
AFI	amniotic fluid index
AFP	alpha-fetoprotein
AFSFO	anterior fontanelle soft, flat, and open
AG	anion gap
AIDS	acquired immunodeficiency syndrome
AIHA	autoimmune hemolytic anemia
ALL	acute lymphocytic leukemia
ALS	amyotrophic lateral sclerosis
ALT	alanine aminotransferase
Alt	alternative regimen
ALTE	acute life-threatening event
AML	acute myeloid leukemia
AMS	altered mental status
ANA	antinuclear antibody
Anti-ENA-4	panel of rheumatologic labs
AP	anteroposterior
AP testing	antepartum testing
APCR	activated protein C resistance
APL	acute promyelocytic leukemia
Appy	appendicitis
APS	antiphospholipid syndrome
AR	aortic regurgitation
ARB	angiotension II receptor blocker
ARF	acute renal failure
ARDS	acute respiratory distress syndrome
AS	aortic stenosis; auris sinister (left ear); ankylosing spondylitis
ASD	atrial septal defect
ASMA	anti–smooth muscle antibody
ASO	antistreptolysin O titer
ASQ	ages and stages questionnaires
AST	aspartate aminotransferase
ATFL	anterior talofibular ligament
ATN	acute tubular necrosis
ATNR	asymmetrical tonic neck reflex
AUB	abnormal uterine bleeding
AV	atrioventricular

AVM	arteriovenous malformations
β-hCG	beta human chorionic gonadotropin
B	bilateral
BAD	bipolar affective disorder
BAL	blood alcohol level
BDD	body dysmorphic disorder
Bicarb	bicarbonate
bid	*bis in die* (twice daily)
bili	bilirubin
BM	bowel movement, stool
BMD	bone mineral density
BMI	body mass index
BMT	bone marrow transplant
BP	blood pressure
BPD	borderline personality disorder
BPM; bpm	beats per minute
BPP	biophysical profile
BRCA	breast cancer gene
BRUE	brief resolved unexplained event
BS	bowel sounds
BSA	body surface area
BUN	blood urea nitrogen
BV	bacterial vaginosis
Ca	calcium
CA	cancer
CA125	cancer antigen 125 test
CABG	coronary artery bypass graft
CAD	coronary artery disease
CAH	congenital adrenal hyperplasia
C-ANCA	cytoplasmic antineutrophil cytoplasmic antibodies
CAP	community-acquired pneumonia
CBC	complete blood count
CBC w/ diff	complete blood count with differential
CBT	cognitive behavioral therapy
cc	cubic centimeter
C/C/E	cyanosis/clubbing/edema
Chem 7	sodium, potassium, chloride, bicarb, BUN, creatinine, glucose
CHF	congestive heart failure
Chol	cholesterol
CHOP	cyclophosphamide, hydroxydoxorubicin, vincristine (Oncovin), prednisone
CHTN	chronic hypertension
ciTBI	clinically important traumatic brain injury
CK	creatinine kinase
CLL	chronic lymphocytic leukemia
CML	chronic myeloid leukemia
CMP	comprehensive metabolic panel
CMT	cervical motion tenderness
CMV	cytomegalovirus
CN	cranial nerves
CNS	central nervous system
COPD	chronic obstructive pulmonary disease
CP	chest pain; cerebral palsy
CPDD	calcium pyrophosphate deposition disease
CPP	cerebral perfusion pressure; chronic pelvic pain

CPR	cardiopulmonary resuscitation
Cr	creatinine
CRF	chronic renal failure
CRP	c-reactive protein
C-section; C/S	cesarean section
CSF	cerebrospinal fluid
CST	contraction stress test
CT	computed tomography, *Chlamydia trachomatis*
CTA	clear to auscultation
CV	cardiovascular
CVA	costovertebral angle, cerebrovascular accident
CVAT	costovertebral angle tenderness
CVS	chorionic villus sampling
CXR	chest x-ray
D5½NS	5% dextrose in half normal saline
D10	a solution with 10% dextrose
D25	a solution with 25% dextrose
D&C	dilation and curettage
DBP	diastolic blood pressure
DBT	dialectical behavior therapy
DDX	differential diagnosis
Derm	dermatology
DES	diethylstilbestrol
DEXA	dual-energy x-ray absorptiometry
DHEAS	dehydroepiandrosterone sulfate
DHP	dihydropyridine
DI	diabetes insipidus
DIC	disseminated intravascular coagulation
DID	dissociative identity disorder
Diff	differential
DIP	distal interphalangeal joint
DKA	diabetic ketoacidosis
dL	deciliter
DLCO	diffusing capacity of the lung for carbon monoxide
DM	diabetes mellitus
DMARD	disease-modifying antirheumatic drug
DNA	deoxyribonucleic acid
DPP-4 inhibitor	dipeptidyl peptidase-4 inhibitor
DRE	digital rectal exam
DTaP	diphtheria, tetanus, and acellular pertussis vaccine
DTR	deep tendon reflexes
DUB	dysfunctional uterine bleeding
DVT	deep venous thrombosis
EBL	estimated blood loss
EBV	Epstein-Barr virus
EC	emergency contraception
ECG	electrocardiogram
ECT	electroconvulsive therapy
ECV	extracellular volume
ED	erectile dysfunction
EDC	estimated date of confinement
EDH	epidural hematoma
EEG	electroencephalogram
EFW	estimated fetal weight
EGA	estimated gestational age
EGD	esophagogastroduodenoscopy

EMB	endometrial biopsy
EMDR	eye movement desensitization and reprocessing
EMG	electromyography
ENT	ear, nose, and throat
EOMi	extraocular muscles intact
EP	electrophysiology
Epi	epinephrine
EPO	erythropoietin
ER	emergency room
ERCP	endoscopic retrograde cholangiopancreatography
ERP	exposure and response prevention
ESR	erythrocyte sedimentation rate
ESRD	end-stage renal disease
ETEC	enterotoxigenic *E.coli*
ETT	endotracheal tube
Ext	extremities
FB	foreign body
FDA	Federal Drug Administration
FEN	fluids electrolytes nutrition
FFN	fetal fibronectin
FFP	fresh frozen plasma
FH	fundal height
FHRT	fetal heart rate tracing
FiO$_2$	fraction of inspired oxygen
FM	fetal movement
FNA	fine-needle aspiration
FRAX	fracture risk assessment tool
FSH	follicle-stimulating hormone
FTA-ABS	fluorescent treponemal antibody absorption
FUO	fever of unknown origin
g	gram
G6PD	glucose 6 phosphate dehydrogenase
GAD	generalized anxiety disorder
GAS	group A streptococcus
GBS	group B streptococcus
GC	gonococcus
GCA	giant cell arteritis
GCS	Glasgow coma scale
GCT	glucose challenge test
GDM	gestational diabetes mellitus
Gen	general appearance of patient
GERD	gastroesophageal reflux disease
GFR	glomerular filtration rate
GI	gastrointestinal
GLP-1	glucagon-like peptide-1
Gluc	glucose
GN	glomerulonephritis
GS	gestational sac
GSUI	genuine stress urinary incontinence
GTC	generalized tonic clonic
GTD	gestational trophoblastic disease
GTT	glucose tolerance test
G-tube	gastrostomy tube
GU	genitourinary
H/A	headache
H&P	history and physical

Hb	hemoglobin
HBsAg	hepatitis B surface antigen
HBV	hepatitis B virus
HCC	hepatocellular carcinoma
HCG	human chorionic gonadotropin
HCO₃	bicarbonate
Hct	hematocrit
HEADSS	home, education, activities, drugs, sex, suicide
HEENT	head, eyes, ears, nose, throat
HELLP	hypertension, elevated liver enzymes, low platelets
Heme	hematologic
HI	homicidal ideation
HIDA	hepatobiliary iminodiacetic acid
HIV	human immunodeficiency virus
HL	Hodgkin lymphoma
HLA	human leukocyte antigen
HOCM	hypertrophic obstructive cardiomyopathy
HONK	hyperosmolar nonketotic coma
HPV	human papilloma virus
hr	hour
HR	heart rate
HRT	hormone replacement therapy
HSP	Henoch-Schönlein purpura
HSV	herpes simplex virus
HTN	hypertension
HUS	hemolytic uremic syndrome
Hz	Hertz
IBD	inflammatory bowel disease
IBS	irritable bowel syndrome
ICH	intracranial hemorrhage
ICP	intracranial pressure
ICSI	intracytoplasmic sperm injection
ICU	intensive care unit
ID	infectious disease
IDM	infant of diabetic mother
IE	infective endocarditis
Ig	immunoglobulin
IHSS	idiopathic hypertrophic subaortic stenosis
ILD	interstitial lung disease
IM	intramuscular
IMA	inferior mesenteric arteries
IMM	intramyometrial
INH	isoniazid
INR	international normalized ratio
I/O	input and output
IPV	inactivated poliovirus vaccine
ISAM	infant of a substance-abusing mother
ITP	idiopathic thrombocytopenic purpura
IU	international unit
IUD	intrauterine device
IUGR	intrauterine growth restriction
IUI	intrauterine insemination
IUP	intrauterine pregnancy
IV	intravenous
IVC	inferior vena cava
IVDA	intravenous drug administration
IVF	intravenous fluid; in-vitro fertilization
IVIG	intravenous immunoglobulin

IVP	intravenous pyelogram
JRA	juvenile rheumatoid arthritis
K	potassium
KD	Kawasaki disease
kg	kilogram
KOH	potassium hydroxide
KS	Kaposi sarcoma
KUB	kidneys-ureter-bladder
L	left, liter
L&D	labor and delivery
L:S	lecithin/sphingomyelin ratio
LAC	lupus anticoagulant
LAD	lymphadenopathy
Lat	lateral
lb	pound
LDH	lactate dehydrogenase
LEMS	Lambert-Eaton myasthenic syndrome
LFT	liver function test
LH	luteinizing hormone
LLQ	left lower quadrant
LMP	last menstrual period
LMWH	low molecular weight heparin
LOC	loss of consciousness
LP	lumbar puncture
LUQ	left upper quadrant
Lytes	electrolytes
MAC	membrane attack complex
MAE	moves all extremities
MAHA	microangiopathic hemolytic anemia
MAOI	monoamine oxidase inhibitor
MAP	mean arterial pressure
M-CHAT	modified checklist for autism in toddlers
MCD	minimal change disease
mcg	microgram
MCHC	mean corpuscular hemoglobin concentration
MCP	metacarpophalangeal
MCV	mean cellular volume; mean corpuscular volume
MDD	major depressive disorder
MDRTB	multidrug-resistant tuberculosis
mEq	milliequivalents
MET	metabolic equivalents
mg	milligram
Mg	magnesium
MG	myasthenia gravis
$MgSO_4$	magnesium sulfate
MI	myocardial infarction
min	minute
mL	milliliter
MMR	mumps, measles, rubella vaccine
MOM	multiples of the mean
Mono	mononucleosis
MPA	medroxyprogesterone acetate; microscopic polyangiitis
MPV	mean platelet volume
MRCP	mental retardation cerebral palsy
M/R/G/C	murmur/rub/gallop/click
MRI	magnetic resonance imaging

MRSA	methicillin-resistant *Staphylococcus aureus*
MS	multiple sclerosis; mitral stenosis
MSAFP	maternal serum alpha-fetoprotein
MSLT	multiple sleep latency test
MTP	metatarsophalangeal joint
MV	minute ventilation
MVA	manual vacuum aspiration
MVP	mitral valve prolapse
Na	sodium
NAFLD	nonalcoholic fatty liver disease
NCAT	normocephalic atraumatic
ND	nondistended
NEC	necrotizing enterocolitis
Neuro	neurologic
NFEG	normal female external genitalia
NG	nasogastric
NHL	non-Hodgkin lymphoma
NICU	neonatal intensive care unit
NIPT	noninvasive prenatal testing
NMDA	N-methyl-D-aspartate
NMEG	normal male external genitalia
NPH	neutral protamine Hagedorn insulin
NPO	*nulla* per os (nothing by mouth)
NPT	nocturnal penile tumescence
NRT	normal rectal tone
NS	normal saline
NSAID	nonsteroidal anti-inflammatory drug
NST	nonstress test
NT	nontender
NTD	neural tube defect
NTG	nitroglycerin
N/V	nausea and vomiting
NVP	nausea and vomiting of pregnancy
O$_2$	oxygen
O&P	ova and parasites
OA	osteoarthritis
Ob/Gyn	obstetrics and gynecology
OC	oral contraceptive
OCD	obsessive compulsive disorder
OCP	oral contraceptive pill
OP	oropharynx; osteoporosis
OR	operating room
OSA	obstructive sleep apnea
OT	occupational therapy
OTC	over the counter
P	pulse
PA	posteroanterior
PALS	pediatric advanced life support
PAN	polyarteritis nodosa
PAP	Papanicolaou smear
PCI	percutaneous coronary intervention
PCOS	polycystic ovary syndrome
PCP	primary care provider; phencyclidine; *Pneumocystis carinii* pneumonia
PCR	polymerase chain reaction
PDA	patent ductus arteriosus
PE	physical exam; pulmonary embolism

PEA	pulseless electrical activity
PEEP	positive end expiratory pressure
PEFR	peak expiratory flow rate
Perf'd Appy	perforated appendicitis
PERRLA	pupils equal, round, reactive to light, and accommodation
PET	positron emission tomography
PFT	pulmonary function test
PGBS	postglucose blood sugar
PGE_1	prostaglandin E_1
pH	negative log of the concentration of hydrogen
PICU	pediatric intensive care unit
PID	pelvic inflammatory disease
PIH	pregnancy-induced hypertension
PIP	proximal interphalangeal joint
PMH	past medical history
PMN	polymorphonuclear neutrophils
PMR	polymyalgia rheumatica
PMS	premenstrual syndrome
PO	*per os* (by mouth)
POC	products of conception
POD	postoperative day
Postop	postoperatively
PPD	purified protein derivative
PPH	postpartum hemorrhage
PPI	proton pump inhibitor
PPROM	preterm premature spontaneous rupture of membranes
PPTL	postpartum tubal ligation
pr	per rectum
preemie	premature baby
prn	*pro re nata* (as needed)
PROM	premature spontaneous rupture of membranes
PS	pain score
PSA	prostate-specific antigen
PSH	past surgical history
pt	patient
PT	prothrombin time, physical therapy
PTB	preterm birth
PTH	parathyroid hormone
PTL	preterm labor
PTSD	posttraumatic stress disorder
PTT	partial thromboplastin time
PTU	propylthiouracil
PTX	pneumothorax
PUBS	percutaneous umbilical blood sampling
PUD	peptic ulcer disease
Pulse ox	pulse oximeter
PVC	premature ventricular contraction
q	*quodque* (every)
qd	*quaque die* (once daily)
qh	*quaque hora* (every hour)
qhs	at bedtime
qid	*quater in die* (four times daily)
R	right, respirations
RA	rheumatoid arthritis
RBC	red blood cell
RDA	recommended daily allowance

RDS	respiratory distress syndrome
RDW	red cell distribution width
Rec	recommended regimen
Resp	respiratory
RF	rheumatic fever, rheumatoid factor
Rh	Rhesus factor
RI	reticulocyte index
RLQ	right lower quadrant
RLS	restless leg syndrome
ROM	range of motion; rupture of membranes
ROS	review of systems
RPL	recurrent pregnancy loss
RPR	rapid plasma reagin
RR	respiratory rate
RRR	regular rate and rhythm
RSV	respiratory syncytial virus
RTA	renal tubular acidosis
RUQ	right upper quadrant
SAB	spontaneous abortion
SAD	seasonal affective disorder
SAH	subarachnoid hemorrhage
SBO	small bowel obstruction
SBP	systolic blood pressure; spontaneous bacterial peritonitis
SCFE	slipped capital femoral epiphysis
SDH	subdural hematoma
Sec	seconds (time)
Ser	serum
SERM	selective estrogen receptor modulator
SG	specific gravity
SGLT-2 inhibitor	sodium-glucose transport protein-2 inhibitor
SH	Salter Harris
SI	suicidal ideation
SIADH	syndrome of inappropriate antidiuretic hormone
SLE	systemic lupus erythematosus
SM	systolic murmur
SMA	spinal muscular atrophy
SNRI	selective norepinephrine reuptake inhibitor
SQ	subcutaneous
SS	systemic sclerosis
SSRI	selective serotonin reuptake inhibitor
STI	sexually transmitted infection
SVC	superior vena cava
TB	tuberculosis
TBI	traumatic brain injury
TCA	tricyclic antidepressant
TD	tetanus and diphtheria toxoids
TEE	transesophageal echocardiogram
TFTs	thyroid function tests
TIA	transient ischemic attack
TIBC	total iron binding capacity
tid	*ter in die* (three times daily)
TIG	tetanus immune globulin
TM	tympanic membrane
TMP-SMX	trimethoprim-sulfamethoxazole
TOA	tubo-ovarian abscess
ToF	tetralogy of Fallot

TOL	trial of labor
TR	tricuspid regurgitation
TS	tricuspid stenosis
TSH	thyroid-stimulating hormone
TSS	toxic shock syndrome
TTN	transient tachypnea of the newborn
TTP	thrombotic thrombocytopenic purpura
TVH	transvaginal hysterectomy
U/A	urinalysis
UC	uterine contraction
UCx	urine culture
UDS	urine drug screen
UOP	urine output
UPT	urine pregnancy test
URI	upper respiratory infection
U/S	ultrasound
UTI	urinary tract infection
UV	ultraviolet
UVJ	urethral-vesicular junction
VCUG	vesiculocystourethrogram
VMA	vanillylmandelic acid
V/Q	ventilation-perfusion
VS	vital signs
VSD	ventricular septal defect
VZV	varicella zoster virus
WBC	white blood cell
WGA	weeks of gestational age
wk	week
WPW	Wolff-Parkinson-White
wt	weight
y/o	years old

NORMAL LAB VALUES

VITALS

Approximate 95% confidence intervals. Means in parentheses where appropriate.

Age	Systolic BP	Diastolic BP	Heart Rate	Respiratory Rate
Term neonate	60–85 (70)	35–60 (55)	93–154 (123)	27–66 (43)
1 yr	70–100 (90)	40–60 (55)	89–151 (119)	20–49 (32)
2 yr	72–105 (90)	40–60 (55)	89–151 (119)	17–39 (26)
3 yr	74–110 (92)	40–65 (58)	73–137 (108)	16–34 (24)
5 yr	78–112 (94)	45–70 (58)	65–133 (100)	16–31 (22)
8 yr	86–117 (100)	45–75 (58)	62–130 (91)	16–24 (20)
12 yr	94–125 (108)	50–80 (60)	60–119 (85)	14–23 (19)
>15 yr	95–130 (115)	50–80 (60)	60–100 (72)	12–20 (16)

A fever is always T ≥100.4°F (38°C) rectally. Rectal can be up to 1°F higher than oral.

HEMATOLOGY—RED BLOOD CELLS AND PLATELETS

Age	Hgb	Hct	MCV	Ferritin	Iron	ESR	Platelets
Preterm	13–15	42–47	118–120				254–290
Term	13.5–18.5	42–60	98–118	25–200	100–250	0–4	290
2 mo	9.4–13.0	28–42	84–106	50–200	40–100		252
6 mo–2 yr	10.5–13.5	33–39	70–86				150–350
2–6 yr	11.5–13.5	34–40	75–86	7–140	50–120	4–20	150–350
6–12 yrs	11.5–14.5	35–45	77–93				150–350
Adolescence							
Male	13–15	36–50	78–98	7–140	65–175	0–10	150–350
Female	12–14.5	37–45	78–98	7–140	50–170	0–20	150–350

HEMATOLOGY—WHITE BLOOD CELLS AND DIFFERENTIAL. CRP NORMAL 0–0.5, ALL AGES

Age	WBC	% Neutrophils	% Lymphocytes	% Monocytes	% Eosinophils
Birth	9–30	55%–87%	11%–37%	6%	2%
12 hr	13–38	64%–74%	9%–29%	5%	2%
24 hr	9.4–34	55%–81%	11%–37%	6%	2%
2 wk	5–20	9%–70%	18%–85%	9%	3%
1 yr	6–17.5	32%–49%	35%–65%	5%	3%
4 yr	5.5–15.5	37%–50%	22%–55%	5%	3%
6 yr	5–14.5	42%–60%	18%–50%	5%	3%
10 yr	4.5–13.5	45%–65%	35%–50%	4%	2%
>12 yr	4.5–13	45%–75%	30%–45%	5%	3%

SERUM SODIUM (NA⁺)

Preterm	130–140 mEq/L
All others	136–145 mEq/L

SERUM POTASSIUM (K⁺)

<10 d old	4.0–6.0 mEq/L
>10 d old	3.5–5.1 mEq/L

Note: Children are notoriously difficult blood draws; hemolysis is a frequent complication and thus potassium is often falsely elevated.

Serum Chloride (Cl⁻)	99–111 mEq/L

SERUM BICARBONATE (HCO₃⁻)

Preterm	18–26 mEq/L
Term	20–25 mEq/L
>2 yr	22–26 mEq/L
Blood Urea Nitrogen (BUN)	7–22 mg/dL

SERUM CREATININE (CR)

Newborn	0.3–1.0 mg/dL
Infant	0.2–0.4 mg/dL
Child	0.3–0.7 mg/dL
Adolescent	Male: 0.6–1.3 mg/dL
	Female: 0.5–1.2 mg/dL

SERUM GLUCOSE

Preterm	45–100 mg/dL
Term	45–120 mg/dL
1 wk–16 yr	60–105 mg/dL
>16 yr	70–115 mg/dL

SERUM CALCIUM (CA⁺²)

Preterm	6–10 mg/dL
Full term	7–12 mg/dL
Child	8–10.5 mg/dL
Adolescent	8.5–10.5 mg/dL

Note: If albumin is low, calcium will be falsely depressed as well. The correction formula is: $[4.0 - (\text{serum albumin})](0.8) + [Ca^{+2}]$.

Serum Magnesium (Mg⁺²)	1.7–2.2 mEq/dL

SERUM PHOSPHORUS (P)

Newborn	4.2–9.0 mg/dL
0–15 yr	3.2–6.3 mg/dL
>15 yr	2.7–4.5 mg/dL

ALKALINE PHOSPHATASE

Infant	150–420 U/L
2–10 yr	100–320 U/L
11–18 yr	Male: 100–390 U/L
	Female: 100–320 U/L

ALBUMIN

Newborn	3.2–4.8 g/dL
1 mo	2.5–5.5 g/dL
3 mo	2.1–4.8 g/dL
6 mo	2.8–5.0 g/dL
1 yr	3.2–5.7 g/dL
2 yr	1.9–5.0 g/dL
3 yr	3.3–5.8 g/dL
5 yr	2.9–5.8 g/dL
8 yr	3.2–5.0 g/dL
>16 yr	3.1–5.4 g/dL

BILIRUBIN (TOTAL)

Age	Preterm	Term
0–1 d	<8 mg/dL	<6 mg/dL
1–2 d	<12 mg/dL	<8 mg/dL
3–5 d	<16 mg/dL	<12 mg/dL
After		0.1–1.2 mg/dL

Direct or conjugated bilirubin should always be <0.4 mg/dL

ASPARTATE AMINOTRANSFERASE (AST/SGOT)

Infant	20–65 U/L
Child/adolescent	0–35 U/L

ALANINE AMINOTRANSFERASE (ALT/SGPT)

Infant	<54 U/L
Child/adolescent	1–60 U/L

CREATINE KINASE (CK/CPK)

Newborn	10–200 U/L
All others	Male: 12–80 U/L
	Female: 10–55 U/L

LACTATE DEHYDROGENASE (LD/LDH)

Neonate	160–1500 U/L
Infant	150–360 U/L
Child	150–300 U/L
Adolescent	0–220 U/L

LIPIDS. HDL SHOULD ALWAYS BE >45 MG/DL

	Desirable	Borderline	High
Total cholesterol (mg/dL)	<170	170–199	≥200
Low-density Lipoprotein (mg/dL)	<110	110–129	≥160

LEAD: NORMAL LEAD IS 0!

Acceptable serum lead level	<10 mcg/dL
Osmolality	285–295 mOsm/kg
Fibrinogen	200–400 mg/dL

ANTINUCLEAR ANTIBODY (ANA)

<1:80	Not significant
>1:320	Significant
Rheumatoid factor	<20 conventional units

SEX HORMONES

	LH (mIU/mL)	FSH (mIU/mL)	Testosterone (ng/dL)	Estradiol (pg/mL)
Prepubertal children	0–1.6	0–2.8	10–20	<25
Postpubertal				
Male	1–10.2	1.4–14.4	275–875	6–44
Female			23–75	
Luteal				15–260
Follicular	0.9–14	3.7–12.9		10–200
Midcycle				120–375
Pregnant			35–195	

SERUM CORTISOL

Pre-ACTH in AM	5.7–16.6
1 hr post-ACTH	16–36

DIABETIC LABS

Insulin (fasting)	1.8–24.6 mcU/mL
C-peptide (fasting)	0.8–4.0 ng/mL
Hemoglobin A1C	4.5%–6.1%

THYROID FUNCTION TESTS

Age	T_4 (mcg/dL)	T_3 (ng/dL)	TSH (mIU/mL)	TBG (mg/dL)
1–3 d	11.0–21.5	100–380	<2.5–13.3	0.7–4.7
1–4 wk	8.2–16.6	99–310	0.6–10.0	0.5–4.5
1–12 mo	7.2–15.6	102–264	0.6–6.3	1.6–3.6
1–5 yr	7.3–15.0	105–269	"	1.3–2.8
6–10 yr	6.4–13.3	94–241	"	1.4–2.6
11–15 yr	5.6–11.7	83–213	"	"
≥16 yr	4.2–11.8	80–210	0.2–7.6	"

HOW TO WRITE A SOAP NOTE

The **SOAP** note was developed by Lawrence Weed, MD, at the University of Vermont as part of the problem-orientated medical record (POMR), intended to standardize the patient's medical record.

SOAP is an acronym for:

- **Subjective:** Document in a detailed, narrative format what the patient, family members, or caretakers are reporting about the patient's health problem.
  - Document the chief complaint (CC) or history of present illness (HPI) with the **SLIDTA** acronym (below is a sample, for pain).
    - **S**everity: Rated on a pain scale of 0 (no pain) to 10 (severe pain)
    - **L**ocation: Location of pain
    - **I**nfluencing factors: Factors that make the pain worse or better
    - **D**uration: How long patient has had pain
    - **T**ype: Description of pain
    - **A**ssociated symptoms: Describe any related symptoms
  - Document past medical history (PMH), past surgical history (PSH), review of symptoms (ROS), medications, and allergies.
- **Objective:** Document the vitals, height, weight, and body mass index (BMI). Document objective observations, physical exam, labs, and studies.
- **Assessment:** Document the diagnosis or differential diagnosis based on your history and physical exam. Document the current status of diagnosis (i.e., stable, unstable, etc.).
- **Plan:** Document how the treatment will be developed to reach the goals or objectives. Document interventions that include:
  - Medications
  - Labs
  - Diagnostic studies
  - Referrals
  - Patient education
  - Follow-up

Daniel C. Maldonado, MD

I

INTERNAL MEDICINE

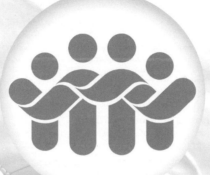

PULMONARY

COMMUNITY-ACQUIRED PNEUMONIA

S **What are the pt's symptoms?**
- Fever   – Cough with or without purulent sputum
- Blood-streaked sputum   – Dyspnea

When was the onset of symptoms?
Strictly defined, symptoms of community-acquired pneumonia begin outside the hospital
- If symptoms begin in the hospital, they must begin within 48 hr to be considered community acquired.
- If greater than 48 hr since admission, or if pt usually resides in a long-term facility, the possibility of nosocomial pneumonia must be considered.

What are the pt's age, gender, and comorbidities?

All of these factors determine points in the PORT classification system (see following):

- Male gender is a risk in pneumonia and thus females receive minus 10 points.
- Age in years equals a number of points.
- Nursing home residence also contributes 10 points.
- Comorbidities also have point values: nondermatologic neoplasias (30 points), liver disease (20 points), congestive heart failure (CHF, 10 points), renal disease (10 points), and cerebrovascular disease (10 points).

Is there any history of recent aspiration?
If so, consider the presence of anaerobic or polymicrobial organisms; choose broader antibiotics.

Does the pt seem able to comply with outpatient antibiotic therapy?
Inability to comply with empiric therapy would mandate hospital admission.

O **Review vital signs**
These provide an idea of the severity of disease.
The following are associated with greater morbidity:
- Temperature greater than 40°C or less than 35°C (15 points)
- Heart rate >125 bpm (10 points)
- Respiratory rate >30 breaths per minute (20 points)
- Systolic blood pressure <90 mm Hg (20 points)
- Altered mental status (20 points)

Perform a thorough pulmonary examination
Bronchial breath sounds, rales, and dullness to percussion are common findings.

Obtain a CBC, Chem 7, CXR, and ABG
Certain values will register points toward the PORT risk classification score:
- Hct <30% (10 points)   – BUN >30 mg/dL (20 points)
- Sodium <130 mEq/L (20 points)   – Glucose >250 mg/dL (10 points)
- Arterial pH <7.35 (30 points)   – pO_2 of >60 mm Hg (10 points)
- Pleural effusion (10 points)

Other values of note would be increased WBC count with a bandemia ("left shift") and an acidosis, either respiratory or metabolic.
Chest x-ray (CXR) often will show one or more areas of lobar consolidations with air bronchograms.

Procalcitonin levels can guide your antibiotic therapy if there is a bacteria infection present or not
Procalcitonin has a high sensitivity and specificity for bacterial infection in the lungs.

A Community-acquired pneumonia

Lung infection that occurs outside of a hospital or other institution. Common organisms are as follows:

- *Streptococcus pneumoniae*   – *Hemophilus influenzae*
- *Staphylococcus aureus*   – *Moraxella catarrhalis*

Assess PORT risk classification

The PORT risk classification system is a point scale, with each risk factor adding up points, as noted above. The classification is as follows:

- Classes I and II ≤70 points

(Class I would be a more obviously well-appearing pt)

- Class III, 71–90 points
- Class IV, 91–130 points
- Class V >130 points

Differential diagnosis

- Nosocomial pneumonia   – Aspiration pneumonia   – Asthma
- Lung cancer   – Tuberculosis   – Pulmonary embolism
- CHF

P Treat pts in risk classes I–III with outpatient antibiotic therapy and follow-up

Prescribe a macrolide, doxycycline, or fluoroquinolone.

Alternatives would include amoxicillin–clavulanate or a second-/third-generation oral cephalosporin.

Stress that the antibiotic regimen must be completed, even if the pt feels better early on in the course of treatment.

Consider treating pts in class III with a brief inpatient observation period if warranted.

Admit pts in risk class IV to the inpatient medical ward, culture, and treat with broad-spectrum antibiotics

Obtain two sets of blood cultures, before treatment with either a fluoroquinolone alone, or a second-/third-generation cephalosporin with a macrolide.

Alternately, consider ampicillin/sulbactam or piperacillin/tazobactam with a macrolide.

Admit pts in risk class V to the intensive care unit, culture, and treat with broad-spectrum antibiotics

Antibiotic choices will include second-/third-generation cephalosporin or β-lactam/β-lactamase inhibitor with a fluoroquinolone or macrolide.

Later, tailor antibiotic treatment based on sputum culture and sensitivities

These will help reduce the emergence of resistant organisms.

Provide high-risk pts with prophylaxis from infections with pneumococcal and influenza vaccines

High-risk pts include those older than 65 years, immunocompromised pts, and those with chronic illnesses mentioned earlier.

Consider CXR follow-up in 6 weeks

This is the minimum time that you would expect to visualize total resolution of a successfully treated infiltrate. Persistence of infiltrates beyond this time warrants additional workup of either incomplete treatment or other etiologies.

ASTHMA

S **Does the pt have episodic dyspnea, cough, wheezing, and/or chest tightness?**
These are classic symptoms of asthma and are often worse at night or in the early morning.
Characterized by reversibility of symptoms following bronchodilator therapy.

How often do symptoms occur? Do they occur at night?
This will help classify the severity of chronic asthma (Table 1-1).

TABLE 1-1 Asthma Classification

Category	Symptoms	Nighttime Symptoms
Mild intermittent	≤2×/wk	≤2×/mo
Mild persistent	>2×/wk, but <1×/d	>2×/mo
Moderate persistent	Daily symptoms	>1×/wk
Severe persistent	Continual symptoms	Frequent

How often is the pt admitted to the ER for asthma? Has the pt been intubated?
This will also give some idea of the severity of the pt's asthma.

Does the pt have exposure to possible triggers of asthma?

- Exercise
- Cigarette smoke
- Sulfates
- NSAIDs
- Sinusitis
- Aspiration
- Nitrates
- GERD
- Smog
- Allergens

O **Conduct a physical examination (PE) and ABG to classify the severity of the current asthma exacerbation (Table 1-2). Order a chest x-ray**

TABLE 1-2 Asthma Exacerbation

	Mild	Moderate	Severe	Impending Respiratory Failure
Speech	Sentences	Phrases	Words	Mute
Body position	Can be supine	Prefers sitting	Unable to be supine	Unable to be supine
Respiratory rate	Normal	Increased	>30/min	>30 min
Breath sounds	Mod. wheezes late expiration	Loud wheezes through expiration	Loud insp. exp. wheezes	Little air movement
Heart rate	<100 bpm	100–120	>120	Relatively slow
Mental status	May be agitated	Agitated	Agitated	Drowsy
Peak expirtory flow (% predicted)	>80	50–80	<50	<50
SaO₂ (% room air)	>95	91–95	<91	<91
PaO₂ (mm Hg, room air)	Normal	>60	<60	<60
PaCO₂ (mm Hg)	<42	<42	≥42	≥42

Although you may see only hyperinflation, bronchial wall thickening, and peripheral lung shadows, you may also be able to rule out pneumonia and pneumothorax.

Asthma

Inflammatory disease of the lung characterized by reversible airway obstruction.

Classify the asthma severity as *mild intermittent, mild persistent, moderate persistent, or severe persistent.*

Also note whether the pt's asthma is stable on this visit or whether the pt is having an exacerbation.

Differential diagnosis

- Foreign body aspiration
- Chronic bronchitis
- Bronchiectasis
- Tracheal stenosis
- Bronchiolitis obliterans
- Allergic bronchopulmonary aspergillosis
- Cystic fibrosis
- Churg-Strauss syndrome

P **If the pt is not currently having an asthma exacerbation, or if it is mild, prescribe the appropriate medications based on the severity of the asthma**

Mild intermittent: Albuterol as needed.

Mild persistent: Add a low-dose inhaled corticosteroid twice daily.

Moderate persistent: Increase the dose of corticosteroids to medium or add a long-acting β_2 agonist. A leukotriene antagonist or theophylline may substitute for the long-acting β_2 agonist daily.

Severe persistent: High-dose inhaled corticosteroids and a long-acting β_2 agonist twice daily. Add oral corticosteroids as needed. Attempts should be made to reduce corticosteroid dosages at every visit during which symptoms are well controlled.

Admit pts with evidence of moderate to severe asthma exacerbation to the hospital

Frequent high-dose delivery of inhaled short-acting β_2 agonists, either as metered-dose inhaler or as nebulizer, with at least three doses in the first hour.

Systemic corticosteroids and mucolytics should also be given to these pts.

Intubate those pts with severe asthma with poor or slow response to treatment and start mechanical ventilation

Further management should ensure adequate oxygenation, avoidance of barotrauma, and hypotension.

Administer inhaled short-acting β_2 agonists and systemic anti-inflammatory medications frequently.

Discharge when

Hypoxia and all other signs of respiratory distress are resolved.

Prescribe a dose of oral prednisone tapered from 60 mg po qd over the next 5 days

Consider outpatient pulmonary function testing when asymptomatic to document severity of disease and response to bronchodilator.

This will also help rule out chronic obstructive pulmonary disease.

TUBERCULOSIS

S Does the pt have risk factors for contracting tuberculosis (TB)?
- Recent contact with TB
- Incarceration
- Homelessness
- HIV (human immunodeficiency virus) infection
- Overcrowded housing
- Immunosuppressive therapy

Does the pt come from Latin America or Southeast Asia? Does he or she have a history of previous incomplete treatment for TB? Has he or she had exposure to someone with documented drug-resistant TB?

These questions are crucial to ask, because they can point out someone who is at risk of carrying multidrug-resistant tuberculosis (MDRTB).

Does the pt have symptoms consistent with TB?
- Malaise
- Night sweats
- Fevers
- Anorexia
- Chronic cough
- Weight loss
- Blood-streaked sputum

Although these symptoms are not specific to TB, together they suggest the possibility of TB.

Weight loss and night sweats are slightly more specific to TB, but the most common presentation is a chronic cough (sometimes blood tinged).

The pt may have no symptoms at all, as in latent tubercular infections.

O Perform PE

Pertinent findings include cachexia, fever, rales, and decreased breath sounds. These are nonspecific findings.

Expect that a pt with latent TB might have an entirely normal PE.

Obtain CXR

Primarily important in distinguishing latent TB from reactivation/active TB

> Primary TB shows infiltrate with hilar lymphadenopathy. It rarely presents as a pathologic state. Often the pt is not even aware of it.
> Residual (healed)/latent TB would show a primary calcified focus (Ghon focus) with or without calcified hilar lymphadenopathy (Ranke complex).
> Calcified foci are sometimes referred to as granulomata.
> Reactivation TB (common active disease) usually presents as infiltrates in the apical posterior segments of the upper lobe or superior segment of lower lobes.

TB can present as multiple nodular densities (military TB), which suggests hematologic and lymphatic dissemination. Other findings include pleural effusion, scarring, and volume loss.

If you suspect active TB, order a sputum sample with a smear for acid-fast bacilli (AFB) and culture for TB. Repeat twice more every 8 hours for a total of three specimens

Although the culture may not grow out for 6–12 weeks, the acid-fast bacilli (AFB) smear, if positive, will confirm the presence of active TB.

Sputum induction may help achieve specimens in pts who cannot provide specimens.

If induction is not an option, bronchoscopy may also be used to obtain samples.

Place a tuberculin skin test or draw QuantiFERON-TB Gold in relevant individuals

This would include pts who have symptoms of TB or asymptomatic people who you are concerned may have latent TB.

Place 5 tuberculin units of protein purified derivative (PPD) on the volar aspect of the forearm, and measure the area of induration (NOT erythema) after 48–72 hours.

Positive tests are interpreted differently for different populations:
- >5 mm: (+) in HIV-positive pts, recent contacts of active TB, signs of previous TB on CXR, and immunosuppressed pts
- >10 mm: (+) in recent immigrants from Asia, Africa, and Latin America, HIV-negative injection drug users, TB laboratory personnel, residents and employees of high-risk settings (e.g., nursing homes, AIDS (acquired immunodeficiency syndrome) facilities, homeless shelters, jails), children <4 years of age, or minors exposed to adults at high risk
- >15 mm: (+) in anyone

A Tuberculosis

The tuberculin bacillus is inhaled and taken to the deepest part of the lungs. In most individuals, primary infection is rapidly contained by the immune system, but the acid-fast covering of the bacillus renders it difficult to be killed by macrophages. This is latent TB infection.

The bacillus can live inside a macrophage for years, waiting for the moment when the host's immune system is less active. Then reactivation occurs, usually in areas of highest oxygen tension (the upper lobes of the lungs).

Reactivation disease is often more severe than primary, and immune activity causes cavitation in the lungs with caseation necrosis on pathology.

Note that reactivation can occur in any part of the body, including the peritoneum, pleura, meninges, and kidneys.

Differential diagnosis

– Pneumonia	– Coccidioidomycosis	– Histoplasmosis
– Sarcoidosis	– Blastomycosis	– Lung cancer

P Immediately isolate those you suspect of having active TB

Respiratory isolation is required to prevent spread of infection.

Obtain three samples of sputum for AFB smears.

If they are all negative, you can remove the pt from isolation.

Begin treatment for those with active TB

Common anti-TB medications include rifampin (R), isoniazid/INH (I), pyrazinamide (P), ethambutol (E), *or* streptomycin (S).

Start R.I.P.E. until culture and sensitivities return.
- If cultures return with INH-sensitive TB, then give R.I.P. for 2 months and then R.I. for an additional 4 months or until follow-up AFB cultures are negative for 3 months, whichever is longer.
- If cultures return with INH-resistant TB, then give R.P. and either E. or S. for 6 months or 12 months of R.E. Remember that streptomycin is given intravenously only.
- If cultures return with MDRTB, a minimum of three drugs (that it is susceptible to) are required with directly observed therapy until culture is negative, and then continue with two drugs for another 12 months.

If pregnant, give R.I.E. for 9 months and do not allow breastfeeding.

Pts with HIV infection are treated in similar fashion as described but require treatment of longer duration and should be given pyridoxine (vitamin B_6) to reduce INH-induced peripheral neuropathy.

Begin treatment for those with latent TB (PPD+, CXR negative, or with evidence of old disease)

I. for 9 months OR

R.P. for 2 months if contact of person with known MDRTB

INTERSTITIAL LUNG DISEASE

 Is there any progressive dyspnea and nonproductive cough?
These are the classic symptoms of interstitial lung disease (ILD).

Are there any occupational and environmental exposures?
The potential causes for ILD number more than 100. A good history is crucial to developing a possible etiology. Possible causes include
- Asbestosis
- Silicosis
- Organic gases
- Pneumoconiosis
- Berylliosis

Is there a history of granulomatous lung diseases?
Sarcoid, fungal, or mycobacterial infections are all associated with ILDs.

What are the pt's past and current medications?
Agents known to cause ILD include
- Bleomycin
- Chlorambucil
- Amiodarone
- Busulfan
- Cyclophosphamide
- Sulfonamides
- Methotrexate
- Carmustine
- Gold salts

Is there any history of connective tissue disorders?
- Lupus
- Wegener granulomatosis
- Rheumatoid arthritis
- Goodpasture syndrome
- Dermatomyositis

Is there any exposure to radiation?
Radiation pneumonitis can also cause ILD.

 Auscultate the lungs
Distinctive dry rales ("Velcro sound") are characteristic for ILD.

Observe for evidence of hypoxemia
Low resting pulse oximetry reading, high respiratory rate, cyanosis, or clubbing

Observe any evidence of right-sided heart failure
Elevated neck veins and edema. Often the result of secondary pulmonary hypertension.

Review the CXR

> Although x-rays may be normal in some pts, very often there are usually early (ground-glass) or late (coarse reticular pattern) findings of ILD. Additional findings may suggest a certain etiology for ILD

- *Pleural disease*: asbestosis, radiation pneumonitis, systemic rheumatic disease
- *Hilar/mediastinal lymphadenopathy*: berylliosis, sarcoidosis, silicosis, amyloidosis, lymphocytic interstitial pneumonia
- *Upper lung involvement*: berylliosis, silicosis, ankylosing spondylitis, chronic hypersensitivity pneumonitis

Perform an ABG and pulmonary function test (PFT)
Although an ABG might be normal, hypoxemia is seen later on.

> PFT revealing a decreased total lung volume and vital capacity with increased diffusion capacity of the lungs are associated with ILD. This is known as a restrictive pattern on PFT.

A Interstitial lung disease
There are many forms of ILD, but they all have one thing in common: progressive, diffuse pulmonary scarring. This scarring reduces the lungs' ability to expand and oxygenate normally, thus producing the restrictive pattern noted above.
The most common form of ILD is idiopathic pulmonary fibrosis, which occurs usually in the sixth decade of life but can occur in any age-group. It is an immune-mediated disease in which injury occurs to the type I alveolar cells, and fibroblast growth and production is stimulated, thus leading to scarring.

Other forms of ILD include

All of the exposures noted above, lupus, rheumatoid arthritis, ankylosing spondylitis, Goodpasture syndrome, sarcoidosis, pulmonary alveolar proteinosis, eosinophilic pneumonias, and lymphangiomyomatosis

Differential diagnosis

Always consider tuberculosis, *Pneumocystis carinii* pneumonia, and lymphangitic metastases of malignancy.

P Perform workup to discover cause of ILD

A thorough workup of ILD should include:

- Cytoplasmic antineutrophil cytoplasmic antibodies to help rule out Wegener granulomatosis
- An antiglomerular basement membrane to rule out Goodpasture syndrome
- Bronchoscopy with bronchoalveolar lavage to look for lymphocytic or neutrophilic dominant cells in the lavage
- Computed tomography (CT) scan of chest, and consider using high resolution
- Biopsy (open lung or transbronchial) to rule out carcinoma and identify the etiologic agent if diagnosis remains in doubt

Begin by treating both the underlying pathophysiology and providing symptomatic relief

Treat/remove underlying agent.

Provide supplemental oxygen to correct hypoxemia. Make arrangements for home O_2 if severe enough.

If an autoimmune cause is suspected, corticosteroids will likely be necessary

Prednisone at 1 mg/kg daily for 8 weeks followed by a maintenance dose of 0.25 mg/kg/d for at least 6 months

If the disease persists, consider selective therapy by case to case basis

Start at 1 mg/kg/d while continuing the prednisone.

Consider risk-benefit ratio with the following therapies:

- Endothelin receptor antagonists, phosphodiesterase inhibitors, tyrosine kinase inhibitors, antifibrotic agents, immunosuppressive agents, and biological response modulators.

Make arrangements for lung transplantation in pts with progressive or end-stage ILD

SOLITARY PULMONARY NODULE

S **Does the pt smoke cigarettes? If so, for how many years and how many packs smoked per day?**

Approximately 25% of all solitary pulmonary nodules noted on CXR are found to be malignant. An accurate smoking history may indicate a level of suspicion of primary lung cancer.

Ask if the pt has any other history of cancer

This nodule may also represent a nonlung malignancy that has metastasized to the lungs, such as colon, breast, cervix, prostate, ovary, stomach, or bladder cancer. Usually, however, these will present with multiple bilateral nodules.

Ask if the pt has any history of tuberculosis, coccidiomycoses, histoplasmosis, or sarcoidoisis

A significant portion of "benign" lung nodules (~75%) can be linked to fungal or mycobacterial infections or granulomatous reactions.

Other benign nodules include hamartomas.

Has the pt had any fevers, night sweats, or weight loss?

These are the common "B" symptoms and are associated with both malignancy and with granulomatous diseases such as tuberculosis.

What is the pt's age?

In general, malignancies are less likely in pts who are younger than 35 years.

O **PE will usually reveal nonspecific findings. Nevertheless, note the following**

Pt's temperature, other vital signs, and overall appearance (cachetic?) Check for palpable lymphadenopathy.

Observation of respirations, palpation, percussion, and auscultation of lungs.

For men, digital rectal examination; for women, breast examination and cervical examination with Pap smear.

Obtain CXR

A current chest radiograph compared with an older film (ideally 2 years ago) can provide important clues regarding the possibility of malignancy.

Size:
- 2–5 mm → 1% chance of malignancy
- 11–20 mm → 33% chance of malignancy
- 21–45 mm → 80% chance of malignancy

Estimation of doubling time:
- <30 days suggests infection
- >2 years suggests benign hamartoma or granuloma

Nodule edge:
- Smooth and well-defined edge suggests benign etiology.
- Ill-defined and lobular edge suggests malignancy.

High-resolution computed tomography of the chest can provide additional clues of etiology and guide management

Calcifications:
- Central and lamellar calcifications suggests benign etiology.
- Sparse and eccentric calcifications suggests malignancy.

Appearance:
- Spiculated, peripheral halos, or thick wall cavitary lesion also suggest malignancy.

Location:
- Peripheral lesions are easier to biopsy with transthoracic needle aspiration.
- Central lesions, especially with mediastinal lymphadenopathy, can be biopsied by bronchoscopy or thoracoscopy.

Consider performing a PET scan if available, but costly

Operates by sensing glucose metabolism of cells.

Prized for its high sensitivity and specificity in detecting malignancy.

Poor sensitivity if lesion is small (<1 cm).

A **Solitary pulmonary nodule**

Although this general diagnosis is sufficient while a workup is in progress, it is a good idea to comment on the likelihood (low, medium, or high) of malignancy.

- A pt younger than 30 years of age with a stable lung nodule over 2 years with a central calcification pattern would be considered a low probability of malignancy.
- A 60-year-old, 40 pack-year smoker with a new lung nodule in the last year, 5 cm in size, with a lobular pattern on CXR and sparse, eccentric calcification pattern would be considered a high probability of malignancy.

P **Pts with a *low* probability of malignancy can be followed with serial CXRs every 3 months for the first year and then every 6 months for the second year**

This follow-up should be sufficient to establish the benignity of the lesion.

Pts with a *high* probability of malignancy can proceed directly to surgical resection without biopsy, so long as it is not contraindicated

Pulmonary function tests will have to be performed to establish that the pt can tolerate lung surgery.

This will allow for biopsy and resection at the same time.

The remaining pts with *intermediate* probability will have to undergo biopsy for definitive diagnosis. Each method has its own benefits and risks

Transthoracic needle aspiration, CT-guided

- Higher diagnostic yield than bronchoscopy for peripherally located masses
- Higher complication rate, such as pneumothorax
- Higher false-negative rate, operator-dependent associated error

Bronchoscopy

- Better suited for centrally located lesions, particularly with lymphadenopathy

CARDIOLOGY

HYPERTENSION

S **Does the pt have a known history of hypertension (HTN)?**
If so, note the age of onset and what previous medications were used to treat it.
Ask if there is a family history of HTN, cardiovascular disease, or strokes.

Does the pt take anything associated with HTN?
These would include alcohol, cocaine, high daily salt intake, cigarette smoking, oral
contraceptives, NSAIDs, steroids, or decongestants.

Does the pt have symptoms that suggest secondary causes of HTN?
Renovascular HTN: abrupt onset in <30 y/o, difficult to control with medicine
Primary aldosteronism: muscle weakness and cramps, and periodic paralysis
Pheochromocytoma: episodic headaches, hypertensive episodes, diaphoresis, palpita-
tions, and weight loss

Does pt report any risk factors associated with poorer prognosis?
- Smoking
- Dyslipidemia
- Sedentary
- Diabetes mellitus
- Obesity

O **What is the pt's blood pressure?**
Obtain at least two blood pressure (BP) measurements with the pt in the supine or
seated position. Each measurement should be at least 2–3 minutes apart. Measure in
both arms and use the highest value.

Look for evidence of end-organ damage
- Left ventricular hypertrophy
- Congestive heart failure
- Renal insufficiency
- Retinal exudates
- Myocardial infarction
- Papilledema
- Stroke

Perform a fundoscopic exam
This exam offers a rare opportunity to directly visualize arteries and veins.
Look for atrioventricular nicking, arterial narrowing, retinal exudates, or hemorrhages.

Examine the heart
Listen for S_4, ventricular lift, murmurs, and a loud aortic component of S_2.

Perform a complete neurologic assessment
HTN can cause both ischemic or hemorrhagic strokes.

Examine the pt for any signs of secondary HTN
Renovascular HTN: abdominal bruit
Cushing syndrome: edema, striae of abdomen
Hyperthyroidism: enlarged thyroid gland, exophthalmos
Coarctation of the aorta: diminished/delayed femoral > upper extremity pulses

**Perform urine and blood tests to screen for secondary causes of HTN or
increased risk of poor outcomes**
Primary aldosteronism: low potassium and high sodium
Renovascular disease: elevated BUN, creatinine, and proteinuria
Poorer prognosis: diabetes (especially if not well controlled) and dyslipidemia

Perform an ECG
Look for evidence of chronic HTN (left ventricular hypertrophy) and evidence of old
infarctions (q waves).

Hypertension

Blood pressure is measured above the normal range on three separate occasions.
Attempt to identify the cause of the hypertension:
  • Most cases (90%) are labeled essential, meaning the cause is unknown.
  • Secondary causes are usually either renal (5%) or endocrine (4%).
Assign the pt to the higher category if diastolic and systolic values fall into different
  categories (Table 2-1).

TABLE 2-1   Hypertension Categories

Category	Systolic (mm Hg)	Diastolic (mm Hg)
Normal	<120	<80
Prehypertension	130–139	85–89
Stage I	140–159	90–99
Stage II	>160	>100

 **Start drug therapy on any pt with at least high-normal HTN or greater with
target organ disease or cardiovascular disease and/or diabetes**

Diuretics: uncomplicated hypertension, heart failure, type 2 diabetes
β-Blockers: uncomplicated hypertension, myocardial infarction, angina, atrial fibrillation, essential tremor, hyperthyroidism, preoperative HTN
ACE inhibitor: diabetes with proteinuria, heart failure, myocardial infarction with
  systolic dysfunction
Calcium channel blockers: type 1 and 2 diabetes with proteinuria
Non-DHP calcium channel blockers: isolated systolic hypertension in elderly, migraine
  headache, atrial tachycardia or fibrillation
α-Blocker: benign prostatic hypertrophy

**Encourage lifestyle modifications in pts with high-normal BP who do not have
diabetes, target organ disease, or cardiovascular disease but have none or
one risk factor**

  – Weight loss   – <1 oz alcohol/day ethanol   – <2.4 g sodium
  – ↓ fats   – Smoking cessation   – Aerobic exercise 30 min/d

**Any pt with stage I HTN with no risk factors or any target organ or
cerebrovascular disease should have a trial of 12 months of lifestyle
modification**

If pt has only one risk factor that is not diabetes, try lifestyle modifications for only
  6 months.
If BP is not normal at the end of this period, initiate drug therapy.

**Start drug therapy in any pt with stage 2 or 3 HTN. Attempt to rule out
secondary causes of hypertension**

Renovascular HTN: Captopril stimulation test of plasma renin activity
Primary aldosteronism: 24-hour urinary aldosterone collection
Pheochromocytoma: urinary test for VMA, metanephrines, and catecholamines
Cushing syndrome: 24-hour collection of urinary free cortisol or overnight dexametha-
  sone suppression test

CHEST PAIN EVALUATION

S **Have the pt describe the pain and where it is located**

Rule out life-threatening causes first before considering more benign conditions.

Myocardial infarction (MI) or unstable angina presents with pain referred over pre-cordium with occasional referral to left arm, jaw, and chin.
- *Unstable angina:* Characterized by chest discomfort that is provoked by less exertion than before. Usually relieved by rest and/or nitroglycerin (NTG).
- *MI:* characterized by chest pain lasting >30 minutes that is not relieved by NTG.

Stable angina presents with similar discomfort, but is consistently provoked by the same level of exertion, lasts only 3–10 minutes, and is relieved with rest and NTG.

Gastroesophageal reflux is usually accompanied by a sour taste in the mouth, worse with reclining or supine position after meals.

Pulmonary embolism (PE), pneumothorax (PTX), aortic dissection, pneumonia, and pericarditis can all present with sharp pain on inspiration (pleuritic).

- *Pulmonary embolism, pneumothorax:* sudden onset with dyspnea
- *Aortic dissection:* sudden onset with tearing sensation to the back between the scapulae
- *Pneumonia:* more gradual in onset with rigors and cough with purulent sputum

What potential risk factors does the pt have for these diseases?
Cardiac diseases:
- Hypertension
- Cigarette use
- Atrial fibrillation
- Past MI
- Diabetes
- Cocaine use
- Aortic stenosis
- Coronary artery disease
- Hyperlipidemia
- History of arrhythmias
- Other valvular abnormalities

Pulmonary embolus:
- Prolonged immobilization or rest
- History of neoplasm/cancer
- Oral contraceptive use
- Recent trauma or surgery

Pneumothorax:
- COPD
- Cigarette use
- Marfan syndrome
- Asthma

The only known risk for aortic dissection is uncontrolled hypertension.

O **Perform a physical exam focused on potential cardiac and pulmonary causes**
Vital signs:
- Rapid heart rate and low blood pressure: acute coronary syndrome, PTX, or PE.
- Hypertension is nonspecific but indicates a potential cardiac cause.
- Tachypnea/poor O_2 sats indicate pulmonary causes such as PE, PTX, or pneumonia, but can also be a sign of cardiogenic shock causing pulmonary congestion and edema.

Neck:
- Holosystolic murmur in the carotids: aortic stenosis
- Elevated neck veins: right heart congestion indicating an acute coronary event, valvular abnormality, pericardial tamponade, pulmonary embolism, or pneumothorax

Chest:
- Decreased/absent breath sounds: PTX; confirm with hyperresonance to percussion
- Rales: left ventricular failure
- Sharp pain to palpation: costochondritis, broken rib (palpation reproduces pain), or herpes zoster (may see vesicles and erythema in a dermatomal pattern)

Heart:
- Displaced apex with sustained heave: left ventricular hypertrophy
- Loud pulmonary component of S_2: pulmonary embolism
- S_3: volume overload
- S_4: pressure overload

- Friction rubs: pericarditis
- Systolic murmur: aortic stenosis, mitral regurgitation, or tachycardia
- Diastolic murmur: mitral stenosis or aortic regurgitation

Ext:
- Peripheral edema: right ventricular failure
- Asymmetric pulses: aortic dissection

A Chest pain

Not all that causes chest pain is cardiac in origin. Consider all of the following sites:

– Skin	– Chest/back muscles	– Ribs/costochondral joints
– Pleura	– Pericardium	– Esophagus
– Aorta	– Ischemic myocardium	

    – Referred pain from stomach, gallbladder, or pancreas

P Order a CXR and stat ECG

ECG:
- ST-segment depression: ischemia
- ST-segment elevation: infarction, or if diffuse, pericarditis
- Right axis deviation, right bundle branch block, and right ventricular hypertrophy: pulmonary embolism

CXR:
- Collapsed lung field/hyperlucency: pneumothorax
- Engorged central pulmonary vasculature: pulmonary embolus
- Widened mediastinum: aortic dissection
- Cardiomegaly: left ventricular hypertrophy, congestive heart failure (CHF), and valvular disorders
- Pulmonary edema: CHF
- Infiltrates: pneumonia
- Rib fractures should be apparent

Begin immediate empiric treatment based on working diagnosis

Stable angina: Give nitroglycerin, β-blocker, aspirin. Order troponin q4h × 3.

Acute coronary syndrome: nitroglycerin, oxygen, morphine, aspirin, β-blocker, and heparin. Order troponin q4h × 3. If ST-elevation MI, consider pts eligibility for cardiac catheterization (see Myocardial Infarction, p. 362 and Unstable Angina, p. 368).

Pulmonary embolism: O_2, heparin, then warfarin; thrombolytics if unstable

Pneumothorax: oxygen followed by chest tube placement
- *Tension PTX:* Place needle in chest on affected side at midaxillary line of second intercostal space.

Aortic dissection: β-blocker, morphine, stat CT chest with IV contrast to confirm diagnosis. Call cardiothoracic surgery.

Costochondritis: NSAID therapy only.

STABLE ANGINA

 Is the pt's pain quality and duration characteristic of stable angina?
The pain classically should be dull tightness, squeezing, or pressure sensation over the
precordium or left side of chest with occasional radiation to left arm, jaw, or chin.
It should last 3–10 minutes and be relieved by rest.
If it lasts greater than 30 minutes, consider an acute coronary syndrome (ACS).

Is the pain precipitated consistently with the same amount of exertion?

Pts with stable angina present with symptoms that are evoked by the same level of activity (e.g.,
climbing two flights of stairs or walking more than 60 feet at a time). The consistency is very
important.

If the pt provides a history of requiring less activity now to evoke the same symptoms,
the pt is experiencing unstable angina, which is treated very differently.

What makes the discomfort better?
Stable angina is usually relieved by rest or with sublingual nitroglycerin.
• These are classic symptoms, and deviation from this pattern is important.
• Pts with symptoms of stable angina who fail to be relieved with three doses of nitro-
glycerin need to be evaluated for an ACS.

Does the pt have any cardiac risk factors?
 – Diabetes mellitus – Hypertension   – Hyperlipidemia
 – Post–myocardial   – Cigarette use   – Cocaine use
  infarction

O **Perform a PE**
Although the PE may be normal in an asymptomatic pt, you might see hypo-/hyperten-
sion, tachycardia, or systolic murmurs or gallops during an ischemic episode.
The PE is also useful for revealing any other evidence of disease that could contribute to
coronary artery disease, such as diabetes mellitus (neuropathy, retinopathy), thyroid
disease, or hypertension.

Obtain an ECG
Although the ECG can be normal in asymptomatic pts, the classic findings are ST-
segment depression of at least 1 mm that is downward sloping during the ischemic
episode and resolves after symptoms disappear.
Findings may be nonspecific, such as T-wave flattening or inversion.
ST-elevations indicate a myocardial infarction (MI), and this needs to be addressed very
differently and immediately.

Consider a stress ECG, echocardiography, or scintigraphic imaging of the heart
These studies may be performed on an outpatient basis to evaluate for level of activity
tolerance, ejection fraction, wall motion abnormalities, valvular dysfunction, or terri-
tories of affected vessels.

Remember not to let any pt with a history of aortic stenosis perform a stress test. Sudden death
may occur.

 Stable angina
Stable angina occurs when there is a fixed narrowing of a coronary vessel. When at
rest, the myocardium is able to obtain all of the blood, and thus oxygen, that it needs
through this stenotic region. However, at increased rates of activity and metabolic
demand, not enough oxygen reaches the myocardium through this lesion, and symptoms of ischemia (angina) occur.
Again, be sure to distinguish this diagnosis from ACS, which includes unstable angina
or ST-elevation MI, which warrants prompt medical attention.

Treat acute symptoms with sublingual nitroglycerin

Administer sublingual nitroglycerin every 3–5 minutes until symptoms resolve for up to three doses. If there is no relief, begin a workup and treatment to rule out ACS.

If asymptomatic, give pharmacologic treatment to prevent further episodes of angina

β-Blockers: These are first-line agents for treating ischemia because they reduce myocardial oxygen demand by reducing heart rate and afterload.
- Avoid in pts with reactive airway disease, bradycardia, or congestive heart failure (CHF) exacerbation.

Long-acting nitrates: Isosorbide mononitrate and dinitrate are examples.
- These doses can be increased and adjusted to reduce symptoms.
- Be sure to watch for hypotension, headaches, and tolerance to nitrates in these pts.
- Nitrates have no effects on mortality in this disease, only on the symptoms.

Sublingual nitroglycerin: Either as a spray or tablet, this medicine can be useful for any "breakthrough" symptoms that may occur during an acute attack or as prophylaxis before strenuous activity.
- A three-dose limit still applies.

Aspirin: This will exhibit antiplatelet activity but should be avoided in those with aspirin-sensitive allergies.
- In those cases, ticlopidine or clopidogrel may be considered.

Calcium channel blockers: These are reserved more as third-line agents, particularly because of their negative effects in pts with a history of CHF or MI.
- They are the first-line therapy in pts with Prinzmetal angina or coronary vasospasm. This phenomenon occurs when the pt has no stenotic coronary lesion but intermittently has angina, usually at rest, caused by coronary spasm.

Modify cardiac risk factors

This means that conditions such as hyperlipidemia, diabetes mellitus, hypertension, smoking, cocaine use, and hyperthyroidism should be medically optimized.

Fasting lipids, glucose, Hgb A1C, TSH may be useful lab studies to order from time to time on your pts.

Consider revascularization for pts who still have symptoms despite maximum medical therapy, in post-MI or unstable angina pts with evidence of ischemia despite symptom control

Revascularization would include the evaluation of coronary artery bypass grafting or percutaneous transluminal, coronary angiography with or without stenting.

CONGESTIVE HEART FAILURE

S **Does the pt have symptoms of congestive heart failure (CHF)?**

- Fatigue
- Paroxysmal nocturnal dyspnea
- Lethargy
- Edema
- Dyspnea on exertion

What amount of exertion induces these symptoms?
With greater than normal activity, with normal activity, with minimal activity, or at rest

If the pt has been stable, has there been a rapid deterioration in condition?
Rapid deterioration in an otherwise stable pt with CHF, think of ischemia or infarction of the myocardium.
Gradual deterioration might occur with noncompliance with medication and diet.

Is there any history of hypertension, dilated or restrictive cardiomyopathy, aortic stenosis, hypertrophic cardiomyopathy, myocarditis, or left-sided infarction?
These are common causes of left-sided heart failure.

Is there any history of mitral stenosis, pulmonary hypertension, endocarditis of tricuspid or pulmonary valve, or right ventricular infarction?
These are common causes of right-sided heart failure.

The most common cause of right-sided heart failure is left-sided heart failure.

O **Review vital signs**
Hypertension is a cause of CHF and is common on presentation.
Tachycardia is a compensatory mechanism for volume overload and hypotension.
Tachypnea can be seen with left-sided heart failure as a result of pulmonary edema.

Look for signs of left-sided heart failure
S_3 gallop, rales, wheezes, and murmurs suggestive of mitral and aortic valves

Look for signs of right-sided heart failure
These include elevated jugular venous pressure, lower extremity edema, abnormal hepatojugular reflux, hepatomegaly, and murmurs indicating right-sided heart valves.

Review ECG for signs of CHF
Left ventricular hypertrophy, Q-waves (indicating old transmural infarction), poor R-wave progression (poor LV function), and right ventricular hypertrophy.

Obtain an echocardiogram
Systolic ejection fraction <40% constitutes moderately reduced systolic function. Can also reveal wall motion abnormalities, show valvular disorders, show atrial and ventricular size, and reveal right ventricular and pulmonary artery pressures.

A **Congestive heart failure**
Inability of the heart to provide enough pressure to move blood. The decreased pressure leads to edema, fluid congestion, and decreased perfusion/oxygen of vital organs.
Most causes include chronic elevated afterload causing weakening of the myocardium.
Symptoms depend on which side of the heart is failing, resulting in either the lungs (left side) or the systemic venous system (right side) being congested with blood.
If possible, further classify whether this represents systolic versus diastolic dysfunction.
Note whether the pt is stable or in CHF exacerbation.

NYHA Classification
Class I: Symptoms only with greater than normal activity
Class II: Symptoms with normal activity
Class III: Symptoms with minimal activity
Class IV: Symptoms at rest

Differential diagnosis

- Acute coronary syndrome
- Pulmonary embolism
- Pneumothorax

- Interstitial lung disease
- Asthma
- Stable angina

P ### Reduce excess intravascular volume

Thiazide diuretics or oral furosemide are suitable for pts with stable CHF.

Consider IV furosemide if pt is in CHF exacerbation.

Avoid diuretics in pts with diastolic dysfunction because these pts have reduced heart relaxation rather than volume overload. Overdiuresis will lead quickly to hypotension.

Reduce afterload

ACE inhibitors are useful in reducing both afterload and the sympathetic nervous system related to cardiac remodeling. When giving an ACE inhibitor, remember to monitor:

- *Renal function:* Do not to give ACE inhibitors to pts with serum creatinine greater than 2.0.
- *Electrolytes:* Hyperkalemia may occur secondary to aldosterone suppression.

Reduce preload

Pts with CHF will benefit from oral long-acting nitrates. Nitroglycerin as needed is unlikely to help.

In pts with CHF exacerbation, consider IV nitroglycerin; for those with exacerbation and hypertension, sodium nitroprusside has been shown to be effective.

Increase cardiac contractility

Digoxin has been used in pts with moderate to severe CHF. Although digoxin has not been shown to actually be of benefit in reducing mortality, it has been shown to improve symptoms and cause fewer admissions related to CHF exacerbation.

Pts with severe CHF admitted to the Cardiac Care Unit with severe hypotension can be treated with IV dobutamine. Use judiciously because oxygen demand can increase with these pts.

Ensure proper oxygenation

As CHF is treated and fluid is removed from the lungs, oxygenation will improve.

Until that time, supplemental O_2 should be given to maintain saturation $\geq 95\%$.

When stable, consider addition of low-dose β-blocker (carvedilol) and increase as tolerated.

Outpatient therapy should consist of furosemide, ACE inhibitors, and a <2 g/d sodium-restricted diet and fluid restriction if indicated

SYSTOLIC MURMUR

S **Does the pt have any risk factors for aortic stenosis (AS)?**
Congenital bicuspid valve or known calcification of aortic valve

Does the pt have any risk factors for mitral valve regurgitation?
Ischemic heart disease:
- Papillary muscle dysfunction
- Left ventricular dilation
- Ruptured chordae tendineae

History of rheumatic fever suggests valvulitis.
Intravenous drug abuse is a risk factor for infective endocarditis.
Illicit diet drugs such as fenfluramine and dexfenfluramine have also been implicated.

Does the pt have angina, syncope, or congestive heart failure?
If the workup reveals aortic stenosis, the average life expectancy is 5, 3, and 2 years, respectively, without intervention.

Are there other medical problems that increase the risk of a systolic murmur?
Systolic flow murmurs, more common over the aortic or pulmonic valve regions, can occur in any hyperdynamic, high-output state (e.g., anemia and hyperthyroidism).

O **Perform a careful exam of the heart. Note where the murmur is best appreciated**

- Right upper sternal border: aortic valve
- Left upper sternal border: pulmonic valve
- Left lower sternal border: tricuspid valve
- Apex: mitral valve

Note if the murmur increases with inspiration
This would indicate a right-sided heart murmur (tricuspid or pulmonic).

Note if the murmur is crescendo-decrescendo or holosystolic
Crescendo-decrescendo is the sound of blood being forced across a stenotic opening, thus implicating the pulmonic and aortic valves.
Holosystolic murmurs indicate that blood is regurgitating without resistance, thus implicating the mitral and tricuspid valves and also ventricular septal defects.

Note any preceding midsystolic click or pop
This is a sign of mitral valve prolapse, a myxomatous degeneration of the mitral valve.
The valve is competent at the beginning of systole, but the central portion of the leaflet pops upward into the atrium in midsystole.
If there is no regurgitation, there will only be the click without the murmur.

Have the pt perform the valsalva maneuver and note if the murmur changes
Murmurs of AS decrease with this maneuver and increase once it is released.
Valsalva decreases blood flow into the heart (by increasing intrathoracic pressures), thus decreasing the volume of blood crossing the stenotic valve.

Note any change with squatting
AS and mitral regurgitation murmurs both increase with this maneuver, whereas IHSS (a type of cardiomyopathy) will decrease.

Continue listening to the pts heart as he or she goes from squatting to standing
IHSS murmurs will actually increase, whereas AS murmurs will decrease.

Continue auscultation while pt performs an isometric handgrip
Mitral regurgitation increases with handgrip, whereas AS and IHSS decrease.

Continue auscultation through the respiratory cycle
Tricuspid regurgitation (TR) murmurs should increase with inspiration. Murmurs of
   pulmonic stenosis and TR should decrease with expiration.

Note if the murmur radiates anywhere
AS should radiate to the carotid arteries.
Mitral regurgitation murmurs often radiate to the axillae.

Note any changes with passive straight-leg raise
AS and TR murmurs tend to increase, whereas IHSS actually decreases.

Palpate the carotid or any other central pulse
AS may have a slow and sustained central pulse (parvus e tardus).

Systolic murmur
Characterize the murmur as either holosystolic or crescendo-decrescendo.

Differential diagnosis
- Aortic stenosis
- Idiopathic hypertrophic subaortic stenosis
- Tricuspid regurgitation
- Hypertrophic cardiomyopathy
- Benign flow murmur
- Mitral regurgitation
- Pulmonic stenosis
- Ventricular septal defect
- Mitral valve prolapse

If you suspect anything other than a flow murmur, order an echocardiogram of the heart
This study should definitively discern the etiology of the murmur.

For pts with aortic stenosis
Send the pt for cardiac catheterization to measure the pressure gradient across the valve.
- Consider valve replacement if gradient is >50 mm Hg or valve area is <1 cm.
- Medically manage with diuretics and sodium restriction.
- Digoxin and calcium channel blockers may be used if atrial fibrillation is present.
Advise pt against vigorous aerobic exercise because sudden death may occur.

For pts with mitral regurgitation
Medical management includes diuretics and afterload reduction.
Digoxin and calcium channel blockers may be used for atrial fibrillation.
Schedule mitral valve replacement before irreversible left ventricular dysfunction
   occurs.

For pulmonic stenosis and tricuspid regurgitation
Intervention is less urgent because right-sided lesions cause less disease.
Refer for replacement when right-sided heart failure symptoms are significant.

For ventricular septal defects
If pulmonary artery pressures are normal on echo, refer these pts for surgery.

For all pts with pathologic murmurs, prescribe antibiotic prophylaxis for dental procedures

DIASTOLIC MURMUR

S **Does the pt have any risk factors for aortic regurgitation (AR)?**
 – History of intravenous drug abuse ≡ infective endocarditis
 – Congenital bicuspid valve   – Syphilis
 – Lupus   – Marfan syndrome
Recent blunt chest trauma (e.g., a steering wheel in a motor vehicle accident) can also be
 a cause of acute AR.

Does the pt have any risk factors for mitral stenosis (MS)?
Rheumatic fever is the most common cause. Lupus and left atrial myxoma are much
 rarer.

O **Listen to the heart murmur. Note where it is best appreciated**
Right upper sternal border: aortic valve
Left upper sternal border: pulmonic valve
Left lower sternal border: tricuspid valve
Left midaxillary line: mitral valve

Note if the murmur increases with inspiration
This would indicate a right-sided heart murmur.

Note if the murmur is high- or low-pitched
High-pitched murmurs tend to implicate pulmonic and aortic valves, whereas low-
 pitched murmurs suggest the mitral valve.

Note change with squatting. AR murmur should increase
This is because squatting increases systemic vascular resistance, thus increasing the
 drive for blood to regurgitate across the aortic valve.

Note change with isometric handgrip
Both AR and MS murmurs should increase.

Note change with breathing
Tricuspid stenosis (TS) murmurs may increase with inspiration and decrease with
 expiration.

Note change with passive, straight-leg raise
TS murmurs should increase. This is because leg raise increases blood return to the
 heart, thus causing increased blood flow across the stenotic tricuspid valve.

Look for evidence of mitral stenosis
 – Prominent jugular A-waves   – Opening snap
 – Diastolic rumble   – Low-pitched
 – At apex in left lateral position – Palpable right ventricular heave
If severe enough, there may also be evidence of right ventricular dysfunction with bilat-
 eral lower extremity edema and ascites.

Look for evidence of aortic regurgitation
Bounding pulses: "water hammer" or Corrigan pulse
Capillary pulsations of nailbeds with lightly applied pressure (Quincke sign)
"Bobbing head" in systole (de Musset sign)
Widened pulse pressure (large difference between systole and diastole)
S_3 on apex
Point of maximal impulse deviated to left and down

Review CXR
Cardiomegaly from left ventricular hypertrophy might be seen with chronic AR.
Pulmonary congestion and edema would be seen with chronic MS.

Diastolic murmur

If enough clinical evidence exists, make a working diagnosis on what you believe is the likely etiology.

Differential diagnosis

Aortic regurgitation

Mitral stenosis

Tricuspid stenosis

Pulmonic regurgitation

Atrial septal defect (ASD)

A congenital ASD can go unnoticed for a lifetime because its characteristic sound, a fixed split S_2, can be difficult to hear, and because as a low-pressure system, it takes a long time for the left-to-right shunt to manifest physical symptoms. However, when enough blood has been shunted to the pulmonary system, the tricuspid valve may experience a relative stenosis. This diastolic murmur may be the first sign of an ASD and may occur relatively late in life.

 Order an echocardiogram of the heart

This study should definitively answer the etiology of the murmur.

If the echo reveals aortic regurgitation, begin with medical therapy

Treat congestive heart failure (CHF) symptoms, if present, with ACE inhibitors, diuretics, and sodium restriction.

If medical therapy fails, or if the pt has acute AR with left ventricular failure, either systolic or diastolic, call a cardiothoracic surgery consult

Surgical replacement of the valve will be necessary.

If the echo reveals MS, again begin with medical therapy

Treat atrial fibrillation with rate control and anticoagulation. If CHF is present (almost certainly would be right-sided), treat with diuretics and sodium reduction.

Call a cardiothoracic surgery consult if mitral valve area is <0.7 cm² or if symptoms persist on maximal medical therapy

It is possible that the stenosis can be relieved without valve replacement, but surgical widening will be necessary. If that fails, the valve will need to be replaced.

Prescribe antibiotic prophylaxis for these pts for all dental procedures

All pts with valvular lesions severe enough to cause a murmur (produced by turbulent blood flow) are at risk for endocarditis.

ATRIAL FIBRILLATION

S **Is the pt experiencing an irregular heart rhythm or palpitations?**

These are the most common symptoms reported by pts.

Asymptomatic atrial fibrillation is even more common.

If the duration is longer than 48 hours or unknown, evaluate for possible atrial thrombus.

Are there symptoms of shortness of breath, chest pain, or altered mental status?

These symptoms may indicate shock, myocardial infarction, or pulmonary edema.

If they are present, strongly consider urgent cardioversion.

Does the pt have a history of hypertension, coronary artery disease, valvular heart disease, atrial septal defect, hyperthyroidism, pericarditis, or chest surgery?

These are common medical and surgical causes of atrial fibrillation.

Is the pt taking any medications? Does he or she use any drugs or alcohol?

Theophylline and β-agonists are common medications that can cause atrial fibrillation.

Excessive alcohol intake ("holiday heart") is a common cause of atrial fibrillation that is often transient and self-resolving.

Does the pt have a history of congestive heart failure, diabetes, hypertension, valvular disorders, or prior stroke? Is he or she older than 75 years?

A "yes" answer to any one of these questions identifies someone who is at significantly increased risk of stroke and should be considered for anticoagulation.

O **Perform a focused PE**

Pulse: A resting heart rate higher than 100 bpm is defined as rapid ventricular rate and warrants rate control with medications or cardioversion.

- Note that not all ventricular beats translate into a palpable radial pulse. The difference between the ventricular and radial pulse is known as the "pulse deficit."

Blood pressure: Without atrial systole and with a rapid ventricular rate, stroke volume can fall dramatically. Severe hypotension is an indication for urgent cardioversion.

Lungs: Pulmonary edema, characterized by rales and bibasilar decreased breath sounds, may be another indication for urgent cardioversion.

Heart: The classic finding is an irregularly irregular heart beat.

- An S4 representing an "atrial kick" is, by definition, absent in these pts.

Examine the ECG

Atrial activity should be disorganized, with an atrial rate between 400 and 600 bpm. This is represented by the "fibrillating baseline." There will be no discernible P-waves, and their presence should lead you to another diagnosis.

The ventricular rate, represented by QRS complexes, should be irregular. It may or may not be rapid (>100 bpm).

If the pt has paroxysmal atrial fibrillation, the ECG may be normal.

Evidence of ischemia or infarction on ECG warrants prompt preparation for urgent cardioversion (see Myocardial Infarction, p. 362 and Unstable Angina, p. 368).

Review the CXR

Evidence of pulmonary congestion or edema warrants urgent cardioversion.

Atrial fibrillation with or without rapid ventricular response

A normally functioning heart should beat approximately 60–100 times per minute. In atrial fibrillation, foci discharge all over the atria and prevent coordinated atrial contraction.

In general, an adult atrioventricular node will not transmit faster than 160–170 bpm, which is why the rate in atrial fibrillation is usually about 160–170.

Differential diagnosis

Atrial flutter: very similar to atrial fibrillation and treated the same (characterized by "sawtooth" pattern on ECG).

Paroxysmal supraventricular tachycardia: A rapid rate requiring a reentry pathway around the atrioventricular node. Although there are no P-waves, it should be regular.

Sinus or junctional tachycardias: Monofocal rapid rhythms. P-waves will be present.

Sinus rhythms with premature beats: Premature atrial or ventricular beats; if frequent enough can make a rhythm seem irregular.

 If the pt is hemodynamically unstable or has pulmonary edema, he or she should be admitted and urgently cardioverted, first electrically and then chemically if unsuccessful

Electrical cardioversion includes an initial synchronized shock at 100 or 200 J followed by another shock at 360 J if unsuccessful.

Chemical cardioversion involves loading and infusion of either ibutilide or procainamide.

If the pt is stable and has a rapid ventricular response, use medications to control the rate

β-Blockers, calcium channel blockers with chronotropic properties (e.g., diltiazem and verapamil), and digoxin are common rate-control agents used.

- β-Blockers are best suited for those pts with ischemia or infarction.
- Diltiazem and verapamil will be better suited for those pts with hypertension or with contraindications for ß-blockers.

These two classes are preferred as initial agents because they can be started intravenously and switched to oral agents. The following medications should be considered adjunctive therapy:

- Digoxin has a slow onset, even with loading.
- Amiodarone is useful as an adjunct, but again has a slow onset.

Two or three agents may be required to achieve a goal rate of 50–100 bpm at rest.

Anticoagulate those pts at risk for thromboembolism

Pts with "lone atrial fibrillation" (<60 years old and without any risk factors for stroke) can be managed without anticoagulation or with aspirin alone.

Other pts should be anticoagulated for a minimum period of 3 weeks with warfarin with an international normalized ratio goal of 2.0–3.0 before elective cardioversion and continued for at least 1 month after successful cardioversion.

Otherwise, anticoagulation should be chronic because of increased risk of stroke from thromboembolism.

PERICARDITIS

 Ask the pt to describe the chest pain

The classic characteristics are a sharp chest pain that is worse with deep inspiration and is relieved with sitting up. Dyspnea and radiation to back, epigastrium, or shoulder are sometimes present.

Does the pt have any medical history associated with pericarditis?

Recent myocardial infarction (MI): Can present as soon as 2–3 days after an MI.
- Pericarditis presenting much later (several weeks to months) is known as Dressler syndrome.

Infection (often initially presents as a respiratory infection):
- *Viral:* influenza, varicella, Epstein-Barr virus, coxsackie, echovirus
- *Bacterial:* pneumococcal, streptococcal, staphylococcal, and gonorrheal
- Tuberculosis
- *Fungal:* coccidioidal, candidal

Renal failure: Uremic pericarditis is a common complication in dialysis-dependent pts.

Malignancy: Lung, breast, and renal carcinomas and lymphoma are common causes. Also, the radiation therapy to treat some of these malignancies can lead to pericarditis as well.

Autoimmune: rheumatoid arthritis and systemic lupus erythematosus

 Review VS

Low blood pressure, pulsus paradoxus, and rapid heart rate may be the first signs of pericardial effusion causing tamponade, a dangerous complication of pericarditis.

Tamponade occurs when the pressure exerted by the pericardial fluid exceeds the pressures inside the heart chambers. The atria collapse first, leading to a lack of blood to be ejected by the ventricles. It is a medical emergency and should be treated with immediate pericardiocentesis.

Fever can be seen but is not specific.

Observe the neck veins

Engorged neck veins might suggest pericardial effusion or tamponade physiology.

Auscultate the heart

Friction rub: The classic PE finding is a three-part friction rub. Actually sounds like rubbing two pieces of leather together with every beat.

Muffled heart sounds: This is the more common auscultatory finding with pericardial effusion.

Obtain an ECG

Nonspecific ST-T wave changes are common.

Classic findings include ST-segment elevation in all leads (uncommon for an MI), which usually causes ST-segment elevation only in contiguous leads.

Low QRS voltage and electrical alternans may be a sign of effusion.

Obtain a stat CXR

Cardiomegaly may be present from pericardial effusion.

 Pericarditis

The pericardium, as the name suggests, is the covering of the heart. It consists of two parts: (1) the visceral pericardium, which sits directly on the heart; and (2) the parietal pericardium, which is a fibrous sac. There is between 15 and 50 mL of pericardial fluid in the sac under normal circumstances. In the case of pericarditis, this amount of fluid is expanded and contains inflammatory cells.

Note the etiology of the pericarditis.

Comment on whether pericardial effusion is present, and if present, if any tamponade physiology is apparent.

Differential diagnosis

Myocardial infarction: substernal chest pain and ECG changes

Pneumonia: pleuritic chest pain

Tension pneumothorax (PTX), restrictive cardiomyopathy, and right ventricular MI can all cause tamponade physiology.

Tension PTX will be characterized by decreased breath sounds on one side of the chest.

> An echocardiogram should be urgently ordered if there is any suggestion of pericardial effusion, to assess for the possibility of pericardial tamponade.

If tamponade is present, the effusion should be drained by pericardiocentesis or surgically, by pericardial window.

Otherwise, treat the underlying problem

For suspected viral pericarditis start NSAIDs

After the pt has been afebrile for 7 days, begin to taper the NSAID dose.

Caution with post-MI pericarditis, NSAIDs can interfere with ventricular healing or remodeling.

If recurrences occur for more than 2 years, refer for pericardiectomy.

If you suspect tuberculous pericarditis, perform a purified protein derivative test. If positive, drain pericardial fluid. If no acid-fast bacilli are present and you still suspect TB, biopsy the pericardium for granulomata

If positive, start anti-TB quadruple therapy (INH, rifampin, ethambutol, and pyrazinamide).

For uremic pericarditis, begin daily dialysis for 2 weeks. Recheck and perform an echocardiogram at that time

NSAIDs will help relieve symptoms.

If effusion persists after 2 weeks, consider drainage.

If the pt has a known malignancy and you suspect neoplastic pericardial effusion, drain the fluid and perform a cytologic study

Consider a partial pericardectomy

Unfortunately, the prognosis for this condition is poor.

PREOPERATIVE CARDIAC CLEARANCE

 Has the pt undergone recent cardiac revascularization (either angioplasty or coronary artery bypass graft) within the last 5 years?

If so, and the pt does not have any new signs or symptoms of ischemia, further cardiac testing before transferring the pt to the OR is not necessary.

Has the pt had a coronary angiogram or stress test in the last 2 years?

If so, and the results were without evidence of ischemia or infarction, and the pt has no new signs or symptoms of ischemia, further cardiac testing before transferring the pt to the OR is not necessary.

Is there any history of _major_ clinical _predictors_ of perioperative risk?

- Myocardial infarction (MI) within the last month
- Unstable angina
- Severe valvular heart disease
- Decompensated heart failure

Are there any _intermediate_ clinical predictors of perioperative risk?

- MI more than 1 mo ago
- Stable angina
- Stable congestive heart failure
- Diabetes mellitus
- Renal failure

Are there any _minor_ clinical predictors?

History of stroke or poor functional capacity (see below) would be minor clinical predictors.

What is the pt's functional capacity?

> Be sure to ask about the pts ability to walk up a hill or a flight of stairs, wash dishes, or perform light housecleaning duties without dyspnea or chest pain. This question is **crucial** because this represents at least 4 metabolic equivalents (METs) of activity.

Low functional capacity is <4 METs.
- Pts who cannot meet at least 4 METs because of noncardiac reasons such as severe arthritis should also be labeled as poor functional capacity.

What type of elective surgery is the pt having?

High cardiac risk:
- Emergent major operations in the elderly
- Aortic or other major vascular (except carotid endarterectomy) surgery
- Prolonged surgeries with anticipated blood loss or fluid shifts

Intermediate cardiac risk:
- Carotid endarterectomy
- Head and neck
- Orthopedic
- Intrathoracic
- Intraperitoneal
- Prostate

Low cardiac risk: breast, cataract, endoscopic, and superficial procedures

O **Obtain an ECG, fasting glucose, Hgb A1C, and creatinine. Note age and BP**

Significant arrhythmias such as high-grade atrioventricular block, supraventricular arrhythmias with uncontrolled rate, and symptomatic ventricular arrhythmias in the setting of coronary artery disease are _major_ clinical predictors of cardiovascular risk.

Evidence of a prior MI on ECG or diabetes or renal insufficiency (Cr >2.0) represents _intermediate_ clinical predictors of risk.

Advanced age, left ventricular hypertrophy, left bundle branch block, rhythms other than sinus, and hypertension are _minor_ predictors of risk.

A __y/o pt with (major/intermediate/minor) predictors of perioperative cardiac events scheduled for (high/intermediate/low) risk surgery

Designate the pt with the highest clinical predictor that you discovered on your evaluation. For example, a pt with three minor clinical predictors and one intermediate clinical predictor is labeled as having an intermediate clinical predictor for perioperative risk for cardiovascular events.

P Refer all pts with major clinical predictors for coronary angiogram before surgery

These pts may require angioplasty or even coronary artery bypass graft before their elective surgery.

If the pt refuses angiogram, he or she should consider delaying or canceling the surgery with medical management and risk factor modification.

Recommend that pts without major but with intermediate clinical predictors with at least MODERATE functional capacity (>4 METs) can undergo low- to intermediate-risk surgeries without further testing

Their functional capacity indicates that despite their clinical predictors, they likely have enough cardiac function to tolerate one of these surgical procedures.

Refer pts without major but with intermediate predictors with at least MODERATE functional capacity going for high-risk surgeries for noninvasive testing first, such as exercise or pharmacologic stress testing

If noninvasive testing reveals high risk for ischemia, then a coronary angiogram is required, with subsequent care dictated by findings and treatment results.

If noninvasive testing reveals low risk, the pt may proceed to the OR.

Also refer pts without major but with intermediate clinical predictors with LOW functional capacity (<4 METs) for noninvasive testing

If these tests reveal low risk of ischemia, the pt may proceed to the OR.

If results show high risk, a coronary angiogram is required, with subsequent care dictated by findings and treatment results.

Pts without major or intermediate predictors with at least MODERATE functional capacity may proceed to the OR without further testing

Pts without major or intermediate predictors with LOW functional capacity undergoing high-risk surgeries should undergo noninvasive testing first; for low- or intermediate-risk surgeries, the pt may proceed to the OR without further testing

GASTROENTEROLOGY

EPIGASTRIC PAIN

S **Obtain a detailed history regarding the quality and timing of pain**
Severe, instantaneous: perforated ulcer, ruptured aneurysm, myocardial infarction
Constant severe pain: acute pancreatitis
Sharp, burning, gnawing, hunger-like pain: peptic ulcer disease (PUD)
Pain that awakens the pt from sleep or 1–3 hours after eating: PUD of the duodenum

> **What is the relationship between food and pain, if any?**
> Gastric ulcer, gastroesophageal reflux disease (GERD): worse after food
>   Duodenal ulcer: tends to be worse before meals

Is there any relief with antacid use?
Duodenal ulcers tend to improve symptomatically after the pt takes antacids.

Is the pt experiencing heartburn or sharp, rising pain in chest?
This type of pain would be typical of GERD.

What medicines is the pt taking? Do they include any NSAIDs?
NSAIDs can cause both duodenal and gastric ulcers.
Antibiotics, especially cyclines, can cause erosive esophagitis.

Ask about any associated symptoms that may raise red flags to rule out cancer
- Family history of cancer
- History of anemia
- Unintentional weight loss
- Hematochezia (bloody stool)
- Feeling of epigastric fullness
- Odynophagia (painful swallowing)
- Hematemesis
- Dysphagia (difficulty swallowing)
- Age older than 45

Any diarrhea, weight loss, or abdominal mass associated with PUD-type symptoms?
This would be consistent with Zollinger-Ellison syndrome, a gastrin-secreting tumor.

Is there any associated nausea or vomiting?
Consider gastric outlet obstruction, which can occur with cancer or chronic PUD.

Is the pt having problems with swallowing? Are liquids easier than solids, or are they the same?
In addition to being symptoms of malignancy, odynophagia and dysphagia may indicate an esophageal constriction, ring, web, or achalasia.
- Early mechanical dysphagia will be worse with solids than liquids.
- Advanced mechanical or motor dysphagia creates problems swallowing both.

Has the pt had any prior radiation therapy to the chest?
Radiation can cause esophagitis.

O **Perform a focused PE**
Vital signs: Always check BP, heart rate, orthostatics, and temperature.
- Perforated ulcer and pancreatitis may present with tachycardia and unstable vital signs.
Cardiac: Check for tachycardia.
Abd: Make sure the pt does not have a surgical abdomen with rigidity, rebound tenderness, tenderness to percussion, and decreased or absent bowel sounds.
- This may indicate perforated ulcer or pancreatitis.
- PUD may have vague tenderness in the epigastrium or left upper quadrant.
Rectal exam: to rule out bleeding

Check labs
A low hematocrit or positive stool occult blood could be signs of PUD.
If you suspect Zollinger-Ellison syndrome, check the fasting gastrin level (normal in PUD).

Obtain an upright CXR
This will rule out free air under the diaphragm, which is indicative of perforated ulcer.

Obtain an ECG
To rule out acute coronary syndrome

If the diagnosis is unclear, perform a barium swallow study
This will help diagnose the presence of PUD in up to 80% of cases.

A Epigastric pain

Differential diagnosis includes
Peptic ulcer disease: gastric ulcer, duodenal ulcer, gastric cancer/lymphoma, Zollinger-Ellison syndrome (rare), perforation GERD
Esophagitis: In immunocompromised pt with difficulty swallowing, consider HSV, CMV, HIV, or *Candida*. Can also have radiation-induced or pill esophagitis.
Esophageal strictures, webs, rings, achalasia, or diffuse esophageal spasms
Pancreatitis: Pancreatic inflammation can occur for any number of reasons.
Acute coronary syndrome: Symptoms may be confused with epigastric conditions.

P Pts with the alarm symptoms listed above should undergo immediate esophagogastroduodenoscopy (EGD)
Best test for malignancy; biopsies performed and other conditions diagnosed visually.

Call an immediate surgery consult for pts with suspected perforated ulcer. For all other pts with ulcers on EGD or suspected ulcers by H&P, start an 8-week course of a proton pump inhibitor
If after 8 weeks symptoms persist, pt should undergo EGD.

Check pts for infection with *Helicobacter pylori*
H. pylori infection is the number one cause of PUD and is extremely common.
The gold standard for diagnosis is histologic exam of antral mucosa via biopsy on EGD.
If not planning EGD, may perform enzyme-linked immunosorbent assay for serum IgG against bacterium.
• If negative, rules out disease. If positive, indicates past exposure, not necessarily active disease.
Urease test: *H. pylori* is a urea-splitting organism. CLO test involves the pt swallowing radiolabeled urea and then the breath is sampled for radioactive material.
• Sensitive and specific.
• Pt may not be taking proton pump inhibitor (PPI) before the test.

Treat *H. pylori* if found
Treatment is 2 weeks with omeprazole, bismuth, and two antibiotics (varies by regimen).

If you suspect esophageal stricture, the pt will need an EGD
Balloon dilation may be necessary.

Treat all pts with suspected GERD with either a PPI or an H$_2$ blocker
Symptoms should improve on this therapy.

RIGHT UPPER QUADRANT PAIN

S Ask the pt to describe the pain

Sharp, colicky pain in the right upper quadrant, often intermittent, causing the pt to double over in pain; radiating to the shoulder should make you think of gallbladder disease.

Are there any associated symptoms?

Fever: Think of acute infectious or inflammatory process
    – Hepatitis   – Cholecystitis   – Ascending cholangitis
Vomiting: obstruction such as gallstone or malignancy
Diarrhea: more common with liver abscess

Is there any relationship of pain with food?

Think of gallstones if pain is worse after fatty meals.

Is the pt an alcohol drinker and has he or she had any alcohol intake recently?

Acute alcoholic hepatitis presents with right upper quadrant (RUQ) pain.

What medications is the pt taking?

Both prescribed and herbal medications may present with drug-induced cholestasis.

Has the pt had any prior surgeries?

Note the reason for surgery and date of surgery.
This will help rule out acute cholecystitis if there has been a cholecystectomy.
It may also point toward a choledocholithiasis (presence of a stone in the common bile duct, retained after the surgery).
Abdominal scars may hurt or cause bowel obstruction secondary to adhesions.

Has there been any recent travel to a Third World nation?

Think of hepatitis A

Has the pt had any unintentional weight loss?

This should always make you think of malignancy.

Is there any clay-colored stool or tea-colored urine?

Seen with bilirubin excretion defect

If female, what is the menstrual history?

    – Ovarian torsion   – Ectopic pregnancy
    – Pelvic inflammatory disease   – Endometriosis

Has there been any history of heart disease?

Rarely, cardiac pain can be referred as RUQ pain.

Any cough, chest pain, shortness of breath?

These symptoms indicate a pulmonary or cardiac cause such as:
    – Pneumonia   – Right-sided heart failure   – Pulmonary embolism

O Perform a focused PE

Vital signs: Fever usually indicates infection.
  • Tachycardia/orthostatics (as an indirect fluid status assessment)
Gen appearance: jaundice/icterus—gallbladder obstruction, acute hepatitis
Abd: absence of bowel sounds—obstruction; check for ascites

- *Murphy sign:* inspiratory arrest during light palpation of right hypochondrium—consider gallbladder pathology
- Masses palpated, hepatomegaly, splenomegaly
- Jaundice, fever, and RUQ pain: triad indicating ascending cholangitis

Pelvic exam if high suspicion that this may be ovarian in origin
Rectal exam for guaiac test

Obtain these labs

CBC: Presence of elevated WBC suggests infection

Liver panel to assess for hepatobiliary causes: bilirubin level, transaminases, albumin, PT/PTT. AST, ALT >1,000, think of acute hepatitis

Check HBsAg, anti-HCV Ab, anti-HAV IgM; if any positive, indicates viral hepatitis

Amylase elevation >500 IU suggest pancreatitis, not as specific as elevated lipase level

Blood cultures: if suspect ascending cholangitis

Pregnancy test

Entamoeba histolytica serum titers to rule out amebic liver abscess, if high suspicion

Obtain radiologic studies

RUQ ultrasound: Helps determine the presence of gallstones, gallbladder obstruction, gallbladder sludge, as well as liver size, abscesses, or tumors

Plain film KUB or abdominal film to rule out obstruction

CXR: to rule out pulmonary causes

CT of abdomen may be needed for pancreatic evaluation, liver abscesses

HIDA scan: if you suspect acute cholecystitis, cystic duct obstruction

 Right upper quadrant pain

Differential diagnosis includes

Gallbladder diseases: acute cholecystitis, ascending cholangitis, common bile duct stone, gallbladder cancer (cholangiocarcinoma)

Liver diseases: hepatitis (alcoholic/viral), abscesses, tumors

Pancreas: gallstone pancreatitis, pancreatic pseudocyst, pancreatic carcinoma

Pulm: pneumonia, pulmonary embolism

Cardiac: right-sided failure with passive hepatic congestion (nutmeg liver on pathology)

Bowel obstruction

Pelvic: ovarian torsion, ectopic pregnancy, pelvic inflammatory disease, endometriosis

 Begin with supportive care

Narcotics for pain control

IV hydration with normal saline

> **Call surgery if pt has acute abdomen or signs of obstruction.**

These include decreased bowel sounds, rigidity, guarding, and tenderness to percussion.

Treat based on the underlying disorder

Cholecystectomy is the treatment for acute cholecystitis/choledocholithiasis and gallstone pancreatitis. Consider prophylactic antibiotics. May need medical stabilization before treatment with nasogastric suctioning and volume resuscitation.

Acute hepatitis: supportive care, may need ICU monitoring

Liver abscess (pyogenic or amebic): antibiotics. Consider drainage if pt has persistent fever or unclear diagnosis.

Ascending cholangitis: antibiotics; endoscopic retrograde cholangiopancreatography or percutaneous drainage may be required. Asymptomatic or intermittently painful gallstone disease does not require surgery.

ABNORMAL LIVER TESTS

S **Does the pt have any other symptoms of biliary disease?**
 – Yellow eyes – Itchiness – Dark urine and light-colored stool

Are there any risk factors for hepatitis?
 – IV drug abuse – Needle sharing – Unprotected sex
 – Tattoos – Blood transfusions (prior surgeries, especially before 1982)

What medications is the pt taking?
 – Tylenol – Antiepileptics – Lipid-lowering medications

Does the pt drink alcohol?
Ask about duration and amount.

Has the pt traveled to or emigrated from a Third World nation?
 – Viral hepatitides – Yellow fever
 – Malaria – Entamoebic diseases

Has there been any recent unexplained weight change?
Unintentional weight loss should lead you to think of cancer.
Rapid weight gain may indicate development of ascites.

Does the pt have diabetes, high cholesterol, and/or obesity?
These conditions are risk factors for nonalcoholic fatty liver disease (NAFLD).

Is there any family history of liver disease?
Both hemochromatosis (a disease of iron overload) and Wilson disease (copper overload)
 are genetic causes of abnormal liver tests.

Does the pt have a history of any autoimmune disease?
Autoimmune diseases can cause autoimmune hepatitis or primary biliary cirrhosis.

O **Check the VS**
Fever, hypotension, tachycardia: infectious hepatic process or end-stage liver disease

Physical evidence of liver disease on the general exam includes
 – Jaundice – Telangiectasias
 – White nail beds – Gynecomastia

Signs of liver disease on the abdominal exam include
 – Flank dullness – Ascites – Hepatomegaly
 – Splenomegaly – Right upper quadrant
   tenderness

Send blood for liver function tests, viral hepatits panel, an antinuclear antibody (ANA) and an anti-smooth muscle antibody (ASMA), serum iron studies, α_1-antitrypsin level, and a serum ceruloplasmin level
Albumin: Many illnesses can affect the liver's production of albumin, but in the presence of known liver disease, this is evidence that function has been affected.
Prothrombin time (PT): The liver produces many of the coagulation factors. When production is affected, PT increases.
Bilirubin: Cholestatic disease presents with an elevation of direct and total bilirubin.
Alanine aminotransferase (ALT): specific for liver, muscle
Aspartate aminotransferase (AST): present in liver, heart muscle, kidney, brain, and red blood cells
  • Moderately elevated enzymes, AST > ALT by >2:1, consider alcoholic hepatitis
  • Otherwise, ALT will usually be > AST.
Alkaline phosphatase (AP): produced in biliary ducts, bone, placenta, and intestines
  • Extrahepatic sources of elevated AP can be differentiated from hepatic by a normal 5'nucleosidase level. It will be elevated with liver disease.

Viral hepatitis panel: Consider anti-HAV IgM, HbsAg, anti-HBc, and anti-HCV as primary tests for active liver disease to rule out hepatitis A, B, and C (see Hepatitis, p. 394).

ANA and ASMA: One or the other should be positive in autoimmune hepatitis.

Ferritin, iron, and iron saturation will all be markedly elevated in the presence of hemochromatosis, which usually presents in the fifth decade of life.

Ceruloplasmin will be elevated in Wilson disease, which usually presents late in the second decade or early in the third decade of life.

α_1-Antitrypsin will be low in its deficiency; another inherited cause of liver disease.

Obtain an ultrasound of the right upper quadrant

Diagnoses presence of gallstones, masses, obstruction, abscesses, or cirrhosis.

A **Liver disease**

Decide if this is hepatocellular injury versus a cholestatic picture.
- ↑↑↑ AST/ALT with ↑ AP and total bilirubin, think of hepatocellular injury.
- ↑↑↑ total bilirubin, AP elevation with ± AST/ALT elevation, think of cholestasis.

Differential diagnosis of hepatocellular injury

Viral hepatitis: A, B, C, D, E, CMV, EBV, HSV, VZV

Autoimmune hepatitis

NAFLD: Fatty degeneration of hepatocytes occurs with metabolic syndrome as noted above

Toxic hepatitis: acetaminophen, alcohol, other medications and toxins

Vascular causes: Budd-Chiari (hepatic vein thrombosis), congestive heart failure, shock liver

Hereditary causes: hemochromatosis, α_1-antitrypsin deficiency, Wilson disease

Differential diagnosis of cholestatic injury

Obstructive: choledocholithiasis, cholangiocarcinoma, pancreatic cancer, sclerosing cholangitis

Nonobstructive: cirrhosis, sepsis, postoperative, primary biliary cirrhosis

P **For most liver diseases, pts will require supportive care and close observation**

Viral hepatitides may improve spontaneously. If they become chronic, refer to hepatology.

For autoimmune hepatitis, give steroids and other immunosuppressive agents as indicated.

For NAFLD, encourage the pt to lose weight. This may reverse some of the damage.

For obstructive lesions, refer pt to a surgeon or gastroenterologist to relieve the lesions.

For pts with cirrhosis or genetic lesions that will cause cirrhosis, consider transplant

Unfortunately, placing a pt on the transplant list may be all that can be done.

Give vitamin K for pts with elevated PT/PTT

This may improve production of clotting factors.

All pts with elevated liver enzymes should be instructed to refrain from alcohol

Repeat abnormal liver tests every 6 months. If no diagnosis is evident, pt may need biopsy

CIRRHOSIS

 Does the pt have any history of drinking alcohol?
Ask about the amount of alcohol consumption: how much for how many years.

Is there a family history of liver cirrhosis?
Genetic causes: hemochromatosis, Wilson disease, α_1-antitrypsin deficiency

Has the pt had increased itching?
Increased bilirubin tends to cause itching but is also the presenting sign of primary biliary cirrhosis.

Does the pt take oral contraceptives or is there a history of a hypercoaguable state?
Hypercoagulability and oral contraceptive use are risk factors for Budd Chiari, a hepatic vein thrombosis.

Ask about more unusual potential diagnoses
Hemochromatosis: Suspect in a pt with diabetes, bronze skin, and hypogonadism.
Wilson disease: Suspect in a young pt with neurologic or psychiatric disease.

 Perform a generalized PE
Vital signs:
- *Low BP:* increased third spacing of fluid
- *Fever:* spontaneous bacterial peritonitis

Gen: Look for gynecomastia, fetor hepaticus, and bilateral parotid enlargement.
Neuro: Assess mental status to determine if hepatic encephalopathy is present. If pt seems altered, have pt hold arms out in front of body, hyperextended at the wrists. If hepatic encephalopathy is present, hands will flap down and back up again; known as asterixis.
Skin: Look for spider angiomas, jaundice, and palmar erythema, all signs of cirrhosis.
Eyes: Conjunctival icterus is the first sign of jaundice. If you suspect Wilson disease, look for a Kayser-Fleischer ring in the iris.
Abd:
- *Ascites:* flank dullness, fullness, distention; check for fluid wave or shifting dullness.
- *Caput medusae:* visible veins on surface of abdomen, surrounding umbilicus.
- *Hepatosplenomegaly:* Splenomegaly is more common because of portal venous. congestion. Cirrhotic livers are usually small/shrunken. Hepatomegaly may indicate malignancy.

Testicles: Check for atrophy.

Perform lab analyses to aid in diagnosis
Transaminases (AST/ALT): Elevation implies ongoing hepatocellular destruction.
Hepatitis B surface antigen: If positive, indicates active hepatitis B infection.
Hepatitis C antibody: If positive, indicates that pt has ongoing chronic hepatitis C.
Ceruloplasmin: If elevated, the pt has Wilson disease.
Iron panel: Elevated ferritin and iron saturation may indicate hemochromatosis.
α_1-*Antitrypsin:* Low level indicates deficiency syndrome.
Antimitochondrial antibody: Indicates primary biliary cirrhosis.
Alpha fetal protein: If elevated, may indicate occult hepatocellular carcinoma (HCC).

Follow-up with lab analyses to aid in management
CBC: Cirrhosis is associated with anemia, leukopenia, and thrombocytopenia.
Chemistry: ↓ Na+ secondary to ascites; elevated NH_3 may indicate encephalopathy.

Obtain a right upper quadrant (RUQ) ultrasound
Detects ascites, cirrhosis, hepatic masses, hepatic/portal vein patency, and biliary dilation.

If unsure of diagnosis, obtain a liver biopsy
This is the gold standard for the diagnosis of cirrhosis, usually done percutaneously.

Cirrhosis

Assess for the Child-Pugh Score: A = 5–6; B = 7–9; C = 10–15. Lower number: better outcome (Table 3-1).

TABLE 3-1   Child-Pugh Score

	1	2	3
Ascites	None	Slight	Moderate/severe
Encephalopathy	None	Slight	Moderate/severe
Bilirubin (mg/dL)	<2	2–3	>3
Albumin (mg/L)	>3.5	2.8–3.5	<2.8
PT (seconds increased)	1–3	4–6	>6

P **All cirrhotics should avoid alcohol. If etiology is known, treat the underlying disorder**

Phlebotomy for hemochromatosis; d-penicillamine for Wilson disease. Give antiviral agents such as interferon alpha and ribavirin for viral hepatitis.

If ascites is present, perform a paracentesis to rule out spontaneous bacterial peritonitis (SBP)

Send fluid for cell count and differential, albumin; consider total protein, LDH, and glucose.

Treat with IV cefepime for SBP if PMN >250 cells/mm or if neutrophil >50% of cells.

Obtain a serum ascites albumin gradient

Subtract ascitic albumin from serum albumin. If >1.1, the pt has portal hypertension.

Restrict dietary sodium to less than 2 g per day

This should decrease ascites development.

Fluid restriction is not necessary unless the pt is severely hyponatremic.

Give oral diuretics if ascites is present

Furosemide 40 mg orally qd and spironolactone 100 mg qd. Always in a 5:2 ratio.

Give lactulose, titrating to three bowel movements per day

Increased clearance of colonic flora should reduce encephalopathy/ammonia level.

Place the pt on the list to be evaluated for a liver transplant screen for HCC q 6 months with RUQ ultrasound and serum alpha fetal protein

DIARRHEA

S **How large are the bowel movements? What is the consistency of the stool?**
Voluminous/watery: Implies small bowel/proximal colon source, osmotic diarrhea. Pt is
  more likely to have electrolyte imbalances.
Small: Think of left colon or rectum source.

What are the associated symptoms?
Inflammatory: pain, tenesmus, fever
Osmotic: cramps, bloating, flatulence

What did the pt eat recently? What does he or she eat regularly?
Preformed bacterial toxicities can come from consuming expired milk products, mayon-
  naise, or old fried rice. These include *Staphylococcus aureus and Bacillus cereus.*
Fruit or milk products may aggravate diarrhea. Fructose or lactose intolerance is
  common.

Does fasting improve the diarrhea?
Osmotic diarrhea stops with fasting, whereas secretory diarrhea will continue.

Is there blood in the stool?
If bloody diarrhea, always think of colitis, infectious versus inflammatory.
Other etiologies of bloody stool (although usually will not be diarrhea) are hemorrhoids,
  colonic malignancy, arterial malformations, and venous mesenteric thrombosis.

Is the stool foul smelling or greasy in appearance?
If there is visible oil, this is known as steatorrhea. It is caused by malabsorption.

What medications has the pt been taking?
Antibiotic usage puts the pt at risk for diarrhea or even *Clostridium difficile* colitis.

Has the pt recently traveled abroad or gone camping?
Traveling abroad puts the pt at risk for parasitic infections.
Drinking from stream water is a risk for *Giardia lamblia,* a small intestinal parasite.

O **Perform a focused PE**
Vital signs: Presence of fever could point to infectious or inflammatory causes. A pt with
  positive orthostatic blood pressure or pulse is hypovolemic.
Gen appearance: Look for rashes, mouth ulcers, flushing, or any other systemic signs.
Abd: Usually nonspecific tenderness, but check for bowel sounds.
Rectal: Check for tone, presence of perianal fistulas/abscesses.

Check stool analyses
| – WBC | – Occult blood | – Fat | – Culture |
| – pH | – Laxatives | – O&P | – *C. difficile* toxin |

Check stool electrolytes and calculate a stool osmotic gap.
  • The osmotic gap is 290-2(stool Na + stool K) mOsmol/kg.
  • In pure osmotic diarrhea, the gap is greater than 125.

Consider other labs for suspected diagnoses
Urine for 5-hydroxyindole acid, the metabolite of serotonin, is the test for carcinoid. For
  malabsorption, send serum for antigliadin and antiendomysial (tests for celiac sprue).

A **Diarrhea**
Defined as greater than 200 g/d of stool; average daily output is 150–180 g/d.
Acute diarrhea is of less than 2 weeks, whereas chronic is greater than 2–3 weeks.

Differential diagnosis of acute diarrhea. Most are infectious
Enterotoxic: These are secretory diarrheas of the small intestine. Occult blood/WBCs are
  negative.
  • Bacterial: *Vibrio cholera* and most types of *Escherichia coli*
  • Viral: Rotavirus, Norovirus (previously called Norwalk agent)
  • Parasitic: *G. lamblia*

Invasive: These are inflammatory diarrheas. Occult blood/WBCs are positive.
- Bacterial: *Campylobacter jejuni, Salmonella, Shigella, E. coli* O157:H7, *C. difficile*
- Parasitic: *E. histolytica,* tapeworm infections

Pts with AIDS may not have fever. Organisms include *Cryptosporidium, E. histolytica, Giardia, Isospora, Strongyloides, Mycobacterium,* cytomegalovirus, etc. Likely if CD4 count <200.

Inflammatory bowel diseases (IBD), ulcerative colitis, Crohn disease can present acutely.

Differential diagnosis of chronic diarrhea

Osmotic diarrheas: Those in which molecules create osmotic load, pulling water into stool

– Celiac sprue	– Intestinal lymphoma	– Bacterial overgrowth
– Drug-induced	– Pancreatic insufficiency	– Lactose intolerance
– Short gut syndrome		

Secretory diarrheas: Water and electrolytes are secreted into the stool.

– Carcinoid	– Zollinger-Ellison	– VIP-oma

Inflammatory diarrheas: Noninfectious causes are fairly limited to IBD. Intestinal wall motion can also be altered. This includes pheochromocytoma, hyperthyroidism, and irritable bowel syndrome.

AIDS enteropathy should always be considered in the differential of chronic diarrhea.

P **If the pt is dehydrated, admit and begin IV fluid/electrolyte replacement**

Then determine the cause of diarrhea and treat accordingly

Acute: For most acute forms of diarrhea, watchful waiting will be all that is indicated. If risk factors indicate, pts may need sigmoidoscopy to rule out ischemia or ulcers.

For chronic diarrheas, start oral loperamide as the cause is investigated

Loperamide decreases intestinal motility. For investigation, consider colonoscopy.

For osmotic diarrheas, dietary changes and oral enzyme therapy may improve symptoms

For IBD, immunosuppressants and NSAIDs, orally and as enemas, should decrease ulcers

If a parasitic infection is detected on the stool ova and parasite study, give specific therapy

NEPHROLOGY

CHRONIC RENAL FAILURE

S **Does the pt have any personal or family history of kidney disease?**
- Diabetes mellitus (DM)
- Systemic lupus erythematosus (SLE)
- Polycystic kidney disease
- Obstructive uropathy
- Focal segmental glomerulosclerosis
- IgA nephropathy
- Hypertension (HTN)
- Glomerulonephritis (GN)
- Alport syndrome
- Interstitial nephritis
- Postinfectious glomerulonephritis

Does the pt have any symptoms of uremia?
- Pruritus
- Vomiting
- Impotence
- Anorexia
- Singultus
- Tremor
- Nausea
- Nocturia
- Leg cramps

Does the pt have any history of volume loss?
Volume depletion from the GI tract or the kidneys can cause acute renal failure.

O **Review VS**
Look for high blood pressure.
Check orthostatics.
Tachycardia and hypotension suggest volume depletion.

Perform PE
Gen: sallow complexion
Skin: ecchymosis, epistaxis (resulting from uremic toxins causing platelet dysfunction)
Neuro: stupor, asterixis, myoclonus
Eyes: fundoscopic exam; pale conjunctiva suggests anemia
Cardio: rubs (pericarditis), murmur, S_3, S_4 suggest fluid overload
Pulm: crackles, decreased breath sounds suggest fluid overload
Abd: palpate for enlarged kidneys
Ext: edema

Check BUN and creatinine
To confirm the diagnosis and compare with previous values if available. This is one of the best ways to differentiate chronic from acute renal failure.

Check Mg^{2+} and phosphorus
These are often high in renal failure because of decreased excretion.

Check Ca^{2+}
Usually low because of decreased GI absorption, resistance to parathyroid hormone, and decreased $1,25 (OH)_2D_3$, which is produced by the kidneys.

Check CBC
CBC shows normocytic anemia caused by decreased erythropoietin.

Estimate glomerular filtration rate (GFR) with 24-hour urine creatinine and creatinine clearance (renal function)

$$\text{Cr Cl(mL/min)} = \frac{\text{Urine Cr(mg/dL)} \times \text{Urine vol.(mL/min)}}{\text{Plasma Cr(mg/dL)}}$$

Normal range of creatinine clearance: 95–105 mL/min

Obtain a renal ultrasound
Size is usually <10 cm in chronic renal failure (CRF).
Diabetes, amyloidosis, and multiple myeloma produce normal to large kidney size.

Review urinalysis
Typical specific gravity is 1.010, and blood and protein are common in CRF.
Waxy casts indicate chronic renal disease.

Check ECG
To evaluate possible pericarditis or changes caused by hyperkalemia

A

Chronic renal failure
A worsening of renal function to a GFR <60 mL/min for longer than 3 months.

Etiologies
- DM
- Cystic kidney disease
- HIV
- HTN
- Interstitial nephritis
- Obstructive uropathy
- Chronic GN
- SLE

P

Treat reversible causes of chronic renal insufficiency
- Infection
- Hypertension
- Obstruction
- Congestive heart failure
- Volume depletion

Monitor I/Os
Many pts will not be oliguric until later in the disease, but it is important to monitor this and start dialysis in a timely fashion.

Prevent hyperkalemia by avoiding foods high in potassium and taking kayexalate when necessary
The kidneys normally excrete excess potassium, but in renal failure they are less effective. As a result, intake of potassium needs to be reduced.

Avoid and treat hyperphosphatemia to prevent renal osteodystrophy
Use calcium carbonate 648 mg po tid with meals when PO^{3-} is less than 6.
Use phosphor binders if PO^{3-} is more than 6.
Restrict foods high in phosphorus such as eggs, dairy products, and meats.
Restrict foods high in potassium such as pinto beans, bananas, tomatoes, and orange juice.

Control HTN and DM to slow progression of renal failure
Tight glycemic control
Recommend using an ACE inhibitor for DM. Avoid ACE inhibitor when Cr >2.0.
Avoid nephrotoxins and IV contrast if possible.
Dialysis after radiocontrast dye does not prevent renal damage.

Restrict sodium intake and maintain adequate nutrition

Treat hyperlipidemia
Cardiovascular disease is the most common cause of death in pts with CRF.

Treat anemia with erythropoietin injections (Epogen), 10,000 U SQ three times per week

Refer for emergent dialysis for severe refractory
- Hyperkalemia
- Acidosis
- Volume overload

Uremia (encephalopathy, pericarditis, or platelet dysfunction)

Prevent and treat uremic bleeding
DDAVP (desmopressin)—causes release of factor VIII
- Cryoprecipitate
- Conjugated estrogens

Treat uremic pruritus with antihistamines

Refer early to a nephrologist for evaluation of dialysis

NEPHROTIC SYNDROME

 What is the clinical presentation?

Edema associated with renal failure

These pts are hypercoagulable because of excretion of anticoagulants into the urine.
- Pulmonary embolism
- Renal vein thrombosis

Does the pt have any conditions that cause membranous glomerulonephropathy?
- Diabetes
- Hepatitis B
- Hepatitis C
- Syphilis
- Amyloidosis
- SLE
- History of cancer: lung, breast, leukemia, lymphoma

Is the pt on any medications that can cause proteinuria?
- Captopril
- NSAIDs
- Probenecid
- D-penicillamine
- Heroin
- Gold

O **Review VS**

Look for hypertension as a sign of possible renal involvement (consider glomerulone-phritis in the differential diagnosis).

Look for hypotension as a sign of decreased intravascular volume.

Perform PE

Gen: lymphadenopathy, malar rash (SLE), pale

HEENT: periorbital edema, doughy earlobes

Pulm: decreased breath sounds, crackles (point to fluid overload and pleural effusion)

Back: check for flank or back tenderness (this may suggest renal vein thrombosis and occurs more with membranous glomerulonephropathy)

Abd: ascites

Ext: pitting edema

Repeat U/A to confirm proteinuria on the dipstick

Proteinuria can be present during high fevers or following vigorous activities.

Protein >300 mg/dL and oval fat bodies are pathognomonic for nephrotic syndrome.

Check a 24-hour urine protein

The pt is instructed to void and discard the first morning urine specimen.

Then begin collecting urine up to and including the next morning's first void.

24-hour urine creatinine is used to ensure a proper collection and to calculate the glomerular filtration rate.
- In females, the creatinine should be from 10–15 mg/kg.
- In males, 15–20 mg/kg.

Check BUN and creatinine to look for renal insufficiency; check serum glucose

In adults, nephrotic syndrome is highly associated with diabetes.

Large proteinuria is often the predecessor of end-stage renal disease in these pts.

Order a lipid panel

To look for hyperlipidemia

Check serum albumin

To look for hypoalbuminemia

Order tests based on clinical suspicion
- RPR
- Hepatitis B/C
- ANA
- dsDNA

Consider imaging and workup if suspect sequelae of hypercoagulability such as deep vein thrombosis, pulmonary embolism, and renal vein thrombosis

Nephrotic syndrome is a hypercoagulable state caused by urinary loss of protein C, S, and antithrombin III.

A   Nephrotic syndrome

A clinical entity, of increased permeability of the capillary basement membranes of the glomeruli, characterized by

- Proteinuria (>3.5 g/1.73 m³/24 hr)   – Hypoalbuminemia and albuminuria
- Hypercholesterolemia
- Edema

Etiology

Membranous glomerulonephritis (most common in adults):
- Idiopathic
- Secondary:

| – Hepatitis B | – Syphilis | – Lymphoma |
| – Leukemia | – Lung CA | – Breast CA |

IgA nephropathy (10% present with nephrotic syndrome)
Minimal change disease (more common in children)
Membranoproliferative glomerulonephritis
Focal segmental glomerulosclerosis:

| – Heroin abusers | – HIV |
| – Reflux uropathy | – Morbidly obese |

SLE
Diabetes mellitus

Differential diagnosis

| – Congestive heart failure | – Cirrhosis | – Renal failure |
| – Severe malnutrition | – Vasculitis | – HIV |

P   Reduce edema with gentle diuresis and salt restriction

Also carefully monitor for signs of intravascular hypovolemia, hypotension.

Reduce proteinuria with ACE inhibitors if creatinine permits

If they have Cr >2.0, do not use an ACE inhibitor (high risk of hyperkalemia in renal failure).

Treat hyperlipidemia with lipid-lowering agents to reduce the risk of cardiovascular disease

Consult Nephrology for renal biopsy and further workup

Biopsy is done when the etiology is unclear.

The treatment of nephrotic syndrome depends on the underlying cause

Primary membranous glomerulonephropathy with prednisone and cyclophosphamide
Focal segmental glomerulosclerosis with prednisone
Hepatitis B with interferon
Syphilis with penicillin
Lupus with steroids

If renal vein thrombosis is suspected, duplex ultrasound of the kidneys should be ordered. Once confirmed, the pt is to be hospitalized and started on heparin

HEMATURIA

S **Is the hematuria at the beginning, end, or throughout urination?**
Hematuria seen at the beginning of urination indicates urethral bleeding.
Terminal hematuria indicates a bladder neck or prostate problem.
Hematuria throughout urination indicates an upper urinary tract problem.

What are the associated symptoms?
Dysuria, frequency, and urgency suggest cystitis.
Flank pain radiating to the groin indicates a kidney stone (rarely painless).
Symptoms such as fever and weight loss may suggest renal cell CA or vasculitis.

Is the pt menstruating?
Menstruation is a common cause of apparent hematuria in women.

Does the pt have a Foley catheter?
Placement of the catheter causes trauma to the lower GU tract.

Is there a family history of kidney disease?
Family history of polycystic kidney disease, Alport syndrome, SLE, sickle cell
History of hemoptysis associated with vasculitis (Wegener granulomatosis)
Recent upper respiratory tract infection suggests IgA nephropathy.

Did the pt recently have a sore throat?
Poststreptococcal GN can occur about 10–21 days after a strep throat infection.
IgA nephropathy causes hematuria a week after a viral infection or with exercise.

What medicine is the pt taking?
NSAIDs and aspirin can increase the risk of bleeding.
Cyclophosphamide causes hemorrhagic cystitis.
Rifampin changes the color of the urine.

O **Review VS**
High blood pressure suggests GN.
Fever suggests infection or malignancy.

Perform a PE
Skin: Malar rash, joint pain suggest SLE; purpura, petechia suggest vasculitis.
Cardio: Atrial fibrillation can cause arterial renal embolism.
Abd: Palpate for any masses, organomegaly.
Back: Check costovertebral angle tenderness (pyelonephritis).
Genitourinary: Check for any trauma, and perform a prostate exam in males.

Check BUN and creatinine to assess renal function

Obtain a 24-hour urine with protein and creatinine
Proteinuria is common with glomerular hematuria caused by leakage through broken
glomerular capillaries.

Check PT and PTT to rule out any coagulopathy

Order a CBC looking for anemia, platelet count, sickle cells

Check electrolytes including calcium, phosphorus, magnesium
Look for any abnormalities such as hypercalcemia suggesting renal stones.

Review urinalysis
Dysmorphic RBCs or RBC casts suggest glomerular disease.
Crystals indicate a renal stone.
Normal-sized/shaped RBCs are a sign of urinary tract bleeding.
A blood clot indicates lower tract disease in general.
Large blood on the dipstick with few RBCs suggests rhabdomyolysis.
Hematuria and pyuria without organisms suggest STD.
Hansel stain for eosinophils in the urine to rule out acute interstitial nephritis

Check urine culture and sensitivity

If suspect infection

Check renal ultrasound to assess renal size and shape

Look for stones, hydronephrosis, or multiple cysts.

Check C4 and C3 complement level

Low complement levels are in a few diseases.

- SLE
- Shunt nephritis
- Membranoproliferative
- Poststreptococcal GN
- Cryoglobulinemia
- Subacute bacterial endocarditis

Order antistreptolysin O or anti-DNAse if poststreptococcal GN is suspected

A **Hematuria**

Urine containing blood (RBCs)

Etiologies

Upper urinary tract (dysmorphic RBCs present):

- Glomerulonephritis from various causes:
  o Poststreptococcal glomerulonephritis
  o IgA nephropathy
  o Membranoproliferative glomerulonephritis
  o Rapidly progressive glomerulonephritides
  o Vasculitis: polyarteritis nodosa, microscopic polyangiitis, Wegener granulomatosis, Henoch-Schönlein purpura
- Renal cell carcinoma

Lower urinary tract:

- Renal stones
- Bladder cancer
- Bladder infection
- Local trauma of urethra or lower

Other causes of red/orange urine

- Rifampin
- Oxacillin
- Pyridium
- yoglobinuriabullet

P **If infection is present, treat and then repeat U/A**

Blood may be present during a urinary tract infection and may clear after treatment.

Consider c-ANCA if Wegener disease is suspected

Consider cryoglobulin when hepatitis C is positive

Consider antiglomerular basement membrane antibody when Goodpasture syndrome is suspected

Order intravenous pyelogram (IVP) if the above tests are negative

IVP shows the anatomy of both the upper and lower urinary tract.

Obtain abdominal CT if mass is present on ultrasound

Spiral CT of the kidneys and ureters is a good way to identify the pathology.

Send urine cytology and order cystoscopy in pts >40 y/o with a negative urine culture, to look for bladder cancer

Risk factors for bladder cancer include:

- Cigarette smoking
- Cyclophosphamide
- Pelvic irradiation

Finally, if you suspect glomerular disease, consider renal biopsy. If all of the above tests are negative, consider an angiogram to rule out arteriovenous malformation

HYPONATREMIA

 S **Does the pt have any history of volume depletion?**

Vomiting and diarrhea cause volume depletion (a decrease in intravascular volume) as well as sodium depletion.

Overuse of diuretics such as furosemide or hydrochlorothiazide

Is the pt on any medications that increase the release of antidiuretic hormone (ADH)?

Antipsychotic agents, narcotics, tricyclic antidepressants

Is the pt taking any medications that can enhance the action of ADH?

– NSAIDs   – Chlorpropamide

Is the pt using any of the vasopressin analogues?

– DDAVP   – Oxytocin

Has the pt recently had surgery?

Most of the time pts are on NS, usually in pain, and on narcotics, all of which can stimulate the release of ADH.

Does the pt have any history of congestive heart failure, nephrotic syndrome, or cirrhosis?

These pts retain more water than sodium.

Ask about history of:

– Myocardial infarction   – Hepatitis   – Alcoholism
– Bilateral LE edema   – RUQ pain   – ↑ abdominal girth

Does the pt have symptoms of adrenal insufficiency or hypothyroidism?

These two endocrine conditions can cause hyponatremia.

Is the pt at risk for syndrome of inappropriate ADH (SIADH)?

Pulmonary processes: cancer, pneumonia

Central nervous system processes: meningitis, tumor, head trauma

O **Check volume status looking for signs of hypovolemia**

– Hypotension   – Tachycardia   – Orthostasis
– Flat neck veins   – Poor skin turgor   – Dry mucous membrane

Look for signs of hypervolemia

– Jugular venous distention   – Hepatojugular   – Ascites
                                     reflex
– Bilateral lower-extremity pitting – Scrotal edema
  edema

Look for any evidence of cirrhosis

– Spider angiomata   – Gynecomastia   – Palmar erythema
– Parotid enlargement
  (alcohol abuse)

Check serum Na⁺. If it is <135 mEq/L, check urine osmolality and electrolytes

Low urine sodium (<10 mEq/L) indicates a nonrenal cause of volume depletion.

High urine sodium (>20 mEq/L) suggests renal solute loss.

Urine osmolality in SIADH is >100 mOsm/kg H_2O.

Check serum glucose

This effectively rules out pseudohyponatremia from hyperglycemia:

$$Na^+_{Corrected} = Na^+_{Serum} + 1.6[(Glucose - 100)/100]$$

Check BUN and creatinine to assess renal function

An elevated BUN correlates with decreased extracellular fluid.

Check serum osmolality

If osmolality is normal, it is pseudohyponatremia caused by:
- Hyperlipidemia (triglyceride >1,000)
- Hyperproteinemia (protein >10)
- Hyperglycemia (see formula above)

Calculate sodium deficit

Na deficit = 0.6 × total body weight × (current serum Na^+ − normal Na^+)

Check TSH and serum cortisol to rule out hypothyroidism and hypoaldosteronism

SIADH is a diagnosis of exclusion.

A **Hypoosmolar hyponatremia**

Low serum sodium in the absence of confoundingly high osmotic agents such as triglycerides, proteins, or glucose.

Normo-/hyperosmolar hyponatremia represents a condition like hyperglycemia where total body sodium is unchanged; it is only redistributed or diluted.

Remember that extracellular volume is determined by total body sodium, and sodium concentration is determined by total body water.
- Therefore, changes in ECV indicate changes in total body sodium.
- And changes in serum Na^+ concentration indicate changes in total body water.

Etiologies

Hypovolemia:
- Vomiting
- Diuretics
- Diarrhea
- Salt wasting
- Adrenal insufficiency

Euvolemia:
- SIADH
- Water intoxication

Hypervolemia:
- Renal failure
- Cirrhosis
- Nephrotic syndrome
- Congestive heart failure

P **If hypovolemic hyponatremia, replace fluids with normal saline**

If diuresis is the cause, discontinue it and replace volume.

If hypervolemic hyponatremia, restrict Na^+ and water intake

Add diuretics to increase sodium excretion if needed.

If euvolemic hyponatremia, restrict fluid to 800–1,000 mL of intake per day

Remember to stop all medications that can cause hyponatremia.

If the pt has hyponatremia with symptoms such as headache, disorientation, confusion, or seizure, treat with 3% NS until symptoms resolve

Symptomatic hyponatremia is an emergency, but never increase at a rate more than 1 mEq/hr to avoid central pontine myelinolysis:
- Flaccid paralysis
- Dysarthria
- Dysphagia

Acutely the goal is to reverse symptoms, not to normalize sodium.

If the pt is asymptomatic, correct slowly with fluid restriction

If fluid restriction does not work, use normal saline, lithium, or demeclocycline.

HYPERNATREMIA

S

Does the pt have any history of volume loss?
- Diarrhea   - Nasogastric suctioning   - Fever   - Excessive burns

Does the pt have access to water and a normal sense of thirst?
- Elderly, bedridden   - Stroke   - Dementia   - Delirium

Is the pt on any medications that can cause hypernatremia?
- Lithium   - Demeclocycline   - Hypertonic NaCl or $NaHCO_3$

Does the pt have conditions that can cause central diabetes insipidus?
- Head trauma   - Neurosurgery   - Meningitis/   - Neoplasm
                                          encephalitis

Does the pt have nephrogenic diabetes insipidus (DI)?
- Hypokalemia   - Hypercalcemia   - Amphotericin B

Has the pt been drinking salt water or ingesting salt tabs?
Salt poisoning leads to a hypervolemic hypernatremia. If hypervolemia is found on
   the exam (edema, hypertension), and the pt is not receiving IV saline, this is the only
   diagnosis.

O

Check BP, heart rate, orthostatics, and I/Os
Hypotension and tachycardia indicate hypovolemia
Polyuria can be caused by DI or primary polydipsia.

Perform a PE
Neuro: focal neurologic deficit, altered mental status, coma
Skin: poor turgor
Ext: edema

If Na^+ >145 mEq/L, check serum Ca^{2+} and K^+
Hypercalcemia and hypokalemia can cause nephrogenic DI.
Hypokalemia and hypertension are associated with hyperaldosteronism, which may
   cause borderline increases in serum sodium concentration.

Check urine osmolality
Urine osmolality <200 mOsm/L indicates central DI.
Urine osmolality between 200 and 500 mOsm/L indicates nephrogenic DI.

Check urine sodium
Random urine sodium can help in assessing the extracellular volume (ECV). Urine Na^+
   <10 mEq/L suggests a low extracellular volume.

Consider administering a water deprivation test if you suspect DI
Give 10 µg intranasal DDAVP after water restriction to differentiate central (urine osmo-
   lality increases by at least 50%) from nephrogenic DI (no change).
Administer this test under close supervision because fluid loss can be excessive.

A

Hypernatremia
Increased serum sodium
Remember that ECV is determined by total body sodium, and sodium concentration is
   determined by total body water.
   • Therefore, changes in ECV indicate changes in total body sodium.
   • And changes in serum Na^+ concentration indicate changes in total body water.

Etiologies
Low ECV: water loss in excess of Na^+ loss
         - Diarrhea   - Vomiting   - Sweat   - GI secretions

Normal ECV: loss of free water with no change in Na^+
  • Diabetes insipidus: central or nephrogenic
High ECV: Na^+ gain in excess of water gain
  • Normally iatrogenic from hypertonic saline infusion

P **If hypovolemic hypernatremia, correct hypovolemia with normal saline (NS)**

Give 500 mL–1 L NS bolus and recheck. Repeat until hypovolemia resolves

After initial boluses have been given, calculate free water deficit.

$$\text{Water deficit:} \frac{\left(\text{Plasma } Na^+ - \text{Desired } Na^+\right)}{\text{Desired } Na^+} \times 0.6 \times \text{body weight in kg}$$

Replace with hypotonic solution (e.g., 1/2 NS or NS).

Also take into account ongoing losses of water (e.g., fever, diarrhea, diaphoresis, urine output) when calculating water deficit.

For example: You have a 70-kg man with a serum Na^+ of 165 mEq/L. You want to calculate the water deficit with a desired corrected Na^+ to be 155 mEq/L in the next 10 hours.
  • Water deficit = (165−155)/155 × 0.6 × 70 = 2.7 L
  • Now, take into account insensible loss (from 0.5 to 1 L/24 hr).
Rate of correction depends on symptoms and the acuity of hypernatremia.
  • If hypernatremia has been present for weeks, correct slower than in a case where the hypernatremia occurred in hrs.
  • Usually give half of the volume in the first 8 hours and then half over the next 16 hours.
  • If rate of correction is too fast, it can cause cerebral edema.

If the pt has isovolemic hypernatremia, evaluate central versus nephrogenic DI
See above.

Treat central DI with intranasal DDAVP
Be sure to replace free water.

Treat nephrogenic DI by removing the offending toxin or medication
Treat with low-sodium diet, thiazide diuretic, and replace free water.

If the pt has hypertonic hypernatremia, identify causes such as hypertonic saline and discontinue them
It is sometimes necessary to use diuretics to excrete excess Na^+, in which case water loss during such therapy needs to be replaced.

HYPOKALEMIA

S **Does the pt have a history of GI potassium loss?**
- Diarrhea
- Vomiting
- Laxatives
- Gastric suctioning

Is the pt taking any medicines that can cause renal potassium loss?
- Hydrochlorothiazide
- Lasix
- Aminoglycosides
- Amphotericin B
- Cisplatin
- Penicillins

Does the pt have any risk factors for transcellular shift of potassium?
- Insulin
- Alkalosis
- Refeeding
- β-Adrenergic drugs such as albuterol, epinephrine
- Hypokalemic periodic paralysis with thyrotoxicosis

Is the pt losing the potassium from the kidneys?
- Type I renal tubular acidosis
- Diabetic ketoacidosis
- Recovery phase of acute renal failure
- Postobstructive diuresis
- Barter syndrome
- Osmotic diuresis

Could this pt have hyperaldosteronism?
Consider this diagnosis in pts with hypertension, hypernatremia, and hypokalemia.
Hypokalemia without any provocation suggests hyperaldosteronism. Remember that
aldosterone causes potassium secretion at the distal renal tubules.

Is the pt at risk for magnesium loss?
Hypomagnesemia causes hypokalemia. Treatment of hypokalemia without replacement
of magnesium can never be achieved. Besides GI losses, renal losses can result from
diuretics, cisplatin, and aminoglycosides.

O **Review VS and perform a PE**
Check for flaccid paralysis and hyporeflexia (can occur with potassium <2.5).
Check for asterixis because hypokalemia can precipitate hepatic encephalopathy.
Abd exam: May have decreased or absent bowel sounds secondary to functional
ileus.

Look for ECG changes
- Flattened T-waves
- Prominent U-waves
- ST-segment depression
- Prolonged QT

Repeat the potassium to verify the abnormality; check BMP, Mg^{2+}, Ca^{2+}, and phosphorus
Prolonged hypomagnesemia can cause hypocalcemia from decreased parathyroid hor-
mone (PTH) secretion, as well as PTH resistance.
Low Mg^{2+} decreases K^+ reabsorption across renal tubules.

Check a CBC
An elevated WBC can cause pseudohypokalemia.

Check urine potassium
To differentiate renal (>40 mEq/24 hr) versus GI potassium (<20 mEq/24 hr) losses

Consider further workup
If you suspect hyperaldosteronism, draw plasma renin (low) and aldosterone levels.
If there is evidence of acidosis (a low bicarbonate), think type I renal tubular acidosis
(RTA).
Urine Cl^- <15 mEq/L indicates GI losses (nasogastric tube suctioning, vomiting).
Urine Cl^- >25 mEq/L suggests renal losses.

Hypokalemia

Low serum potassium

Etiologies

GI loss:

- – Diarrhea
- – Laxatives
- – Vomiting
- – Gastric suctioning

Renal loss:

- • Type I RTA
- • Diabetic ketoacidosis
- • Recovery phase of acute renal failure
- • Postobstructive diuresis
- • Barter syndrome
- • Osmotic diuresis
- • Medicines that can cause renal potassium loss:
    - – Thiazide diuretics
    - – Aminoglycosides
    - – Cisplatin
    - – Furosemide
    - – Amphotericin B
    - – Penicillins

Transcellular shift of potassium

- – Insulin
- – Alkalosis
- – Refeeding

β-Adrenergic drugs: albuterol, epinephrine

Hypokalemic periodic paralysis with thyrotoxicosis

P **Eliminate and treat conditions that can cause transcellular shifts of potassium**

Replace potassium.

- • Oral replacement is preferred and is much safer than the IV route.
- • In symptomatic, severe hypokalemia, IV KCl (10 mEq/L/hr).

Treat low Mg^{2+} with $MgSO_4$ IV or MgO po depending on severity

It is nearly impossible to replace the K^+ if the Mg^{2+} is not replaced.

In addition to replacing potassium, the underlying cause of hypokalemia should be addressed and corrected as follows

Control diarrhea, vomiting.

Discontinue diuretics.

Use a standing dose of potassium in pts on cisplatin, aminoglycosides.

Treat chronic hypokalemia (such as Barter syndrome) with KCl supplement or potassium-sparing diuretics: spironolactone, triamterene, or amiloride

If hypokalemia is caused by hyperaldosteronism, a CT scan of the abdomen should be ordered to evaluate for adrenal mass

Treat hyperaldosteronism with spironolactone.

Consider consulting Endocrinology.

HYPERKALEMIA

S **Does the pt have a personal or family history of kidney disease?**
Renal insufficiency decreases the excretion of K+ (potassium).

Briefly review the pt's diet
Some salt substitutes (KCl) are high in potassium.
Foods that contain K+ include pinto beans, bananas, tomatoes, and oranges.

Is the pt taking any medications that can cause hyperkalemia?
Spironolactone is a competitive inhibitor of aldosterone, which causes an increase in
absorption of sodium and an increase in secretion of potassium.
ACE inhibitors also decrease renal excretion of potassium.
NSAIDs inhibit production of renin and aldosterone synthesis.

Does the patient use albuterol?
β-Agonists such as albuterol can cause potassium to shift out of the cells.

Does the pt have any conditions that could cause hyperkalemia?
Rhabdomyolysis: trauma, statins, cocaine, alcohol
Volume contraction: With rehydration, K+ will drop to normal or even low levels.
  – DKA   – Sepsis   – Severe dehydration

Does the pt have a history of malignancy?
Can cause tumor lysis syndrome with death and leakage of internal contents of rapidly
overturning cancer cells into the bloodstream

Is the pt diabetic?
Diabetes mellitus can cause type IV RTA because of the defect of H+-ATPase pump in the
collecting tubules.
Other causes of type IV RTA include obstructive uropathy and interstitial nephritis.

Is the pt fasting?
In pts who are dependent on dialysis, prolonged fasting decreases insulin secretion,
which promotes potassium shift from intracellular to extracellular space.
In a normal individual, this amount of potassium is excreted. In a pt dependent on
dialysis, the potassium cannot be excreted, potentially causing life-threatening
arrhythmia.

Was it a difficult blood draw?
Hemolyzed blood specimen can cause falsely elevated K+.
This is a diagnosis you should confirm with a repeat test showing a normal K+.

O **Review VS and perform a general PE**
Look for evidence of muscle weakness, paralysis, or arrhythmia.

Order an ECG
ECG shows peaked T-waves, flattening or absence of P-waves, widened QRS, and pro-
longed PR interval. This results in an ECG with the appearance of a sine wave.
Do not rely on ECG findings.
As the K+ increases, the T-waves increase and then begin to decrease again.
So although the absence of peaked T-waves does not exclude significant hyperkalemia,
their presence is nearly diagnostic.
Arrhythmia includes ventricular fibrillation and asystole.

Repeat potassium to verify result or see effect of acute treatment
Traumatic venipuncture can cause hemolysis. Look for a comment of hemolysis.

Check BUN and creatinine to assess renal function
Decreased renal function increases the risk of hyperkalemia caused by poor excretion.

Check Ca²⁺ level
It is often low in renal failure but high in conditions such as multiple myeloma.

Check CBC for anemia, leukocytosis, and thrombocytosis
Both leukocytosis and thrombocytosis can cause pseudohyperkalemia from leakage of K+ from these cells.

Check U/A
Rhabdomyolysis: Myoglobin tests as large blood in the dipstick without any RBCs on microscopy.

Check urine potassium
Hyperkalemia with urine K⁺ >30 mEq/L suggests transcellular shifts.
Hyperkalemia with urine K⁺ <30 mEq/L indicates impaired excretion.

Consider ordering a blood gas
This is a fast way to check serum potassium. Stat chemistry may take up to 1 hour to come back. Blood gas chemistry often comes back in 5 minutes.

 Hyperkalemia
High serum potassium

Etiologies
Decreased cellular potassium uptake
Increased cellular potassium release

– Insulin deficiency	– Rhabdomyolysis	– Tumor lysis syndrome
– Aldosterone deficiency	– Hyperosmolality	
– β-Adrenergic blockers	– Volume contraction	

Decreased renal clearance
Acute or chronic renal failure

Differential diagnosis
Hemolyzed blood specimen: Lysis of RBCs releases the internal contents of the cells, which are high in potassium.

 Quantify serum potassium level and check an ECG for changes; if there are ECG changes, give 10 mL of IV calcium gluconate over 1 minute
Stabilizes the myocardium (does not affect the potassium level).
Works in <5 minutes and lasts for 30–60 minutes. Repeat prn q 3–5 minutes.

If K⁺ >7, place a cardiac monitor and give meds to move K⁺ intracellularly
10 U insulin IV with an amp of D50 W (monitor serum K⁺ and glucose)
NaHCO₃ 2 mEq/kg IV over 5–10 minutes (monitor K⁺)

If K⁺ >6, place a cardiac monitor and give meds to increase K⁺ excretion
Give kayexalate with sorbitol to enhance clearance through the GI tract.
Use IV diuretics like furosemide.

If K⁺ does not improve with above management, consult renal for dialysis

Avoid meds that can cause hyperkalemia, such as NSAIDs and ACE inhibitors

Avoid foods that contain high K⁺, including pinto beans, bananas, tomatoes, and orange juice

URINARY TRACT INFECTION

S **Does the pt have any symptoms of a lower urinary tract infection (UTI)?**
- Urgency   – Frequency   – Dysuria   – Suprapubic pain

Does the pt have any evidence of an upper UTI?
Pyelonephritis: flank pain, fever/chills, nausea/vomiting

Does the pt have any risk factors for UTI?
- Recent sexual   – Diabetes   – Pregnancy
  intercourse
- Foley catheter   – Anal sex   – Anatomic abnormality

O **Check VS and orthostatics**
Look carefully for any evidence of urosepsis:
- Hypotension   – Tachycardia   – Fever

Perform a general PE
Abd exam: suprapubic tenderness
Back: Check costovertebral angle for tenderness (suggests pyelonephritis).

Check a urinalysis
Positive leukocyte esterase suggests infection.
Positive nitrite also suggests infection, but some bacteria do not produce nitrate.
WBC >5 = pyuria
RBCs are often but not always present in UTI.

Order a urine Gram stain and culture and sensitivity
Escherichia coli is one of the most common causes of UTIs.
Look for 10^2 colonies in symptomatic females or 10^3 in symptomatic males.

Other common organisms are the following:

Klebsiella	*Proteus*	*Enterobacter*
Pseudomonas	*Serratia*	*Citrobacter*

Staphylococcus aureus is a rare cause of UTI, and if isolated from the urine, it is normally a result of hematogenous spread.
Isolating *Streptococcus bovis* from the urine is an indication that the pt may have a colonic malignancy.

If there is fever, tachycardia, hypotension, flank pain, vomiting, or other signs of systemic or upper UTI, consider blood cultures
Try to obtain these before administering antibiotic

Check the CBC
Look for leukocytosis and bandemia, both of which suggest a systemic infection.

A **Urinary tract infection**
Usually bacterial (but other infectious agents such as fungal and viral also occur) infection of the upper (kidneys) or lower (bladder) urinary system

Differential diagnosis
Lower UTI:
- Prostatitis   – Epididymitis   – Interstitial   – Urethritis
  cystitis

Upper UTI:
- Appendicitis   – Meningitis   – Pneumonia
- Endocarditis   – Renal stone   – Sepsis

If it is an uncomplicated lower UTI, treat with a 3-day course of TMP/SMX

In pregnant women, avoid TMP/SMX (in third trimester) and quinolones. Suggest a 7-day course of nitrofurantoin or first-generation cephalosporin.

For a woman with recurrent simple UTIs, prophylactic measures should be considered:
- Postcoital antibiotic; TMP/SMX, one single-strength tablet.
- Pt self-administered treatment.
- Continuous low-dose antibiotic.
- Void after intercourse.
- Drink cranberry juice.
- Avoid use of diaphragm with spermicide.

Do not treat asymptomatic bacteriuria except in pts with diabetes mellitus or pregnancy.

If there is evidence that the pt has pyelonephritis, treat with 7 days of quinolone, or 14 days with TMP/SMX, or amoxicillin–clavulanate. Admit and treat for 1–2 days with IV antibiotics if the pt has nausea, vomiting, and is unable to keep any liquid down

If the pt is not tolerating oral fluids, then he or she may not survive at home. Once the pt is afebrile, switch to oral antibiotic.

If the pt continues to have fever after 48 hours of starting IV antibiotics, consider CT abdomen to rule out renal abscess

Also consider emphysematous pyelonephritis, a rare, but fatal disease if not detected early, especially in poorly controlled diabetics. It is caused by a gas-producing organism, usually *E. coli*. A KUB is usually diagnostic. Its management is antibiotics and nephrectomy.

If the pt is a male with a UTI, treat with 7 days of antibiotics and perform a urologic workup if no risk factors are present (e.g., unprotected anal intercourse)

UTIs are distinctly rare in men, so when they occur, the cause needs to be investigated. Most commonly, prostate enlargement will be the cause.

If *Candida* is cultured from the urine in a pt with a Foley catheter, remove the Foley

If funguria persists, fluconazole 100–400 mg/d for 7 days is recommended. Alternatively, one can order amphotericin B bladder wash (50 mg/L continuously for 5 days).

If there is pyuria without bacteriuria or hematuria, culture for *Chlamydia* and gonorrhea. Also consider tuberculosis

HEMATOLOGY/ONCOLOGY

ANEMIA

S **Does the pt have any symptoms of anemia?**
- Fatigue/weakness
- Dizziness
- Decrease in work capacity
- Headache
- Dyspnea
- Palpitations or anorexia

Does the pt report blood loss?
- Hematemesis
- Melena
- Hemoptysis
- Trauma
- Hematochezia
- Postop
- Hematuria
- Menorrhagia

Does the pt have unusual cravings (pica) such as starch, clay, or ice?
A common sign of underlying anemia is strange food cravings.

Does a female pt report an abnormal menstrual cycle?
Ask about last menstrual period, duration, flow, and number of pads.

Does pt have conditions associated with anemia?
HIV risk factors
Environmental exposure (lead)
Alcohol use or intravenous drug abuse
Parasitic infection (malaria)
Chronic disease (autoimmune, infection, thyroid, liver or renal)
GI surgery (iron absorbed by distal duodenum)

Is there a family history of blood disorders?
- Sickle cell
- Thalassemia
- Kidney disease
- Autoimmune disorders

Review medications (some can cause bone marrow suppression)
- Chemotherapy
- Antibiotics
- Antiseizure medications

O **Does the pt have VS associated with hemodynamic instability?**
Tachycardia, hypotension, and positive orthostatics suggest acute blood loss.

Perform a PE
Gen: Assess nutrition and fluid status, cachexia, temporal wasting, and skin turgor.
> *HEENT*: conjunctival pallor
> *Heart*: murmur
> *Abd*: splenomegaly
> *Rectal exam*: stool guaiac, hemorrhoids
> *Skin changes*: brittle nails, jaundice
> Lymph nodes

Evaluate the results of a CBC with differential
Normal Hb and Hct is 13.5 and 42, respectively, for females; 15 and 45 for males.
Mean corpuscular volume (MCV) = (Hct × 10)/RBC; normal is about 90.
- If it is microcytic anemia (MCV <80), check a microcytic (iron) panel.
- If it is macrocytic anemia (MCV >100), check a macrocytic panel.
Mean corpuscular hemoglobin concentration (MCHC) = Hb × 100/Hct
- Hypochromic (MCHC <30): iron deficiency, thalassemia
- Hyperchromic (MCHC >37): spherocytosis, newborns
RDW normal range is 11.5–14.5. Helpful in distinguishing thalassemia and anemia of chronic disease from the following conditions with increased RDW (>14.5):
- Iron deficiency
- Megaloblastic anemia
- Hemoglobinopathies
- Immune hemolytic anemia
Reticulocyte count to assess function of bone marrow; it comes as a percentage.
- Reticulocyte count is usually given as reticulocyte percent (normal 0.5%–1.5%)
- Calculate the reticulocyte index (RI) to interpret:
  o RI = Retic % × (pt's Hct/45) = (normal is about 1). For example, severe anemia 1 × 21/45 = 0.467 (inappropriately normal reticulocyte count). To have a normal RI with this level of anemia requires a reticulocyte percent of about 2.2 → 2.2 × 21/45 = 1 = Normal
    • High RI suggests increased production; low RI suggests decreased production.

Look at RBC morphology (sizes, shapes, and inclusions) (see Appendix A).

Look for markers of hemolysis

- Increased lactate   – Increased bilirubin   – Schistocytes
  dehydrogenase

Anemia

A low level of circulating RBCs (Hb <12 in females or 13.5 in males). The etiologies of anemia can be summed as uncompensated blood loss, destruction, and lack of production. Time course can be chronic to acute.

Differential diagnosis/etiology

Check MCV and decide whether it is microcytic, normocytic, or macrocytic.

- Microcytic (MCV <80):
  o Iron metabolism: iron deficiency, chronic disease
  o Globin synthesis: thalassemia, hemoglobinopathy
- Normocytic (80–100)
  o Increased loss/destruction: posthemorrhagic, hemolytic
  o BM infiltration: malignant, myelofibrosis, storage disease
  o Decreased erythropoietin production: renal, liver, endocrine
- Macrocytic (MCV >100): B_{12} or folate deficiency

After identifying the type of anemia, investigate the cause. It is not enough to say iron-deficiency anemia or anemia of chronic disease. In the case of iron deficiency, at least ensure that it is not caused by chronic losses from GI cancer. One way of investigating is to check iron studies if the anemia is microcytic.

- Serum iron: normal 70–170
  o Increased: hemolysis (thalassemia, acute leukemia), iron poisoning, transfusion, liver disease, nephritis, hemochromatosis
  o Decreased: iron deficiency, chronic blood loss, chronic disease (systemic lupus erythematosus, rheumatoid arthritis, infection), decreased iron absorption
- Total iron binding capacity (TIBC): normal 250–450
  o Increased: iron deficiency, blood loss, pregnancy, liver disease
  o Decreased: anemia of chronic disease (infection, renal, liver), burns, malnutrition, iron overload
- Iron saturation = (serum iron × 100)/TIBC → normal 10%–50%
  o Increased: iron therapy, thalassemia, hemochromatosis
  o Decreased: iron deficiency, cancer, chronic disease

If the pt is hemodynamically unstable, admit to a monitored bed

If there are signs of acute blood loss, the pt should be monitored closely. If the pt is bleeding and you fluid resuscitate him or her, you should see a response in the pulse and blood pressure (correction of tachycardia and hypotension).

Place two large-bore IVs, provide aggressive fluid resuscitation, type and cross, and monitor serial CBCs

Two IVs are needed to assure that IV access is not lost if one of them fails. They are large bore so that you can give IV fluid boluses quickly and so RBCs pass smoothly. After three boluses of IV fluids, consider transfusing blood, especially if the hematocrit is low.

If hemodynamically stable, work up the underlying cause and treat it

Transfuse only if pt is symptomatic and there is no evidence of hemolysis.

THROMBOCYTOPENIA

S **Does the pt have bleeding with fever or altered mental status?**
Suspicious for thrombotic thrombocytopenic purpura (TTP)/hemolytic uremic syndrome (HUS), which requires immediate attention

Does the pt report any mucocutaneous bleeding?
The following suggest low platelets:
- Spontaneous gum bleeding
- Menorrhagia
- Epistaxis
- Easy bruising or rash
- GI or GU bleeding

Review medications
Many medications cause decreased platelets
- Sulfonamides
- Heparin
- Thiazides
- INH
- Quinine

When was the pt's last alcohol use?
Alcohol causes direct toxicity to bone marrow.
Chronic abuse may cause liver disease and splenomegaly (sequestration).

Does the pt have medical problems associated with low platelets?
History of HIV: Consider autoimmune-mediated etiology.
History of chronic liver disease or hepatitis: Consider splenic sequestration.

Does the pt report recent blood transfusions or fluid replacement?
After massive transfusions or fluid resuscitation, platelet counts may be low because of dilution.

O **Review VS and perform a PE**
Gen: Assess level of consciousness
Skin: petechiae, purpura, ecchymosis, rash, pallor, jaundice, lymph nodes
Heart: prosthetic valve
Abd: splenomegaly, hepatomegaly

Review the results of a CBC
Thrombocytopenia is defined as platelets <150,000.
Multiple cell lines affected (anemia, leukopenia) suggests a problem with decreased production.
Consider bone marrow aspirate/biopsy: Low number of megakaryocytes indicates decreased platelet production. Increased number of indicates likely increased destruction.

Review peripheral smear
In a pt with disease associated with accelerated destruction, look for the following:
- Fragmented RBCs (schistocytes) suggests TTP or MAHA.
- Large platelets suggests idiopathic thrombocytopenic purpura (ITP).

Consider further lab tests
Consider PT, PTT, and disseminated intravascular coagulation (DIC) panel to rule out DIC.
Consider lactate dehydrogenase, bilirubin as markers for hemolysis.
Consider a comprehensive metabolic panel to rule out renal failure.
Consider antinuclear antibody, Coombs test if suspect autoimmune mediated.
Consider HIV, hepatitis panel if pt has risk factors.

Consider further imaging
Spleen size is often difficult to interpret, consider abdominal ultrasound.
Consider CT head in pt with altered level of consciousness.

Thrombocytopenia

Low platelet count is usually defined as platelets of <150,000.

Etiologies

Splenic sequestration

Increased destruction

- Immune causes: ITP, AIHA (Evan syndrome), drugs, systemic lupus erythematosis (SLE), HIV
- Nonimmune causes: TTP/HUS, sepsis, DIC, prosthetic heart valve

Decreased production

- Bone marrow infiltration: lymphoma, leukemia, other malignancy, myelofibrosis
- Bone marrow toxicity: alcohol, vitamin B_{12}, folate deficiency

Differential diagnosis

- DIC   – Malignant hypertension   – Vasculitis
- Severe preeclampsia   – HUS   – Infectious colitis

 Identify and treat hematologic emergencies immediately. Admit the pt to a monitored bed if you suspect any of the following

- TTP   – ITP   – DIC

Consider the following pentad for diagnosing TTP. You do not need all five to make a diagnosis!

- Fever   – Altered mental status   – Thrombocytopenia
- MAHA   – Renal failure

If high suspicion of TTP, treat with plasmapheresis, prednisone 1 mg/kg, but DO NOT give platelet transfusion unless life threatening

Giving platelets in TTP can make the condition worse.

If high suspicion of ITP, treat with prednisone 1 mg/kg; may use IVIG or WinRho (if Rh-positive) if platelets <10,000 or <20,000 with bleeding

Do not give prednisone in HIV or lymphoma/leukemia if possible.

If suspect DIC, identify and treat the underlying etiology

DIC can be associated with sepsis.

Consider transfusion of platelets if platelet count is <10,000 or <20,000 with evidence of bleeding. Implement conservative measures in hemodynamically stable pts

Implement all of the following measures to minimize the risk of bleeding:

- Bed rest, stool softener, cough suppressants, padded bed rails
- Avoid NSAIDs and aspirin.

Withdraw any medications that could potentially be causing the problem (see above).

Vitamin supplementation for pts with decreased production includes:

- Thiamine 100 mg bid, folate 1 mg qd, and multivitamins

POLYCYTHEMIA

S **Does the pt report bleeding?**

One of the most common reasons pts seek medical treatment is for spontaneous bleeding (e.g., nosebleeds, hematemesis, melena).

This bleeding commonly represents platelet dysfunction.

Does the pt have symptoms related to hyperviscosity?

Increased blood volume and sticky cells cause stasis.

- Vertigo   – Tinnitus   – Headaches
- Visual changes   – Recurrent thrombosis

Does the pt have pruritus, especially after a warm shower?

Pruritus is a common complaint and is often caused by an increased release of histamine.

Does the pt report skin changes?

Erythromelalgia, defined as painful burning and erythema of the hands, is common.

Does the pt have a medical history suggestive of a secondary cause?

A pt with any of the following is at risk for secondary polycythemia:

- Smoker   – Chronic lung disease   – Congenital heart disease
- Renal disease   – Recent relocation to high-altitude region

Is the pt taking any medications?

Diuretics cause contraction of plasma volume and increased hematocrit.

O **Look for VS suggestive of secondary causes of polycythemia**

Obese pts with high blood pressure and large necks are at risk for obstructive sleep apnea (OSA). Pulse oximetry:

- <92% suggests lung or heart disease.
- Normal measurement is typical of smoker polycythemia.

Perform a PE

HEENT: funduscopic exam (engorged retinal veins)

Abd: splenomegaly

- Lack of splenomegaly suggests a secondary cause.
- *Skin*: ruddy complexion, plethora or cyanosis

Review the CBC with differential

Common abnormalities include overproduction of cell lines.

- Leukocytosis (basophilia, eosinophilia)
- RBC
  o Males: Hgb >17; Hct >50%
  o Females: Hgb >15; Hct >45%
- Thrombocytosis

What are the results of RBC mass and erythropoietin (EPO) levels?

A pt with elevated Hct should have RBC mass measured.

- Normal RBC mass: males 26–34; females 21–29.
- High normal RBC mass suggests spurious polycythemia.

If RBC mass is elevated, check EPO level to differentiate between primary versus secondary causes:

- EPO low or absent suggests polycythemia vera.
- EPO high suggests a secondary cause.

Consider checking venous blood gas

Smoking causes elevated carboxyhemoglobin.

Consider alkaline phosphatase, uric acid, and vitamin B$_{12}$

These markers are commonly elevated in polycythemia vera.

Consider a renal ultrasound or CT abdomen/pelvis

A pt suspected of an EPO-secreting mass should have further imaging to look for hepatoma or renal mass.

Consider pulmonary function test and/or sleep study

A pt with risk factors for chronic obstructive pulmonary disease (COPD) or OSA should have further diagnostic studies to rule out underlying lung disease.

 ### Polycythemia

Increased number of RBCs in the blood

Etiologies

Polycythemia vera

Polycythemia from secondary causes

- Smoking (normal pulse oximetry, high EPO, COHb high)
- Hypoxia pulse oximetry <92% suggests coronary heart disease, right-to-left shunt, chronic lung disease
- EPO-secreting mass

Hepatoma, uterine leiomyoma, renal cyst, cerebellar angioma

Renal disease (polycystic kidney disease)

 ### Identify pts with secondary causes of polycythemia

Treat underlying cause

– Smoking cessation	– Continuous positive airway pressure or
– Home oxygen (COPD)	– BiPAP (OSA)
	– Surgical resection (EPO-secreting mass)

Treat polycythemia vera with pt education and minimize risks of hyperviscosity

Phlebotomy is the treatment of choice.

- One unit removed per week for goal Hct <45
- Low-iron diet
- Allopurinol for hyperuricemia
- Benadryl, H_1 blocker for pruritus
- Anagrelide used for thrombocytosis

Consider using hydroxyurea (myelosuppressive agent)

If increased phlebotomy requirement, thrombocytosis, intractable pruritus.

COAGULOPATHY

S **Does the pt report any easy bleeding?**

Pts with congenital coagulation disorders bleed easily, especially after trauma, surgery, tooth extractions, or any invasive procedure.

Bleeding into joints and muscles is common in hemophiliacs with minor trauma.

Does the pt have a family history of bleeding disorders?

Hemophilia A and B are both X-linked disorders.

Does the pt report recent bleeding?
- Hemoptysis   - Melena   - Hematochezia
- Hematemesis   - Menorrhagia   - Hematuria
- Easy bruising   - Epistaxis   - Gum bleeding

Does the pt have joint pain?

Hemophilia pts may have hemarthrosis with pain in weight-bearing joints.

Review medications

Ask specifically about medicines such as warfarin or heparin.

Does the pt have risk factors for developing an acquired coagulopathy?

Disseminated intravascular coagulation (DIC): Fever/chills, fatigue, or weight loss suggests infection or malignancy; also consider complication of pregnancy/retained abortion.

History of liver or renal disease.

Vitamin K deficiency: Assess nutritional status (anorexia, weight loss, malabsorption, homeless).

O **Does the pt have VS suggestive of infection or sepsis?**
- Fever   - Tachycardia   - Hypotension

Perform a good general PE, looking specifically for the following

Abd: splenomegaly

Joints: hemarthrosis

Skin:
- Ecchymosis
- Petechiae/purpura
- Evidence of chronic liver disease (spider angiomata, jaundice)
- Bleeding from venipuncture or catheter sites

Review the pt's CBC

Leukocytosis, especially with left shift, indicates infection.
- Blood, urine, sputum cultures, and CXR to investigate source

Thrombocytopenia (common in DIC and sepsis)
- Check fibrinogen level (low or inappropriately normal in DIC). Pts with anemia should have a further workup (see Anemia, p. 56).

Evaluate the PT and PTT results

Review the coagulation cascade: PT (**W**arfarin: **E**xtrinsic) → 7\10—2(5)—1—Clot/PTT (**H**eparin: **I**ntrinsic) → 12—11—9(8)
- Factor 8 is a cofactor for factor 9, and factor 5 is a cofactor for factor 2.
- The figure demonstrates that PT and PTT have factors 10, 5, 2, and 1 in common (when these factors are involved, both will be elevated).

Prolonged PT, normal PTT = Low factor 7
- Coumadin therapy   - Mild liver disease   - Early vitamin K deficiency

Prolonged PTT, normal PT = Low factor 12, 11, 9, or 8.
- Heparin therapy   - Lupus anticoagulant
- Hemophilia A or B   - Von Willebrand disease

Prolonged PT and PTT = Low factor 10, 5, 2, or 1.
- DIC   - Liver or renal disease
- Primary fibrinolysis   - Vitamin K deficiency (vitamin K dependent factors
                               are 2, 7, 9, 10)

What do the liver and renal function tests reveal?
Liver and renal disease are common causes for coagulopathy resulting from decreased
  synthesis or retention of coagulation factors.

Consider factor VIII, IX level
Males with a family history of easy bleeding should be evaluated for hemophilia.

A Coagulopathy
A condition in which an abnormality of the clotting cascade leads to an increased risk of
  bleeding and is reflected in abnormal PT and/or PTT

Differential diagnosis
Congenital disorders
- Factor VIII deficiency (hemophilia A)   - Factor IX deficiency (hemophilia B)
- Von Willebrand disease
- Platelet dysfunction disorders

Acquired disorders.
- DIC   Vitamin K deficiency   - Leukemia
- Liver disease   - Coumadin or heparin   - Primary fibrinolysis
                            therapy
- Renal disease   - ITP   - TTP/HUS

P If you suspect a life-threatening condition, admit the pt to a monitored bed
Carefully review vital signs for signs of hypovolemia.

Look at a peripheral smear for fragmented RBCs to decide whether this is hemolysis or blood loss
Transfusion is not always the answer. In cases of hemolytic anemia, it can actually
  exacerbate the problem.

If you suspect DIC, treat the underlying cause and give necessary supportive care
Common underlying causes are sepsis; deliver fetus.
Can give fresh frozen plasma (FFP), cryoprecipitate, and platelets in cases of
  hemorrhage.
Use IV heparin for thrombotic events.

After ruling out DIC, consider primary fibrinolysis and uncontrolled bleeding
May use aminocaproic acid to optimize platelet action and promote clotting.

Avoid ASA and other antiplatelet factors hemophilia A involves replacement of factor VIII and ddAVP
Prophylactic infusions of factor VIII before dental procedures and joint replacements

Hemophilia B is treated with FFP
FFP contains, among other things, Factor IX.

Optimize treatment of liver or renal disease treat vitamin K deficiency with 10 mg SQ

DEEP VEIN THROMBOSIS

S **Is there any shortness of breath or chest pain?**

> The greatest complication of deep vein thrombosis (DVT) is pulmonary embolism (PE), which warrants prompt action.

Has there been any recent prolonged bed rest or immobility?
Risk factors for DVT include:
- Recent surgeries (especially orthopedic)
- Stroke
- Myocardial infarction
- Air or bus travel of long duration

Are there any risk factors for hypercoagulable states?
Malignancies: prostate, lung, ovary, cervical, colon, stomach, pancreas
Nephrotic syndrome
Oral contraceptives usage

Is there a known family history of DVT?
Inherited causes of hypercoagulable states include:
- *The Factor V Leiden mutation*: Factor V is normally degraded by activated protein C. This mutation is also known as activated protein C resistance (APCR), an autosomal-dominant trait carried by 5% of the population. It is most common in whites.
- *Hyperhomocysteinemia*: Mutation may lead to an excessive amount of this amino acid metabolite, leading to both arterial and venous thrombotic episodes. It occurs in approximately 5%–7% of the population and usually presents in the third or fourth decade.
- Deficiencies of antithrombin III, protein C, and protein S do occur but are far more rare than the previous two conditions.

Are there any prior episodes of a DVT?
Include information about confirmation of diagnosis and prior treatment with anticoagulation and duration.
Recurrent DVT after proper anticoagulation mandates lifelong anticoagulation or filter placement to prevent further DVT and PE.

O **Check VS**
Low blood pressure ≡ think of pulmonary embolism.
- Tachypnea
- Tachycardia
- Low O_2 saturation

Check pt's leg(s) for signs of DVT. Physical findings are usually nonspecific.
- Leg pain
- Erythema
- Tightness
- Palpable cord
- Edema
- Homans sign (pain with dorsiflexion of ankle); sensitivity is only about 50%.

Perform duplex ultrasound of affected leg, looking for evidence of DVT
Highly specific and sensitive for DVT.
Signs include lack of spontaneous flow in vein, absence of increased flow velocity with compression veins more distally, and inability to collapse vein with compression.

Check to see if one or both legs are involved
Bilateral leg involvement suggests either a cardiac (heart failure), hepatic, or renal (nephrotic syndrome) etiology rather than DVT.

Deep vein thrombosis

The Virchow triad for risk of DVT is immobility, vascular damage, and hypercoagulability.

Although it usually occurs in the legs, it should be considered in any extremity.

The use of duplex ultrasound is diagnostic. History aids more in discovering the etiology. Physical exam is not always useful in these pts.

Differential diagnosis

- Lymphedema   – Myxedema   – Cellulitis
- Muscle strain   – Baker cyst rupture

P **First, decide whether to anticoagulate this pt**

Contraindications to anticoagulation include:

- Recent GI bleed
- Stroke
- Recent craniotomy

Otherwise, begin anticoagulation with heparin

Unfractionated heparin starting with an IV bolus of 100 U/kg (maximum 5,000 U) and continue at a rate of 10 U/kg/hr. Check PTT after 6 hours and adjust for a goal PTT of 1.5–2.0.

OR

Low-molecular-weight heparin, such as enoxaparin, at 1 mg/kg SQ bid. This method is becoming more popular because of less need to monitor PTT.

Monitor platelets daily. If decreasing, consider heparin-induced thrombocytopenia.

Then, administer oral warfarin

Start with warfarin 5 mg po qd. Monitor international normalized ration (INR) and adjust for a goal rate of 2.0–3.0.

Warfarin is a difficult drug to maintain in the therapeutic range because effects are not seen until 2 days after each dose, it has multiple drug interactions, and it even interacts with certain foods. Therefore, INR must be checked frequently.

Continue heparin (in either form) until warfarin reaches therapeutic levels, and then discontinue.

Arrange for outpatient appointment with an anticoagulation clinic before discharge to continue monitoring INR and adjust warfarin dose accordingly.

Continue treatment for 3–6 months on initial episode of DVT; if this is not the first event, administer warfarin lifelong.

If indicated, factor Xa inhibitors may be an option

If anticoagulation is contraindicated, consider vena caval filter placement to prevent a PE.

Send off blood tests to assess for the genetic hypercoagulable states noted above.

LYMPHOMA

S **Does the pt have any "B" symptoms?**
The presence of any of the following is associated with a worse prognosis:
  • Fevers known as Pel-Ebstein occur in a cyclic pattern
  • Drenching night sweats to the point of having to change the sheets
  • Unintentional weight loss, 10% or more of body weight over 6 months

Does the pt report any painless lymphadenopathy?
Common in Hodgkin lymphoma (HL) and non-Hodgkin lymphoma (NHL)

Does the patient have any systemic symptoms?
  – Malaise   – Weakness   – Marked fatigue

Does the pt report pruritus?
Common with HL (especially the nodular sclerosing) usually worse after bathing/
  showering

Does the pt report any respiratory symptoms?
A pt may present with a dry cough or shortness of breath.

Does pt have abdominal pain?
Early satiety or abdominal pain may suggest splenomegaly.

Does pt report diffuse body pain with alcohol ingestion?
Thought to be caused by eosinophil infiltration of tumor sites (HL).

Does the pt have any risk factors for HIV?
AIDS is common with B-cell lymphomas.

Does the pt have a history of a previous infection?
History of any of the following infections increases the likelihood of lymphoma:
  – Epstein-Barr virus: HL and NHL   – Hepatitis C: NHL
    (African Burkitt lymphoma)   – *Helicobacter pylori*: gastric lymphoma
  – Human T-lymphotropic virus:
    T-cell lymphomas

Is there a history of autoimmune disorders?
Pts with RA, SLE, and Sjögren syndrome are at increased risk for developing lymphoma.

O **Review VS and perform a PE**
Abd: splenomegaly, hepatomegaly
Skin: lymph nodes (size, consistency, tenderness)

Review CBC with differential
Malignancy of cell lines vary in presentation.
  – Lymphopenia   – Leukocytosis   – Thrombocytosis
  – Eosinophilia   – If there is bone marrow invasion, expect pancytopenia

Look for abnormal liver and renal function tests
Abnormal values suggest organ involvement.

Check a lactate dehydrogenase (LDH) and uric acid level
LDH serves as a marker for the bulk of tumor.
High uric acid level suggests high cell turnover and risk for tumor lysis (see below).

Evaluate chemistry panel, phosphorus, and calcium
Common abnormalities with tumor lysis are high K, high P, and low Ca.

Consider CXR
Look for pleural effusions and hilar or mediastinal lymphadenopathy.

Consider CT of the chest, abdomen, and pelvis
To evaluate extent of disease

Consider excisional node biopsy
Entire node is needed to evaluate architecture and type of lymphoma.
Fine-needle aspiration is not sufficient for diagnosis.

Consider bilateral bone marrow biopsy
To evaluate whether bone marrow is involved

Consider lumbar puncture in HIV pts or if you suspect Burkitt lymphoma
consider MUGA scan to evaluate ejection fraction (prechemotherapy)

A Lymphoma
Cancer of lymphoid tissue is often divided into NHL and HL (Tables 5-1).

TABLE 5-1   Types of Lymphoma

Non-Hodgkin Lymphoma	Hodgkin Lymphoma
Low grade	Lymphocyte predominance
Small lymphocytic/CLL	Mixed cellularity
Follicular, small or mixed	Nodular sclerosing
Intermediate	Lymphocyte depleted
Follicular, large cell or small cleaved	
Diffuse, mixed or large	
High grade	
Immunoblastic or lymphoblastic	
Small noncleaved (Burkitt and non-Burkitt lymphoma)	

P Identify life-threatening complications
- Acute leukemia (see Leukemia, p. 68)   – Tumor lysis syndrome

Identify and treat tumor lysis syndrome promptly
Tumor lysis syndrome is the result of rapid death of tumor cells.
IV fluid resuscitation, allopurinol, alkalinize urine (add HCO_3 to fluids), loop diuretics
as needed, management of electrolyte abnormalities.

Treat NHL based on histologic grade
Low-grade NHL:
• Watch and wait or chemotherapy with or without radiation
Intermediate or high-grade NHL:
• Chemotherapy (CHOP) plus radiation or chemotherapy alone (at times monoclonal
antibody rituximab may be added)
• HLA-matched allograft bone marrow transplant

HL stages
Stage I: single lymph node
Stage II: 2 or more lymph nodes same side diaphragm
• "B" indicates "B" symptoms.
• "A" indicates absence of "B" symptoms.
Stage III: more than 1 extranodal sites (liver, bone marrow, brain, and lung)
Stage IV: Diffuse involvement

Treat HL based on staging
Stage I and IIA: radiation alone
• With large mediastinal mass, radiation plus chemotherapy
Stage IIB or IIIA: radiation +/– chemotherapy
Stage IIIB or IV: chemotherapy (MOPP, ABVD)
• Consider autologous bone marrow transplant.

LEUKEMIA

 Does the pt have any risk factors for leukemia?

Previous treatment for malignancy is one of the largest risk factors for leukemia.
  • Use of alkylating agents (cyclophosphamide, melphalan)
  • Irradiation
Other risk factors include radiation exposure (Hiroshima, Chernobyl) and smoking.
Down syndrome (trisomy 21), neurofibromatosis, and Fanconi syndrome also increase
  the risk.

Is the pt experiencing any systemic symptoms?

Malaise, weakness, fever, weight loss, and night sweats are common "B" symptoms.
  Often they confer a worse prognosis.

Ask the pt about bruising, epistaxis, gum bleeding, hematochezia, or menorrhagia

As malignant cells infiltrate the bone marrow, cellular production decreases. Often
  symptoms of thrombocytopenia will be the first sign of malignancy.

Ask the pt about recurrent infections

This would be a sign of immune system impairment, also common in leukemia.

 Review VS

Low-grade fevers are common in leukemia. In neutropenia, fever indicates infection.
Hypotension, tachycardia, and orthostatics indicate an unstable pt; transfer to the ICU.
Tachypnea and hypoxia are signs of pulmonary leukostasis.

Perform a PE

Gen: Assess level of consciousness; pts should not be altered.
HEENT: Look for conjunctival and mucosal pallor. Retinal hemorrhages and gingival
  hyperplasia indicate AML.
Neck: Cervical lymphadenopathy may indicate chronic lymphocytic leukemia (CLL).
Lungs: Rales may indicate leukostasis or a pneumonia.
Heart: Tachycardia and a systolic ejection murmur are common in anemic pts.
Abd: Hepatosplenomegaly likely indicates myeloid leukemias either acute or chronic.
Skin: Petechiae and ecchymoses are common findings of thrombocytopenia. Be sure to
  check the axillae, groin, and epitrochlear for lymphadenopathy.

Check CBC with differential with a peripheral smear

Although leukemia can be seen with any CBC, pancytopenia or anemia/thrombocytope-
  nia with leukocytosis are the most common findings.
Presence of circulating blasts on the smear is virtually diagnostic of leukemia.

Check a complete chemistry panel

Serum potassium, phosphorus, lactate dehydrogenase, and uric acid may all be elevated,
  sometimes markedly, as indicators of large cell volume turnover.
As serum phosphorus increases, serum calcium tends to decrease.

Check PT/PTT, fibrinogen, and D-dimer studies

Disseminated intravascular coagulation (DIC) is common in APL.

Order a CXR

This will rule out mediastinal involvement and pulmonary leukostasis.

Perform a bone marrow biopsy

Biopsy is required for the diagnosis of leukemia. It should be hypercellular with more
  than 30% blasts. Immunohistochemical stains can be performed to complete the
  diagnosis.

Leukemia (Table 5-2)

TABLE 5-2   Types of Leukemia

Lymphocytic	Myeloid
Acute lymphocytic leukemia (ALL)	**Acute myelogenous leukemia (AML)**
Childhood pre-B cell (L1)	Undifferentiated (M0)
Adult pre-B cell (L2)	Myeloblastic (M1)
B-cell (Burkitt type) (L3)	Myeloblastic with differentiation (M2)
T-cell (L1, L2)	Promyelocytic (M3); t(15:17)
Chronic lymphocytic leukemia (CLL)	Myelomonocytic (M4)
B-cell T-cell	Monoblastic (M5)
Large granular lymphocytic	Erythroleukemia (M6)
Hairy cell	Megakaryoblastic (M7)
	Chronic myelogenous leukemia (CML)
	Almost always Philadelphia chromosome
	(t(9; 22)) positive

Literally means "white blood," an old term given to those diseases that may increase
   circulating white blood cells. Can be acute or chronic and lymphocytic or myeloid.
Both ITP and aplastic anemia can look like leukemia on the initial CBC.

P   **Identify and treat hematologic emergencies; admit pt to monitored bed**

Blast crisis: blood blasts >100,000; causes leukostasis (pulmonary, cerebral, or GI).
  • Perform cranial irradiation for cerebral involvement.
  • Perform leukapheresis and start hydroxyurea and allopurinol; alkalinize the urine.
  • Avoid blood transfusion because this may increase viscosity.
DIC (acute promyelocytic leukemia). Give IV cryoprecipitate, fresh frozen plasma, and
   platelets to stop bleeding.
Consider Amicar, an agent that stimulates production of von Willebrand factor.
Tumor lysis syndrome (see Lymphoma, p. 66)
For suspected sepsis, panculture the pt, start broad-spectrum antibiotics, and give
   pressors as needed.

Refer all pts to heme, but chemotherapy for ALL generally includes daunorubicin, prednisone, vincristine, and asparaginase. Most AML theraples include Ara-C + daunorubicin. There is one special case

APL (M3): Ara-C + trans-retinoid acid (ATRA): leads to high remission/cure rate!

For pts with CML, allogenic BMT or an allogenic stem cell transplant are the only hope of cure

Without BMT, CML will eventually result in blast crisis and death.

For CLL, symptomatic treatment is indicated for lymphadenopathy, organ involvement, cytopenias, or systemic symptoms

Fludarabine, cyclophosphamide, and rituximab can be used.
Newer targeted immunologic therapies in all leukemias are available.

BREAST MASS EVALUATION

S **Does the pt report changes in a breast mass?**

Most breast lesions are first detected by self-examinations (>90%).
Details of mass should include:
- When the mass was first detected
- Changes in size, consistency, tenderness, skin
- History of abnormal breast mass in past (fine-needle aspiration [FNA], biopsy, surgery)

Does the pt have risk factors for breast cancer?

Family history of breast cancer (BRCA-1 or BRCA-2), Li-Fraumeni syndrome
Female gender (150:1 F:M)
Early age of menarche, late age of first pregnancy, late age of menopause
Diet may play a role, but this is currently controversial
Moderate alcohol intake (mechanism unclear)
Use of oral contraceptives (OCPs) or hormone replacement therapy (HRT)
Previous radiation exposure

Is the pt currently breastfeeding?

Nursing predisposes to infections that may cause breast mass.

Does the pt give a history of recent trauma to breast?

Fat necrosis is common after trauma; may present as skin changes and breast mass.

Has the pt had a breast surgery?

If so, consider complications such as scarring or rupture of implant.

Has the pt had menopause or removal of her ovaries?

If the pt has functioning ovaries, then many of the benign masses are still on the differential: fibrocystic change, fibroadenoma, and phyllodes tumor.

O **Does the pt have VS suggestive of infection such as fever?**

A breast abscess is a common cause of breast mass.

Perform a PE

Breast (examine pt sitting and supine): skin changes (induration, dimpling, erythema), nipple discharge, palpable mass (note size, consistency, tenderness)
Lymph nodes: axillary or supraclavicular lymph nodes.

A **Breast mass**

Common finding in women of all ages. The goal of the workup is to differentiate benign breast masses from breast cancer.

Differential diagnosis of breast mass

Breast carcinoma: a very common cause of cancer in women.
Fibrocystic breast disease: presents as intermittently painful mass/masses during premenstrual cycle. Usually occurs in women receiving some form of estrogen either from ovaries, OCPs, or HRT.
Fibroadenoma: 1–5 cm, nontender, round, rubbery, mobile, benign mass of the breast that does not change during menses, and generally resolves after menopause. As with fibrocystic disease, usually occurs in women on estrogen.
Phyllodes tumor: rapidly growing fibroadenoma-like mass that can be either benign or malignant, usually treated with local excision and no lymph node dissection in either case (malignant form metastasizes to the lungs, not the lymph nodes). Will recur if not completely excised.
Fat necrosis: a rare cause of breast mass, with dimpling or induration of overlying skin, usually caused by trauma; important because it is clinically very similar to breast carcinoma.

Breast abscess/cellulitis: an infection causing an erythematous, tender area with or without induration, underlying mass, or fluctuance. Usually caused by *Staphylococcus aureus*. More common in breastfeeding women.

Lymphadenopathy: should be worked up carefully to differentiate benign from malignant causes: infection, metastases of solid tumors, lymphoma.

Complication of breast surgery: scar, keloid, ruptured breast implant.

P **If a questionable mass is found, first do an ultrasound in young women or a mammogram in postmenopausal women**

An ultrasound is more effective in evaluating younger women because of the higher amount of connective tissue in their breasts.

If a questionable mass is found on imaging or exam, perform a biopsy

For cystic masses use FNA, but for more suspicious masses refer to surgery.
- Simple cyst: fluid-filled requires no further workup
- Everything else: requires FNA, core-needle, or excisional biopsy

Cystic lesion with no residual mass: examine color of fluid.
- Clear or green color, repeat breast exam in 4–6 weeks
- Bloody fluid or abnormal cytology: proceed to excisional biopsy
- Malignant cells (see Breast Cancer, p. 72)

If the mass is suggestive of fibrocystic disease, consider FNA and recommend a supportive bra and avoidance of caffeine. Consider danazol if the pain is severe

Consider biopsy if the FNA is bloody, the mass persists, or recurs.

Danazol suppresses FSH and LH and is also used in endometriosis.

If lesion is consistent with fibroadenoma, then nothing needs to be done

For an unclear diagnosis, excision is warranted.

If phyllodes tumor is diagnosed, it should be excised

If fat necrosis or breast abcess is diagnosed, biopsy should still be performed to confirm diagnosis

Treatment with antibiotics that cover *S. aureus* (oxacillin or dicloxacillin)

Educate all pts about breast cancer and benign breast masses. Give reassurance when appropriate and explain how to perform breast exams

Explain that the breast exam should be performed once a month about 1 week after menses (when the breasts are generally less tender).
- Examine the entire breast from sternum to midaxillary line from ribs to clavicle, with special attention to not miss the "tail of the breast," the upper outer quadrant (which extends into the axilla), because this is where more than half of breast cancers occur.
- The breasts should also be examined in the mirror, looking for dimpling of overlying skin.

BREAST CANCER

 S **How old is the pt?**
Two-thirds of pts with breast cancer are older than 50 years.

What were the pt's ages of menarche and menopause (if postmenopausal)?
Early menarche and late menopause are associated with an increased risk of breast cancer.

Has the pt ever had breast cancer in the past?
If there is a personal history of breast cancer, there is a risk of recurrence.

Has the pt ever had a breast biopsy before and, if so, what were the results?
A finding of atypical hyperplasia on previous biopsy is also an increased risk of cancer.

Has a first-degree relative had breast cancer and, if so, how old was she?
The presence of breast cancer in a first-degree relative increases the risk some 300%–400%.
A diagnosis of breast cancer at a young age (<60 years) could indicate a genetic mutation in either the BRCA-1 or BRCA-2 genes. Carriers of these genes have an extremely high risk.

Has the pt noticed a mass in either breast or puckering or dimpling of the skin?
These can be physical signs of active malignancy.

Has the pt had any nipple discharge and, if so, what kind?
Bloody nipple discharge has a high concordance with infiltrating ductal carcinoma. Other types of nipple discharge may or may not be associated with malignancy.

O **Perform a breast exam: visualize the breasts with the arms overhead and on the hips with the shoulders forward, to examine the axillae, and then to palpate the breasts**
Early findings: palpable firm irregular nodule or breast mass, or sometimes no findings at all
Late findings: axillary lymphadenopathy, edema, immobile breast mass, bone pain, skin or nipple retraction

Order a mammogram
Routine screening each year after 40 years of age, and earlier with those with higher risk factors.
Abnormal findings most often occur (60%) over the upper lateral quadrant of breast mass.

Order and follow up on ultrasound-guided needle biopsy results
Infiltrating ductal carcinomas are the most common (85%), but other possible histologic types include invasive lobular (6%–8%) and noninvasive intraductal or lobular in situ (5%).

Consider ordering the following laboratory analyses
CBC: May present with anemia.
Liver function test: Elevation could signify hepatic metastases.
Estrogen receptor, progesterone receptor on tumor: If positive: less aggressive cancer; may be more amenable to hormonal treatment.
Human epidermal growth factor receptor-2 (her-2) status on the tumor. If positive: pt may respond to Herceptin, a monoclonal antibody therapy.

Continue workup to look for metastases when clinically indicated
Chest x-ray for pulmonary metastases
CT of brain or liver if suggestion of metastases is present
Bone scan to assess for bony metastases or elevated alkaline phosphatase or calcium

Carcinoma of the breast

Be sure to classify the stage of the cancer, because this has implications on treatment and prognosis, and survival. Also, determine the type of carcinoma (e.g., ductal, lobular).

TNM classification for breast cancer

Tumor
- T1: tumor ≤2 cm
- T2: tumor 2–5 cm
- T3: tumor > 5 cm
- T4: tumor of any size that extends to chest wall or skin

Lymph nodes
- N0: no lymph node metastases
- N1: axillary lymph nodes are (+) on biopsy, but mobile on palpation
- N2: axillary lymph nodes are (−) on biopsy, fixed on palpation
- N3: internal mammary lymph nodes are (+)

Metastases
- M0: no distant metastases present
- M1: (+) distant metastases present

Confirm suspected metastases with biopsy; many diseases can mimic metastatic breast on a scan

Staging of breast cancer based on TNM classification

Stage I: T1,N0,M0
Stage IIA: T0,N1,M0; T1,N1,M0; T2,N0,M0
Stage IIB: T2,N1,M0; T3,N0,M0; T2,N2,M0; T3,N1/2,M0
Stage IIIA: T0,N2,M0; T1,N2,M0
Stage IIIB: T4, any N,M0; any T,N3,M0
Stage IV: M1, any T/N

Await tumor histology for other prognostic variables

Estrogen/progesterone receptor (+) tumors: less aggressive, likely to respond to hormones.

Her-2-neu receptor (+): more aggressive tumor, will likely respond to Herceptin.

High-grade tumors have a poorer prognosis than low-grade tumors.

Lobular carcinoma in situ: cancer likely in the contralateral breast; do bilateral mastectomy.

 Treat based on staging

For stages I, II, or III, the pt will require:
- Lumpectomy with axillary lymph node dissection and postoperative radiation

OR
- Modified radical mastectomy with adjuvant chemotherapy and hormonal therapy such as anastrozole, letrozole, or tamoxifen (for hormone receptor (+) tumor)

Chemotherapy regimens vary, but they will likely include doxorubicin, cyclophosphamide with +/− docetaxel versus cyclophosphamide, methotrexate, and fluorouracil.

Trastuzumab, a monoclonal antibody to HER2 can be used.

Pts with stage IV disease are considered incurable. Remission may occur with palliative radiotherapy and hormonal therapy.

LUNG CANCER

 Is there a history of smoking?

Carcinoma of the lung is strongly associated with smoking and can be dose-dependent.

> Multiply the number of packs of cigarettes smoked per day by the number of years smoking to come up with "pack-years" of smoking, a useful way to quantify pt's smoking.

Is there any past exposure to asbestos, radon gas, arsenic, chromium, or nickel?

These are all environmental risk factors for developing lung cancer.

Is there a history of pulmonary fibrosis, sarcoidosis, or chronic obstructive pulmonary disease?

There is a higher associated risk of lung cancer with these diseases.

Does the pt have any general or specific symptoms associated with lung cancer?

In addition to weight loss and anorexia, chronic cough and hemoptysis can often be seen.

Bony pain in the chest, back, or pelvis is an ominous sign of possible metastasis.

Headaches, nausea, vomiting, altered mental status, or seizures suggest brain metastasis.

 Perform a PE

Cachexia: Muscle wasting that is most noticeable in the temporal area of the face (temporal wasting) is more likely to be seen with advanced or long-standing history of carcinoma.

Superior vena cava syndrome: Engorgement/erythema of the head and upper extremities, caused by obstruction of the superior vena cava, requires prompt attention.

Horner syndrome: The triad of ptosis, miosis, and anhidrosis of one eye stems from involvement of the inferior cervical ganglion and sympathetic chain on the ipsilateral side. Lung cancer causing Horner syndrome is often called a Pancoast tumor.

Digital clubbing can also be seen.

Pleural effusion, characterized by decreased breath sounds and dullness to percussion, can be seen in advanced lung cancer, as can findings of obstructive pneumonia.

Obtain a CXR

Lung cancer is often represented as a white mass on the x-ray.

Obtain and review chest and liver CT, PET scan, MRI of the brain, and bone scan

Elements of special note include the size of tumor, number of nodules, presence or absence of effusion, and location of affected lymphadenopathy.

Once tissue confirmation of malignancy is confirmed, PET scan can identify metabolically active sites of metastases in mediastinal nodes.

MRI of the brain and a bone scan can identify areas of distant metastases.

Obtain pathologic tissue evidence of carcinoma

> Centrally located lesions can be biopsied by bronchoscopy, whereas transthoracic needle biopsy assisted by CT will be more appropriate in a more peripherally located lesion.

If a pleural effusion is present, consider thoracentesis to obtain possible malignant cells.

Carcinoma of the lung

If pathology is available, be sure to characterize the carcinoma as either small cell or non–small cell carcinoma. Small cell is associated with an aggressive course and poor prognosis.

TNM classification for non–small cell carcinoma of lung

Tumor:
- T1: <3 cm in size
- T2: >3 cm, or in main bronchus but >2 cm from carina or invades visceral pleura
- T3: in chest wall, diaphragm, or pericardium or in main bronchus ≤2 cm from carina
- T4: involving mediastinum, heart, trachea, esophagus, vertebral body; malignant pleural, or pericardial effusion

Lymph nodes:
- N0: No evidence of regional lymph nodes
- N1: Lymph node metastasis to peribronchial or ipsilateral hilar region
- N2: Metastasis to ipsilateral mediastinal lymph nodes or subcarinal lymph nodes
- N3: Metastasis to any contralateral lymph node group

Metastases:
- M0: No evidence of distant metastasis
- M1: Distant metastasis present

Staging of non–small cell carcinoma, based on TNM classification

Stage IA: T1,N0,M0
Stage IB: T2,N0,M0
Stage IIA: T1,N1,M0
Stage IIB: T2,N1,M0 or T3,N0,M0
Stage IIIA: T3,N1,M0 or T1–3,N2,M0
Stage IIIB: any T,N3,M0 or T4, any N,M0
Stage IV: any T, any N, M1

Classification for small cell carcinoma of lung

Limited disease: Tumor is confined to unilateral hemithorax.
Extended disease: Tumor extends beyond hemithorax, or there is a pleural effusion.

Differential diagnosis

Includes nonlung metastasis (colon, prostate, cervical), tuberculosis, or benign pulmonary nodule. Biopsy will help resolve these possible alternative diagnoses.

 For non–small cell carcinoma, treat based on stage. For stages I or II malignancy, order pulmonary function tests (PFTs) to decide if the pt is capable of living with only one lung. If the PFTs indicate a possibility, arrange for surgical resection

This stage of lung cancer is curable. Although only a lobe may need to be resected, pts should be capable of living with only one lung, in case surgical complications require complete resection.

All stage III pts will require chemotherapy and radiation. Stage IIIA may be amenable to surgical resection, whereas stage IIIB will not. Pts with stage IV are incurable and should receive palliative treatment only

For small cell carcinoma, all pts require chemotherapy with a cisplatin/etoposide-based regimen

Use radiation for cerebral metastases, and surgery may be effective for very limited disease. Newer immunologic targeted therapies are now available.

COLON CANCER

 Does the pt have any GI symptoms?

Although pts can present with nonspecific symptoms (e.g., weight loss, anorexia, and fatigue) or no symptoms at all, certain symptoms can suggest on which side of the colon the cancer is located:
- Anemia and dull vague abdominal pain are associated more with right-sided rather than left-sided colon cancers.
- Left-sided colon cancers more typically exhibit constipation, diarrhea, change in stool caliber, rectal bleeding, and intestinal obstruction.

Is the pt at any increased risk of developing colon cancer?

Age: Incidence increases after age 45.

Race: Higher incidence exists among African-Americans than whites.

Personal or family history of neoplasm, including benign polyps: Consider more periodic screening in these pts.

Inflammatory bowel disease: The cumulative risk can reach up to 20% after 30 years.

O Perform PE

Gen: Cachexia can be seen in pts with advanced or long-standing history of carcinoma.

Abd: Advanced disease may present with a palpable abdominal mass or hepatomegaly.

Rectal: A digital rectal examination can reveal mass in about half of rectal cancer cases. Stool will often be positive for occult blood on a guaiac card.

Otherwise, most pts will have a normal PE.

Consider ordering the following laboratories

CBC: May present with anemia.

Liver function test: Elevation could signify hepatic metastases.

Carcinoembryonic antigen (CEA): Often elevated in pts with colon cancer. Measure in all pts with confirmed colon cancer to monitor treatment.

Obtain a CXR

Although a negative CXR does not rule out metastatic disease, nodules on CXR are likely to represent metastases.

Obtain colonoscopy and consider imaging study

Colonoscopy is the diagnostic procedure of choice.
- Allows for biopsy of lesion at the same time as direct visualization.
- If the pt refuses colonoscopy, or for some reason will not tolerate the procedure, barium enema and CT colonography can be used in lieu of colonoscopy to detect cancers with great reliability.

If biopsy from colonoscopy reveals colon cancer, CT scan of the chest, abdomen, and pelvis should be ordered to evaluate for metastases.

A Carcinoma of the colon

Be sure to classify the stage of the cancer, because this has implications on treatment and prognosis, and survival.

TNM classification for colon cancer

Tumor:
- Tis: Carcinoma in situ, confined to epithelium or lamina propria
- T1: Invasion of submucosa
- T2: Invasion of muscularis propria
- T3: Invasion into subserosa or pericolic or perirectal tissue
- T4: Invasion of other organs or structures

Lymph nodes:
- N0: No evidence of regional lymph nodes metastases
- N1: Metastasis in 1–3 pericolic or perirectal lymph nodes
- N2: Metastasis in ≥4 pericolic or perirectal lymph nodes
- N3: Metastasis in any lymph node along the course of a vascular trunk

Metastases:
- M0: No evidence of distant metastasis
- M1: Distant metastasis present (liver most common, followed by lung)

Staging of colon cancer based on TNM classification

Stage I: T1,N0,M0; T2,N0,M0
Stage II: T3,N0,M0; T4,N0,M0
Stage III: any T,N1–3,M0
Stage IV: M1, any T/N

Differential diagnoses for the symptomatology include

– Inflammatory bowel disease	– Irritable bowel syndrome
– Infectious colitis	– Diverticulosis/diverticulitis

P **Treatment is based on the given stage**

Stage I: Surgical resection of the tumor with end-to-end anastomosis.
Stage II: Resection-anastomosis with postoperative adjuvant chemotherapy
   (5-fluorouracil and leucovorin), radiotherapy, OR immunotherapy.
Stage III: Resection-anastomosis with postoperative adjuvant chemotherapy, radiotherapy, AND immunotherapy.
Stage IV: Chemotherapy for palliative treatment (fluorouracil, leucovorin, and irinotecan). There is no known cure for stage IV disease.

As noted above, after treatment, pts should have CEA levels monitored to rule out recurrence. Elevations in the levels likely mean metastatic disease

PROSTATE CANCER

 What is the pt's age and ethnicity?

Nearly all pts with prostate cancer are 65 y/o or more. *African-Americans tend to be at higher risk than other ethnicities for prostate cancer.*

Does the pt have a father or a brother who has had prostate cancer?

Those with a family history of prostate cancer are also at a higher associated risk.

Are there any symptoms of advanced disease?

Extensive local involvement:

- Dysuria   - Urinary retention   - Increased frequency
- Back pain   - Hematuria   - Outflow obstruction

Metastatic disease:

- Bone pain   - Fractures   - Deep vein thromboses
- Lower extremity weakness (cord compression)   - Pulmonary emboli

More than 80% of pts with prostate cancer are asymptomatic at the time of diagnosis.

 Perform a PE

Cachexia can be seen in pts with advanced or long-standing history of carcinoma.

Digital rectal exam (DRE) may reveal an enlarged, indurated prostate with focal nodules.

A normal prostate exam does not argue strongly for or against prostate cancer because pts with prostate cancer can have elevated prostate-specific antigen (PSA) and a normal DRE.

Perform a complete neurologic exam of the lower extremities to rule out cord compression.

Obtain a PSA tumor marker test

A normal PSA is less than 4 ng/mL; a value greater than 10 ng/mL has about a 2 in 3 chance of being associated with prostate cancer.

Obtain a transrectal ultrasound of the prostate with or without MRI

Ultrasound findings will help stage the tumor.

Systematic biopsy can be done during ultrasound if malignancy is suspected.

If tissue biopsies confirm prostate cancer, an MRI is the more accurate way to visualize both the prostate and regional lymph node involvement.

Order a radionuclide bone scan to detect any bony metastases

Prostate cancer has a high propensity to metastasize to the bone. It causes what are known as blastic lesions, called that because osteoblastic activity is stimulated. Osteoblasts increase the formation of new bone and thus cause increased uptake of radionuclides.

There is little usefulness in CT scan for staging of prostate cancer

 Carcinoma of the prostate

Gleason score should be available by pathology

In adenocarcinoma of the prostate, the part of the tumor with the highest histologic grade determines its biologic activity. Higher scores = more likely metastatic disease.

To determine a Gleason score, the pathologist assigns a number to the histologic grade of two areas of the tumor, and each is scored from 1 to 5 (1 is best differentiated, 5 is worst). The two scores are added up to give a Gleason score of 2–10.

TNM classification for prostate cancer

Stage T1: cancer not detectable by DRE

- T1a: with cancer in ≤5% of tissue resected, usually found at autopsy or on resection for prostatic hyperplasia
- T1b: with cancer in >5% of tissue resected, usually found at autopsy or on resection for prostatic hyperplasia
- T1c: cancer found on biopsy indicated by elevated PSA

Stage T2: cancer palpable on DRE but confined to prostate
- T2a: single nodule in only one lobe, surrounded by normal tissue
- T2b: tumor in the majority of one lobe
- T2c: tumor involves both lobes of prostate

Stage T3: palpable tumor extends beyond the prostate without distant metastases
- T3a: unilateral extracapsular extension
- T3b: bilateral extracapsular extension
- T3c: tumor invades seminal vesicles

For all T stages M (metastases) are either (+) or (−).
- M1–2: only pelvic nodes are involved
- M2+: distant metastases

Any T stage can have M+. Metastases can only be diagnosed by pelvic lymphadenectomy.

Approximately 10% of all tumors with a Gleason score <5 have lymphatic metastases, whereas they exist in 70% of all tumors with scores ≥9. However, a PSA of <10 ng/mL carries only a 10% chance of lymphatic spread. Based on these numbers, a pt and his physician must make the decision to perform a pelvic lymphadenectomy.

P **Refer the pt to a urologist**

Simple prostatectomy may be curative in T1a and T1c disease.

Radical prostatectomy (removal of prostate and seminal vesicles) improves survival for stages T1b and all of T2.

Radical prostatectomy may be useful in stages T3 with or without M+, in that morbidity from the tumor will likely be reduced. However, benefit on mortality is uncertain.

If the pt refuses surgery or is not a candidate, radiation is a viable option

External-beam radiation is likely to cause impotence (60% of all pts remain sexually functional following surgery).

Radioactive seed implantation seems best suited for T2a disease.

Useful in pts with high-grade malignancies and in pts with positive surgical margins.

For pts with M+ tumor, androgen deprivation tends to slow the rate of growth

Androgen deprivation can be accomplished surgically (castration) or medically. Gonadotropin-releasing hormone antagonists to prevent luteinizing hormone secretion seems to be the preferred method.

Chemotherapy is a last resort for palliation

Only 10% of M+ pts have an objective partial response.

INFECTIOUS DISEASE

FEVER OF UNKNOWN ORIGIN

S **Does the pt have symptoms that fit the criteria of fever of unknown (FUO)?**

To remember the criteria, remember the number 3.
Fever should be greater than 101.0°F (38.3°C) for ≥3 wk followed by 3 consecutive days of hospitalization OR 3 outpatient visits without a confirmed diagnosis.

The 3 weeks are not necessary for diagnosis of FUO if the fever begins in a pt already hospitalized for a noninfectious problem (nosocomial FUO), if the pt is neutropenic (neutropenic FUO), or if the pt is HIV positive (HIV-associated FUO).

Does the pt have a history of any autoimmune diseases?
Any autoimmune disease can be associated with others, and these may present with fevers.

Has the pt had any exposure to tuberculosis (TB)?
TB is a common cause of FUO.

Does the pt practice unsafe sex or use injection drugs?
HIV can also cause an FUO.
IV drug usage is also a risk factor for endocarditis, another common cause of FUO.

Does the pt have any history of recent travel?
Third World nations carry a risk of parasitic (e.g., malaria) or chronic bacterial (e.g., brucella) infections.

Has the pt noticed any masses or lumps on the body?
Malignancy is a common cause of FUO. Lumps may represent lymph nodes or tumors.

Is the pt taking any medications?
Many medications can produce fever.

Does the pt have any other physical symptoms that may lead you to a diagnosis?

– Headaches	– Night sweats	– Weight loss
– Anorexia	– Rashes	– Arthritis
– Cough/hemoptysis	– Diarrhea	– Swelling

Ask if the pt is on chronic immunosuppression
If so, consider organisms such as cytomegalovirus, fungi, or *Pneumocystis carinii*.

O **Document the actual severity and frequency of fevers**
This will rule out factitious disorder/malingering and may show a pattern consistent with certain diseases:
- *Two daily spikes*: consistent with Still disease (the systemic form of juvenile rheumatoid arthritis [JRA], which can also occur in adults)
- *Fever every third or fourth day*: consistent with malaria

Conduct a thorough PE to look for any potential causes of the fever
Rash: malar rash of systemic lupus erythematosus, cellulitis, JRA, or polyarteritis nodosa (PAN)
Petechiae: leukemia, endocarditis
Lymphadenopathy: HIV, lymphoma, other malignancy
Systolic murmur: endocarditis
Decreased breath sounds: pneumonia, empyema, TB
RUQ tenderness: liver abscess
Thyromegaly: thyroiditis, Grave disease (with thyrotoxicosis)

Fever of unknown origin

With criteria as noted above, it is now the practitioner's job to ascertain the actual cause.
- For nosocomial FUOs, note that septic thromboembolism is a common event and that medications may cause fever either on their own or by allowing for opportunistic infections.
- For HIV-associated FUO, seek out opportunistic infections.
- For neutropenic FUO, ascertaining the cause is less important than keeping the pt alive until the neutrophil count recovers.

For a differential diagnosis of all other FUOs (a.k.a. Classic FUO), remember ABCs!
Autoimmune diseases, bugs (infections), and cancer will account for some 60%–80% of all causes of FUOs. The following are some common diseases that cause fever:

Autoimmune: lupus, JRA, PAN, cryoglobulinemia, polymyalgia rheumatica, Still disease
- *Bugs* (infections): pneumonia; urinary tract infection; cellulitis; sinusitis; meningitis; endocarditis; abscess of liver, spleen, kidney, or bone; tuberculosis; fungi; HIV; malaria; viral infections
- *Cancer*: Consider solid tumors as well humoral malignancies.
- *Drugs*: steroids, amphetamines, antibiotics, atropine, isoniazid, procainamide, quinidine
- *Endocrine*: hyperthyroidism, thyroiditis
- *Embolism*: deep vein thrombosis or pulmonary embolus
- *Factitious or familial* Mediterranean fever
- *Granulomatous*: sarcoidosis, Crohn disease, ulcerative colitis

P **Perform cultures on the pt at all sites**

Blood cultures times 2, sputum, urine cultures are indicated in all pts with FUO.
Cerebrospinal fluid and peritoneal cultures if relevant.
Be sure to send blood and sputum in special media to look for fungal and TB species if clinical suspicion is raised during history and physical.

Order radiographic studies as clinical suspicion warrants

A CXR should be done on all pts with FUO as part of the initial workup. However, the following studies should only be done based on clinical suspicion:
- KUB
- CT chest/abdomen/pelvis
- RUQ ultrasound
- Echocardiography
- Upper GI series

Administer empiric antibiotics if the pt appears ill or unstable

Broad-spectrum antibiotics for bacterial infections are a good initial choice. If the pt fails to improve after a few days, consider empiric use of antifungal medicines.
Steroids have not been shown to be of empiric benefit in pts with FUO and may in fact worsen the condition of pts with occult infections.

Send off other serum studies

CBC with differential, antinuclear antibody, rheumatoid factor

Realize that up to 15% cases of FUO resolve or persist without a confirmed diagnosis

ACUTE BACTERIAL ENDOCARDITIS

 Does the pt have fever, fatigue, muscular pain, or malaise?
These are very general complaints, but these are the common complaints in endocarditis.

Does the pt have a history of valvular heart disease or rheumatic fever?
Any abnormality of the heart valves increases the risk of endocarditis.
Rheumatic fever (RF) is one of the primary causes of mitral valve stenosis.

Does the pt have a prosthetic heart valve?
Treatment differs considerably based on whether it is a native or prosthetic valve (see below).

Has the pt ever used IV drugs?
IV drug use is a huge risk factor for endocarditis. It also changes the treatment approach (see below).

Does the pt report any new dyspnea on exertion or decreased exercise tolerance?
Congestive heart failure resulting from valvular disease is one of the sequelae of endocarditis, as well as a reason to consider surgery as a treatment option.

 Review VS and perform a PE
Look for fever (temperature >100.4°F = 38°C)
Neuro: defects as a sign of possible stroke from septic emboli
Cardio: murmur, especially one consistent with valvular regurgitation
HEENT: Roth spots (round white spots surrounded by a retinal hemorrhage)
Skin:
- *Janeway lesions*: painless hemorrhagic macules/nodules on the palms, soles
- *Osler nodes*: painful pea-sized subcutaneous nodules in the fingers, toes, palms, soles

Obtain serial blood cultures
These are necessary not only to help make the diagnosis but also to decide on treatment.

Review the CBC with differential
Look for clues suggesting bacterial infection, such as high white count with left shift.

Check U/A for signs of hematuria or RBC casts
Glomerulonephritis is a well-known immunologic effect of endocarditis.

Order rheumatoid factor
Helps to make the diagnosis because it is one of the minor criteria.

Review the echocardiogram
Look for signs of intracardiac mass, abscess, or other abnormalities, particularly around a valve.

If transthoracic echo is negative or inconclusive, consider transesophageal
Often a better view of the heart can be obtained using transesophageal, but it is more invasive and requires sedation, so it should only be used if transthoracic echo is inconclusive and clinical suspicion of endocarditis remains high.

 Acute bacterial endocarditis
Bacterial infection of the inner wall (endocardium) of the heart
Diagnosis is often made using Duke criteria:
- Major criteria
  - Two or more positive blood cultures
  - New murmur or echocardiogram showing endocardial involvement

- Minor criteria
  - History of previous valvular abnormality, heart surgery, or IV drug use
  - Fever
  - Evidence of septic emboli
  - Immunologic signs: glomerulonephritis, RF positive, Osler nodes, Roth spots
  - Single positive blood culture

For diagnosis, you need two major or one major and three minor or five minor

For possible endocarditis, you need one major and one minor or three minor

Differential diagnosis

Vasculitis: PAN, MPA, Wegener disease, HSP

Infectious: meningitis, sepsis, pneumonia, myocarditis, pericarditis, malaria, HIV, syphilis, EBV, CMV

Oncologic: paraneoplastic syndrome, metastases

Endocrine: hyperthyroid, hypothyroid, DKA

Rheumatic: SLE, RA, MCTD, JRA

This disease can be subtle, so using the duke criteria can be helpful in determining the likelihood that this is endocarditis

Draw blood cultures and treat first empirically and then based on sensitivities

Vancomycin or ampicillin with aminoglycoside (plus rifampin if prostatic valve is present) is a good choice for empiric treatment.

Duration of treatment is usually about 6 weeks.

Consult cardiothoracic Surgery for possible surgery if pt has congestive heart failure, abscess, or failure of antibiotics

In these cases, surgery may be the only option.

Consider consulting Cardiology and infectious disease for more advice

Advice from the experts is an important component of care. This can be a difficult disease to treat, and even if treated correctly, more than half of these pts require valve replacement eventually.

Provide prophylaxis with amoxicillin or clindamycin 1 hour before invasive procedures like dental procedures

If the pt is high risk and will undergo GI or GU surgery, give IV/IM ampicillin and aminoglycoside.

HIV WITH FEVER

S **What is the pt's last CD4 count and viral load?**

Infections like *P. carinii* pneumonia (PCP), Cocci, and cytomegalovirus are more common with lower CD4 counts.

Does the pt have a history of opportunistic infections?

Previous PCP infection increases the risk of recurrence.

Examples of organisms that cause opportunistic infection are as follows:
- Fungal (candida, histoplasma, cryptococcus, coccidioides, aspergillus)
- Protozoal/fungal *(P. carinii)*, protozoa (cryptosporidia, microsporidia, isospora), and sporozoa (toxoplasma).

Does the pt have risk factors for exposure to known infection?

Sick contacts: TB exposure, homelessness, incarceration, IV drug abuse

Recent travel: Southwest United States, Arizona (cocci); Ohio/Mississippi river valleys (histo)

Employment: farmers: aspergillus; hunters: blastomycosis

Animal contacts: bird droppings (crypto); cats (toxo); bat droppings (histo)

What medications is the pt taking? Is he or she on HAART or prophylaxis?

If the pt is on TMP/SMX or azithromycin prophylaxis, for example, he or she is less likely to have PCP or membrane attack complex (MAC), respectively.

Does the pt have symptoms suggestive of infection?

CNS: changes in mental status, headache, neck stiffness, and fever (meningitis). HIV pts do not have typical symptoms, may be subtle: fatigue and fever.

Respiratory symptoms such as cough, exertional dyspnea, pleuritic chest pain, night sweats, and fever may reflect conditions like sinusitis, bronchitis, and pneumonia. As CD4 counts decrease, PCP, TB, fungal, lymphoma, or Kaposi sarcoma (KS).

GI symptoms include odynophagia or dysphagia suggesting esophagitis; abdominal pain, diarrhea, and fever suggesting infectious etiology.

O **Review VS, looking for signs of hemodynamic instability**

Sepsis: fever, hypotension, tachycardia

Dehydration: positive orthostatics

Pneumonia: increased respiratory rate, low pulse oximetry

Perform a PE

Gen: assess level of consciousness, nutritional status

HEENT: funduscopic, ulcers, thrush, meningismus, lymph nodes

Abd: hepatomegaly, splenomegaly (histo, TB)

Skin: subcutaneous nodules, ulcers

Evaluate CBC with differential

Leukocytosis with left shift suggests infection; consider urine, blood, sputum, stool cultures, lumbar puncture (LP), and CXR (cultures should include bacteria, fungal, and acid-fast bacillus [AFB]).

Anemia (chronic disease, parvovirus B-19) also occurs often.

Thrombocytopenia: common in HIV

Obtain a CD4 count

Some infections are more common at lower CD4 counts:
- CD4 >500 cells/mm^3: sinusitis, bronchitis, oral thrush
- CD4 200–500 cells/mm^3: pneumonia (bacterial)
- CD4 100–200 cells/mm^3: PCP, histo, cocci, miliary TB, lymphoma
- CD4 <100 cells/mm^3: toxo, crypto, MAC, KS
- CD4 <50 cells/mm^3: CMV infections

Consider further diagnostic studies

If predominant CNS symptoms, consider:
- CT head: Ring-enhancing lesions suggest toxoplasma or lymphoma
- LP: opening pressure, cell count, protein, glucose, Gram stain, culture, AFB, VDRL test, cryptococcal Ag
- Serum crypto Ag, toxoplasma Ab

If predominant pulmonary symptoms, consider:
- Sputum Gram stain, cx: fungal, AFB, PCP (expectorated or induced)
- Place purified protein derivative (PPD)
- LDH: increased with PCP, TB, lymphoma
- ABG: hypoxemia and high A-a gradient common with PCP
- CXR: Normal CXR does not indicate absence of disease
  - Bilateral interstitial infiltrates common with PCP, histo, cocci
  - Upper lobe cavitary lesion with TB or pentamidine-treated PCP
  - Pleural effusions common with TB or KS
- Consider CT chest or bronchoscopy

If predominant GI symptoms, consider:
- Send stool WBC, culture, ova and parasites, *Isospora* and *Cryptospora*. If any suspicious skin lesions, biopsy.

 HIV and fever

Infection in HIV-positive pts requires special consideration because they are immunosuppressed and therefore at increased risk from not only normal pathogens but also a wide range of opportunistic infections.

Etiologies

CNS infections *(Streptococcus pneumoniae, crypto*, HSV, VSV, toxo)

Pulmonary infections (*S. pneumoniae, Haemophilus influenzae*, TB, PCP, *Rhodococcus equi*)

GI infections (*Candida*, HSV, CMV, crypto-/iso-/microspora, MAC)

Malignancy (lymphoma, KS, cervical or anal cancer)

P **Ensure that the pt is on appropriate prophylaxis**

If CD4 count <200, start PCP prophylaxis with TMP/SMX.

If CD4 count <100, start MAC prophylaxis with azithromycin.

Treat based on source of infection

Esophagitis: fluconazole (*Candida*)

Sinusitis or bronchitis: amoxicillin or augmentin

TB: see TB, p. 6

MAC: clarithromycin 500 mg twice per day

PCP: TMP/SMZ DS (or pentamidine if allergic) for 21 days
- If PaO_2 < 70, a-A gradient >35, give steroids
- Lifelong prophylactic therapy with TMP/SMZ DS or dapsone if allergic; cryptococcal meningitis: amphotericin B

Histoplasmosis: mild-moderate disease: itraconazole; severe disease: amphotericin B; maintenance therapy: itraconazole

Coccidioidomycosis or aspergillosis: amphotericin B

Toxoplasmosis: pyrimethamine and sulfadiazine

CELLULITIS

S **Does the pt report any recent breaks in the skin?**

Many things can cause a break in the skin and be a portal of entry for infection:

- Abrasions
- Bites (insect, dog, cat)
- IV drug abuse (IVDA)
- Cuts
- Surgical wound
- Preexisting skin conditions
- Burns
- IVs

Does the pt have any preexisting skin problems?

These conditions can also cause a break in the skin and lead to cellulitis:

- Eczema
- Athlete's foot
- Psoriasis
- Venous stasis
- Pemphigus
- Pressure ulcer

Does the pt have diabetes?

Increased risk, especially in poorly controlled diabetes mellitus:

- Poor immune system activity, especially with hyperglycemia
- Decreased peripheral sensation, may not notice foot injuries like stepping on a piece of glass

Is the pt using IV drugs or skin popping?

Intravenous or subcutaneous use of drugs or other substances is another risk factor for infection.

Is the pt homeless or alcoholic?

These pts tend to be at increased risk for skin infection resulting from poor hygiene.

Does the pt have any other medical problems?

Renal failure, especially end-stage renal failure, also leads to poor healing and increased risk of cellulitis and other infections.

Similarly, hepatic failure/cirrhosis can lead to poor healing.

Malnutrition from any cause can lead to poor healing.

Pts with cancer have an increased risk from things like chemotherapy, which can weaken the immune system, to central venous catheters, which can be portals of entry for the infection.

Review the medicines the pt is taking

It is important to note immune-suppressing medicines like prednisone.

Does the pt have any other preexisting immune deficiency?

Neutrophil (both acquired and congenital) defects like neutropenia and chronic granulomatous disease (CGD) place the pt at particularly increased risk.

HIV can also lead to immune deficiency and a variety of opportunistic infections.

O **Review the VS and perform a PE**

Look for fever, which may indicate infection with *Staphylococcus pyogenes* or that there is more than cellulitis: abscess, toxic shock syndrome, endocarditis.

Skin:

- Look specifically at the lesion for redness, warmth, swelling, and pain.
- Note if the cellulitis overlies any bones or joints.
- Palpate carefully for any crepitus or fluctuance.
- Look for signs of underlying trauma, such as:
  - Abrasion
  - Bites
  - Burns
  - Cuts
- Look for signs of underlying skin disease, such as:
  - Tinea
  - Folliculitis
  - Herpes
  - Venous stasis
  - Eczema
  - Pressure ulcers

Look in the ear, especially in diabetics who are prone to infections like otitis externa.

Examine the lower leg (one of the most common sites).

Ask IV drug abusers to show you where they inject.

Feel for lymph nodes in the area.

Consider biopsy/culture of the inflamed skin
This may give you the diagnosis as well as the best treatment if you can get sensitivities from the culture.

Consider obtaining an x-ray or MRI if the lesion overlies superficial bone
Look for signs of periosteal elevation suggesting osteomyelitis.

A ## Cellulitis
Acute inflammation of the skin caused by bacterial infection leading to warmth, redness, swelling, and local pain

Etiologies
Staphylococcus aureus: usually spreads from a local infection like an abscess caused by a foreign body. Associated with IVDA. Consider possible endocarditis.

Streptococcus pyogenes: usually diffuse and rapidly spreading associated with lymphangitis as well as fever

Streptococcal (groups A, B, C, or G): associated with venous stasis/peripheral vascular disease and pts with diabetes

H. influenzae: associated with infections above the neck (sinusitis, otitis) and people with diabetes

Pseudomonas aeruginosa: diabetics, hot tub folliculitis, and people who step on a nail while wearing tennis shoes

Pasteurella multocida: associated with cat and dog bites

Vibrio vulnificus: associated with shell fish/ocean

Mycobacterium marinum: associated with fish tanks and swimming pools

Differential diagnosis
- Necrotizing fasciitis
- Osteomyelitis
- Folliculitis
- Elder abuse
- Toxic shock syndrome
- Mucormycosis
- Gangrene
- Eczema
- Abscess
- Burn
- Lyme disease
- Cryptococcus
- Herpes
- Viral exanthem
- Tinea
- Endocarditis
- HIV
- CGD

P ### In general, empiric therapy can begin with Keflex or oxacillin
These drugs will cover most of the common causes of cellulitis (Group A Strep and Staph aureus).

If empiric therapy fails or the pt has an underlying immunodeficiency, consider admission for IV antibiotics
If the pt fails outpatient empiric therapy, then he or she may have:
- Unidentified immune deficiency (HIV, ESRD, cancer).
- MRSA or other resistant organisms: Admit for IV vancomycin.
- Osteomyelitis, endocarditis, or other underlying infections/conditions.
- Diabetes: Make sure there is good anaerobic coverage because of the increased risk of anaerobic coinfection.

Carefully identify pts who need surgical intervention
Some pts may need surgical debridement:
- Necrotizing fasciitis
- Abscess—Pyomyositis

Pts with osteomyelitis will need Orthopedic consultation.

Consult Dermatology in cases that are not clear

ENDOCRINOLOGY

DIABETES

S **Does the pt have any risk factors for diabetes?**
– Obesity   – Polycystic ovarian syndrome   – Gestational diabetes
Multiple first-degree relatives with diabetes
• Type 1 DM associated with HLA-DR3 or HLA-DR4
Ethnicity
• Type 1 DM: Scandinavians are at highest risk
• Type 2 DM: African-Americans, Mexicans, Native Americans

What is the pt's age?
Type 1 DM is common in children 10–14 years of age or in older nonobese pts.
Type 2 DM is common in those older than 40 years.

Does the pt experience the three P's (polyuria, polydipsia, polyphagia)?
Type 1 DM often presents with polyuria and weight loss.

O **Review VS**
Obesity (BMI >30), calculate using: BMI = (Wt in kg)/(Ht in m)^2
• So a 100-kg (220-lb) person who is 1.83 m (72 in or 6 ft) tall has a BMI of: 100/$(1.83)^2$ = 29.8.
High blood pressure (risk for micro- and macrovascular complications)
Orthostatics (assess volume status)

Perform a complete PE, looking specifically for
Gen: Assess mental status.
HEENT: Perform a funduscopic exam; inspect dentition.
Ext: Document integrity of skin, edema or deformities, strength of pulses.
Neuro: Assess sensation using monofilament if possible.

Review renal function tests
Obtain creatinine to assess renal impairment. Some medications such as metformin (if
Cr >1.6 men or >1.5 women) are contraindicated in this case.

Perform diagnostic test
Criteria for diagnosing DM include:
• Random blood sugar (BS) >200 mg/dL (two separate occasions)
  o 110–200 mg/dL = impaired glucose tolerance
• Fasting blood sugar (FBS) >126 mg/dL (two separate occasions)
  o 110–126 mg/dL = impaired glucose tolerance
• 2-hour plasma glucose >200 mg/dL (oral glucose tolerance test, OGTT)
  o 140–200 mg/dL = impaired glucose tolerance

Check HbA1c
Typically, RBCs live about 110 days in the bloodstream, and during that time they can
become glycated. For this reason, this test can be used to estimate the level of glycemic
control in the last approximately 3 months. Normal HbA1c is 6.
You can calculate a corresponding BS using the HbA1c:
• Average BS = ([HbA1c−4]35) + 65
• So HbA1c of 7 = avg BS of = ([7−4]35) + 65 = 170

Review results of a fasting lipid panel
Pts commonly have triglycerides >200 mg/dL and HDL <35 mg/dL.

Check urinalysis
Glucosuria occurs when the threshold for reabsorption of glucose is exceeded.
Ketonuria suggests diabetic ketoacidosis (DKA) or starvation.
Send urine specifically for microalbumin.

Look for evidence of the metabolic syndrome

Pts with metabolic syndrome have a higher prevalence of coronary artery disease.
The metabolic syndrome is defined by the presence of three or more of the following:
- Obesity: waist circumference >40 inches in men, >35 inches in women
- Dyslipidemia:
  o Fasting triglycerides >150 mg/dL
  o HDL cholesterol <40 mg/dL in men, <50 mg/dL in women
- Hypertension: blood pressure >130/85 mm Hg
- Diabetes: fasting plasma glucose >110 mg/dL

A Diabetes mellitus

Type 2 Diabetes: poor glycemic control resulting from insulin resistance and decreased insulin secretion in response to hyperglycemia

Type 1 Diabetes: poor glycemic control resulting from absence of endogenous insulin secretion (>90% autoimmune)

Secondary diabetes:
  – Pancreatic disorders   – Genetic (hemochromatosis)
  – Cushing syndrome   – Drugs (steroids)

P Identify and treat pts with DKA/HONK (see p. 90). Educate all pts before initiating medications

Diabetic teaching (e.g., pathophysiology, complications, lifestyle)
Glucometer for home glucose monitoring
Log of adverse effects, especially of symptoms such as sweating, tremulousness, and confusion because these may be a sign of overmedication
Nutrition, exercise, smoking cessation, immunizations (pneumococcal, influenza)

Keep treatment goals in mind at each visit

  – HbA1c <7.0%   – LDL <70 mg/dL   – Blood pressure <130/80 mm Hg
  – HDL >40 mg/dL   – Triglycerides <150 mg/dL

Begin with oral medications such as biguanides or sulfonylurea

Begin with monotherapy and then a combination of oral agents before insulin.
  – Sulfonylureas   – Thiazolidinediones
  – Biguanides   – α-Glucosidase inhibitors
  – Dipeptidyl peptidase-4 inhibitor   – Glucagon-like peptide-1
  – Sodium-glucose cotransporter-2
    inhibitor

Begin insulin if the pt fails to reach goals with oral medications

In general, the amount of insulin can be estimated based on the pt's weight. Use about 0.6 per kg to estimate the units needed, and then use two-thirds in the morning and one-third in the evening. Of the morning dose, two-thirds should be intermediate and one-third short-acting. In the evening, use one-half intermediate and one-half short-acting.
  – Ultra-short-acting (lispro, aspart)   – Intermediate (NPH, lente)
  – Short-acting (Novolin, Humulin,   – Long-acting (glargine, detemir)
    regular)
  – Mixed combinations (70/30, 50/50)

Refer the pt annually to ophthalmology, dentistry, and podiatry

Such referrals will help reduce the number of complications, such as blindness, tooth loss, and amputation.

DIABETIC KETOACIDOSIS AND HYPEROSMOLAR NONKETOTIC COMA

S What is the pt's age?
Certain age groups are more likely to present with DKA versus HONK.
- DKA is common in young type 1 DM, also seen with type 2.
- HONK is common in older pts, seen in type 2.

Does the pt report any of the three P's (polyuria, polydipsia, polyphagia)?
Common clinical manifestations of uncontrolled hyperglycemia:
- Polyuria: frequent urination caused by glycosuria
- Polydipsia: frequent drinking driven by dehydration and hyperosmolarity
- Polyphagia: increased food intake often with weight loss

Does the pt report recent illness?
Decompensated glycemic control results from underlying infections:
- Urinary Tract infection   – Pneumonia   – Pancreatitis

Other factors that may precipitate hyperglycemia:
- Myocardial infarction (MI)   – Cerebrovascular accident
- Alcohol binge   – Pregnancy   – Trauma

Does the pt have a history of lack of adherence to medications or nutrition?
Nonadherence is one of the most common causes of poorly controlled sugars.

Review medications
Diuretics and steroids can increase blood sugars.

O Does the pt have VS suggestive of hemodynamic instability?
Consider the following in a pt who presents with severe hyperglycemia:
- *Sepsis*: fever, hypotension, tachycardia
- *Respiratory distress*: tachypnea (Kussmaul respirations)
- *Severe volume contraction*: orthostatics

Perform a PE
Gen: Assess level of consciousness (obtunded); evaluate for acetone breath.
Look for signs of infection.

Perform diagnostic tests to differentiate DKA from HONK
Check finger stick.
Check arterial blood gas (ABG).
- Low pH in DKA, normal in HONK

Check serum electrolytes, including calcium, magnesium, and phosphorus.
- Calculate anion gap.
  - High in DKA, normal in HONK.
- Check serum ketones.
  - High in DKA, none/decreased in HONK.
- Calculate serum osmolality: increased in HONK.
  - $2 \times$ (observed $Na^+ + K^+$) + glucose/18 + BUN/2.8

What is the result of the CBC with differential?
Leukocytosis with left shift indicates infection.
Consider U/A, blood, urine and sputum cultures, and CXR.

What are the results of the pt's renal and liver function tests (LFTs)?
Pts who are severely volume contracted typically have a rise in BUN and creatinine.
Abnormal LFTs suggest infection or alcohol-induced.

Consider the ECG
MI is a common precipitant of a severe hyperglycemic state.
Arrhythmias are common with electrolyte abnormalities.

A **Severe hyperglycemia**

Diabetic **K**etoacidosis
- DM: *hyperglycemia (glucose >300 mg/dL)*
- *Ketonuria, ketonemia, or both*
- *Acidosis pH < 7.35, bicarbonate <15*

Hyperosmolar **N**on**k**etotic coma
- Hyperglycemia (glucose >400 mg/dL)
- Impaired mental status
- High plasma osmolality (>340 mOsm)
- Lack of significant ketosis

P **Admit to a monitored bed**

DKA and HONK are life-threatening conditions.

Treat precipitating factors

As mentioned above, many things can cause or precipitate DKA/HONK; look for these causes and treat them or the pt will not get better.

Provide aggressive fluid resuscitation immediately, even before insulin

These pts (HONK > DKA) are very volume depleted.

Estimated free water deficit = 0.5 × body wt (kg) × (corrected Na^+−140/140).

Initial volume replacement with normal saline (NS). Replace 1 L in first hour, second L in next 1–2 hours, and then continue 1/2NS 500 mL/hr.

Add D5 to IV fluid when glucose levels approach 250 mg/dL

To avoid rebound hypoglycemia

IV insulin therapy: load 0.1–0.2 U/kg IV and then continuous infusion 0.1 U/kg/hr

This will decrease serum glucose concentration.

Continue until anion gap (AG = Na−[Cl + HCO_3]) is closed (AG <15).

SQ dose of regular insulin 30 minutes before stopping infusion.

Make a flow sheet of important electrolytes and glucose to carefully follow and replace electrolytes

In hyperosmolar states, the electrolytes K, Ca, Mg, and P will be artificially high in the serum because of the lack of insulin. So it is important to monitor them carefully in order to avoid dangerous sequelae of low serum electrolytes (such as arrhythmia) as the insulin is replaced.

Finger sticks every hour initially

Carefully avoid hypoglycemia (remember to add D5 when the blood sugar approaches 250) and make sure your interventions are working.

Electrolytes, anion gap q2 hours initially. P, Mg q6 hours initially

As mentioned above, treatment is not over until AG <15, and these pts will nearly always require electrolyte replacement.

Repeat ABG after 4 hours

Another way of verifying that your interventions are working

HYPOTHYROIDISM

S **Does the pt experience symptoms related to a hypothyroid state?**
- Fatigue
- Weakness
- Cold intolerance
- Weight gain
- Constipation
- Dyspnea
- Brittle hair/nails
- Dry skin
- Muscle cramps
- Depression
- Difficulty concentrating
- Loss of hearing (fluid accumulation in the middle ear)

Does the female pt report changes in her menstrual cycle?
Evaluate thyroid function with any menstrual irregularity or history of infertility.

Does the pt have a history of Graves disease?
Previous radioablation and thyroidectomy are risks for primary hypothyroidism.

Does the pt have risk factors for central hypothyroidism?
Pts with central nervous system (CNS) lesions are at risk for a hypothyroid state.
- Head trauma
- Pituitary tumors
- CNS radiation

Does the pt have symptoms associated with other pituitary hormones?
Consider other hormones of the pituitary gland as being affected:
- Stunted growth (growth hormone)
- Hypogonadism, dysmenorrhea (FSH/LH)
- Decreased libido/lactation (prolactin)

Does the pt have a history of autoimmune disease?
- Pernicious anemia
- Type 1 diabetes mellitus
- Myasthenia gravis
- Vitiligo

Does the pt have a history of infiltrative disease?
Places the pt at risk for developing hypothyroidism:
- Hemochromatosis
- Sarcoidosis
- Amyloidosis

Review medications
Medications may affect thyroid hormone secretion or metabolism.
- Propylthiouracil
- Methimazole
- Lithium
- Amiodarone

O **Review the pt's VS for signs of hypothyroidism**
- Bradycardia
- Diastolic hypertension
- Hypothermia

Perform PE
Gen: assess level of consciousness
HEENT: alopecia, periorbital edema, thinning outer eyebrow, goiter, hoarseness
Skin: nonpitting edema (myxedema), dryness, pallor
Ext: cool to touch
Neuro: delayed relaxation of deep tendon reflexes

Review CBC and renal function
Abnormal lipids may affect RBC morphology, causing macrocytic anemia.
Pts with elevated BUN and creatinine suggests volume contraction.

Evaluate the pattern of TSH and thyroid hormone
Elevated TSH, decreased free T4 (primary hypothyroidism)
Decreased or normal TSH, decreased free T4 (central hypothyroidism)
Elevated TSH, normal free T4, T3 (subclinical hypothyroidism)

Consider antithyroid peroxidase or antithyroglobulin
Obtain antibodies in a pt suspected of autoimmune disease: subclinical hypothyroidism
with positive antibodies has a 4% risk of hypothyroidism.

Hypothyroidism
Inadequate secretion of thyroid hormone

Etiologies
Primary (thyroid):

– Hashimoto Thyroiditis	– Radiation	– Thyroidectomy
– Subacute thyroiditis	– Drugs	– Iodine excess
– Iodine deficiency	– Congenital	

Secondary (pituitary):
- Tumor   – Infiltrative disease   – Sheehan (postpartum)

Tertiary (hypothalamic):
- Tumor   – Radiation   – Infection

Identify pts with myxedema coma
A pt who presents with altered level of consciousness, hypothermia, hypoxia, bradycardia, and hypotension with known hypothyroidism must be treated promptly.

Myxedema coma is a medical emergency. Admit to monitored bed
Load L-thyroxine 400 µg IV, then 100 µg IV qd.

Avoid aggressive rewarming
Causes vasodilation worsening hypertension.
Respiratory support may be needed because of decompensation with shock and coma.
Support respiratory status as needed. Look for precipitating cause:

– Infection	– GI bleed	– Congestive heart failure
– Myocardial infarction	– Cerebrovascular accident	– Trauma

Have low threshold for starting IV antibiotics. Check cortisol level and replace as needed. Identify pts with thyroiditis and treat them symptomatically
Pts with thyroiditis usually do not require hormone replacement. Monitoring and symptomatic care is sufficient because this condition is usually self-limited.

Identify primary hypothyroidism and treat with ʟ-thyroxine 1.7 µg/kg/d
- Older pts and those with coronary artery disease should start at lower doses.
- Titrate slowly until TSH is normal, and then reevaluate in 6–8 weeks.
- Increase dose with pregnancy.
- Many drug–drug interactions require higher doses.

Identify central hypothyroidism and monitor free T4 levels
This is to assess adrenal function because replacement therapy may precipitate an adrenal crisis.

Subclinical hypothyroidism is usually monitored and not treated
Treatment is controversial; some indications include dyslipidemia or pregnancy.

HYPERTHYROIDISM

S | **Is the pt experiencing any symptoms of hyperthyroidism?**

Most pts with hyperthyroidism are symptomatic. Common symptoms include:

– Tremors	– Heat intolerance	– Diaphoresis
– Anxiety	– Weight loss	– Diarrhea

Pts older than 70 years may not manifest the same typical symptoms as younger pts; common clinical manifestations in those older than 70 years include:

– Atrial fibrillation	– Congestive heart failure (CHF)	– Wasting
– Anorexia	– Fatigue	

Has the pt had any fevers?
Rarely, low-grade fevers may occur.

Ask women about changes in their menstrual cycles
Common manifestations include oligomenorrhea and amenorrhea.

Has the pt noticed any weakness?
Often, despite having increased energy, pts could have trouble climbing stairs, secondary to proximal muscle weakness.

Other than weight loss, has the pt noticed any physical changes?
Goiter might be the most common physical change.

Pts may complain of eye enlargement or a "bug-eyed" appearance. This is known as exophthalmos or proptosis and is common in Graves disease.

Some pts may complain about changes of the skin on their shins. It may be thickened, hyperpigmented, and itchy. This is dermopathy, a myxedema also associated with Graves disease.

Is there a family history of thyroid disease?
Family histories of hypo- and hyperthyroidism are common.

O | **Review VS**

Low-grade fever may be present. Temperature >41°C is a sign of thyroid storm.
Tachycardia, increased pulse pressure (high systolic, low diastolic) are common.

Perform a PE
Gen: Wasting, fidgeting, and pressured speech are common. Note if the pt has altered mental status. This is a sign of thyroid storm.
Eyes: Many common findings may occur.
  • Exophthalmos: Common but only occurs in Graves disease.
  • Staring, lid lag, and lid retraction may occur with all types of hyperthyroidism.
Neck: These pts will likely have a goiter.
  • Diffusely enlarged, smooth, nontender: think of Graves disease.
  • Nodular: Think of toxic multinodular goiter versus malignancy.
    ○ Auscultate over a goiter for a bruit; also common in Graves disease.
Cardiac: Atrial fibrillation is extremely common; systolic murmurs, signs of CHF.
Neuro: A fine tremor is extremely common.
Skin: Commonly, skin will be warm, smooth, and moist. Look for pretibial myxedema with an orange-skin appearance. Pts may also have vitiligo.

Send serum for thyroid-stimulating hormone (TSH), free T4, and T3 levels
TSH is the most sensitive test for screening. Low in the presence of hyperthyroidism.
High free T4 classical, but some pts will have T3 toxicosis.

Order thyroid radioiodine uptake if you cannot delineate the etiology by H&P
High uptake, homogenous distribution suggests Graves disease.
Low uptake suggests thyroiditis.
Patchy areas of increased and decreased uptake suggests multinodular goiter.

Obtain an ECG
This will rule out atrial fibrillation.

Hyperthyroidism (thyrotoxicosis)
A syndrome of increased metabolic rate secondary to overproduction of thyroid hormone

Differential diagnosis
Graves disease (most common): an autoimmune condition resulting in an antibody that, instead of destroying thyroid tissue, binds to the TSH receptor and stimulates it.

Toxic multinodular goiter: happens in pts who have had long-standing simple goiter. More common in the elderly.

Thyroiditis (subacute, painless): an autoimmune condition in which thyroid tissue is destroyed. May be a precursor to Hashimotos thyroiditis or may be self-limiting.

Hyperfunctioning thyroid malignancy: Cancer should always be ruled out by biopsy.

Identify pts with thyroid storm
Pts have a high mortality rate. Admit to a monitored setting immediately. Identify and treat precipitating factors (usually infection or dehydration):
- Methimazole or propylthiouracil
- Iodide (Lugol's solution)
- Propranolol IV
- Hydrocortisone

Identify pts with thyroiditis
In these pts, there is no role for antithyroid medications or radioactive iodine (RAI) because the hyperthyroidism is caused by release of preformed thyroid hormone and not overproduction.
Generally resolves spontaneously after 2–4 months.

Hyperadrenergic symptoms can be treated with β-blockers
Oral propranolol is the drug of choice.

Excessive thyroid secretion can be treated with antithyroid drugs
Methimazole or propylthiouracil.
Monitor for potential side effects: agranulocytosis, hepatitis, lupus-like syndrome.

Indications for radioiodine ablation therapy
Adverse reaction to oral medications
Severe cardiac manifestations
Toxic multinodular goiter
Contraindications: pregnancy, breastfeeding

Indications for subtotal thyroidectomy
Pregnant pts or children with adverse reaction to oral medications
Large goiters with compressive complications

Monitor treatment by following free T4 levels

If the pt has atrial fibrillation or CHF, treat as noted in SOAPs on these illnesses

Refer pts with exophthalmos to Ophthalmology. Orbital radiation may be necessary

HYPERPARATHYROIDISM

S **Does the pt have symptoms associated with hypercalcemia?**

– Fatigue	– Weakness	– Lethargy	– Polyuria—AMS
– Nausea	– Vomiting	– Constipation	– Polydipsia

Review medications

Thiazide diuretics may exacerbate underlying hyperparathyroidism.
Long-term lithium may also cause hyperparathyroidism.

Does the pt have recurrent UTI or kidney stones?

Hyperparathyroidism increases the risk for calcium-containing stones because of the
  increased filtered load of calcium by kidney.

Does the pt have joint pain?

Oligo- or polyarticular pain may suggest underlying pseudogout or gout.

Is there a family history of similar symptoms?

MEN type I: primary hyperparathyroidism, pituitary adenoma, ZE
MEN type IIa: primary hyperparathyroidism, medullary thyroid carcinoma and
  pheochromocytoma
Familial hypocalciuric hypercalcemia (FHH)

O **Review VS**

Hypertension is commonly associated with hyperparathyroidism.

Perform a PE

Gen: Assess level of consciousness.   *Skin*: vitiligo
HEENT: slit lamp (corneal   *Ext*: joint effusions
  calcifications)
Neuro: proximal muscle weakness

Review CBC and BUN/Cr

Leukocytosis suggests infection (UTI).
Assess for ARF (increased BUN/Cr) caused by UTI, dehydration, or calculi.
  • Consider urinalysis to assess presence of hematuria or pyuria.
  • Consider abdominal film and then renal ultrasound to rule out calculi.

Check total calcium, albumin, or serum ionized calcium

Majority of calcium bound to albumin, correct for changes in serum albumin
  • Corrected calcium = ([4.0–Alb] × 0.8) + Measured calcium

**To rule out possible lab error, consider checking an arterial blood gas for
ionized calcium**

Serum ionized calcium levels are most indicative of actual serum calcium levels.

Check parathyroid hormone (PTH) level to assess gland function

PTH high, calcium high indicates primary hyperparathyroidism.
PTH normal, calcium high suggests primary hyperparathyroidism.
PTH high, calcium low suggests secondary hyperparathyroidism.
PTH low, undetectable, look for another cause of hypercalcemia.

Check phosphate, alkaline phosphatase

PTH increases renal excretion of phosphate, causing low serum phosphate.
PTH increases osteoblast activity, causing high alkaline phosphatase.

Consider 24-hour urine collection for calcium

Increased with primary hyperparathyroidism
  • Men >300 mg/24 hr; women >250 mg/24 hr
  • Decreased excretion indicates FHH (<150 mg/24 hr)

Consider a DEXA scan (see Osteoporosis, p. 102) to rule out osteoporosis

Consider ECG

Hypercalcemia increases risk for arrhythmia or sudden death; look for short QT.

A Hyperparathyroidism

Condition in which there is increased secretion of PTH or PTHrP, leading to increased serum calcium, decreased serum phosphorus, and increased excretion of both in the urine. This can lead to urinary calcium stones as well as bone demineralization.

Etiologies

Primary hyperparathyroidism
- Parathyroid adenoma
- Parathyroid hyperplasia

- Parathyroid carcinoma
- MEN type I or IIa

Secondary hyperparathyroidism
- Chronic renal failure

Tertiary hyperparathyroidism
- FHH

- Postrenal transplant

Differential diagnosis

Malignancy (PTHrP), multiple myeloma, iatrogenic, renal failure

P Admit pts with symptomatic hypercalcemia

Pts with hyperparathyroidism are at risk for severe increases in calcium (>12 mg/dL). With severe hypercalcemia, pts are at risk for seizure, arrhythmia, and sudden death.

Administer aggressive IV fluid resuscitation if the pt has symptomatic hypercalcemia

Use caution with elderly, cardiac, or renal pts.

Increased serum calcium often causes a diuresis, and on admission many of these pts are intravascularly depleted.

Aggressive fluid hydration also helps reduce the serum calcium by dilution.

Give loop diuretics once the pt is euvolemic

The loop diuretic such as furosemide will increase excretion of calcium.

Give calcitonin and bisphosphonates if aggressive IV fluids or loop diuretics are contraindicated or not working

Works at the level of the bone rather than the kidneys to reduce the serum calcium

Educate pts to avoid dehydration, diuretics, and excess calcium. Monitor asymptomatic pts closely

Every 6–12 months calcium, PTH, renal function measurements, and DEXA scan.
Surgical indications include:
- Calcium >11.5 mg/dL or episode of life-threatening hypercalcemia
- Creatinine clearance decreased by 30%
- Evidence of kidney stones or nephrocalcinosis
- 24-hour urine calcium excretion >400 mg
- Decreased bone density: T-score below −2.0

For pts who decline surgery or have contraindications, medical management includes:
- Bisphosphonates   - Calcitonin   - Phosphate replacement

Secondary hyperparathyroidism caused by chronic renal failure

Vitamin D supplementation and calcium salts.
Some pts require parathyroidectomy.

ADRENAL INSUFFICIENCY

 Has the pt had weakness, fatigue, dizziness, polyuria, or excessive thirst?
These symptoms are associated with cortisol and aldosterone deficiency.

Has the pt had any other symptoms suggestive of adrenal insufficiency?
- Nausea or vomiting   - Abdominal pain   - Anorexia
- Diarrhea   - Weight loss   - Salt cravings

Has the pt noticed any changes in skin color?
Skin hyperpigmentation (classic in primary AI and absent in secondary AI) occurs at scars, areolae, and creases, such as in the palms and groin area.

When did these symptoms begin?
The duration of symptoms can be either acute or chronic.
- Acute symptoms suggest things such as hemorrhage, thrombosis, or necrosis.
- Chronic symptoms suggest autoimmune, TB, or adrenoleukodystrophy.

Does the pt or anyone in the family have autoimmune problems such as thyroid disease, type 1 diabetes, vitiligo, or lupus?
Increases the probability that the pt has autoimmune AI

If the pt is a woman, has she noticed any changes in menstruation?
Amenorrhea may suggest secondary AI.

Does the pt have any headaches or visual changes?
These are symptoms associated with other pituitary hormones:
- Polyuria, polydipsia (diabetes insipidus)
- Headaches, visual changes (space-occupying lesions)

Ask the pt about HIV risk factors
Look for a history of AIDS or risk factors for HIV. Pts with AIDS are at risk for AI, especially because of infections (TB, fungal).

Has the pt ever developed a leg clot?
Antiphospholipid syndrome is associated with AI as well as thrombosis.

What medicines does the pt use?
Any of the following medications pose a risk for AI:
- Warfarin therapy   - Long-term steroid   - Ketoconazole   - Phenytoin

Does the pt have cancer or a history of previous cancer?
Metastatic tumors (lung, breast, kidney) or lymphoma cause AI (adrenal cortex).

 Review VS
Sepsis, hemorrhage: fever, tachycardia, hypotension
Aldosterone deficiency: orthostatic hypotension

Perform a PE
Altered mental status is commonly seen.
Look for signs of pituitary involvement.
- Stunted growth (growth hormone)
- Delayed puberty or depression, weight gain (hypothyroid)
Also look for signs of AI and its associated diseases:
- Hyperpigmentation   - Vitiligo
- Thinning of axillary or pubic hair   - Thyroid enlargement

What are the results of CBC and chemistry panel?
Common abnormalities: normocytic anemia, low sodium, high potassium, elevated BUN/creatinine, low glucose

Perform diagnostic tests

Check cortisol, adrenocorticotropic hormone (ACTH)
- Primary AI = low cortisol, high ACTH (>100 pg/mL)
- Secondary/tertiary AI = low cortisol, low ACTH

Cosyntropin test = an ACTH stimulation to evaluate adrenal response:
Check AM cortisol, give 250 µg cosyntropin IV, repeat cortisol after 60 minutes.
- Normal = poststimulation cortisol at least 18 µg/dL more than initial
- Primary AI = no increase in cortisol

If you suspect secondary AI, consider a metyrapone test, insulin-induced hypoglycemia.

Consider imaging studies

CXR to look for evidence of TB or lung mass.
Head MRI to rule out pituitary tumor.
Abdominal CT to look for enlarged adrenal glands or calcifications.

Consider biopsy of adrenal mass for definitive diagnosis

 Adrenal insufficiency

Can be primary (adrenal) or secondary (central: CNS). Corticotropin-releasing factor
is released from the hypothalamus, stimulating ACTH release from the pituitary,
stimulating the adrenals to release cortisol. The adrenals also make aldosterone and
androgens.

Primary AI causes include:		*Secondary AI*
– Autoimmune	– Lymphoma	– Pituitary tumors
– Tuberculosis	– Hemorrhage	– Craniopharyngioma
– AIDS	– Necrosis	– Long-term steroid use
– Fungal infections	– Thrombosis	– Postpartum (Sheehan)
– Metastatic tumor	– Adrenoleukodystrophy	– Head trauma

Tertiary AI: hypothalamic tumors

Differential diagnosis and possible comorbidities

Acute: dementia, liver failure, acute renal failure, septic shock, diabetic ketoacidosis
Chronic: delirium, chronic fatigue syndrome, depression, dark skin, acanthosis nigricans, paraneoplastic syndrome

P **Determine if the AI is acute or chronic**

The dose of hydrocortisone depends on this.

If acute AI, initiate workup but do not wait for results, because this condition is life-threatening. Give hydrocortisone 100 mg bolus, then 100–200 mg IV over 24 hours and fluid resuscitation with IV fluid

Without cortisol replacement (hydrocortisone), the pt is less likely to respond appropriately to stressors (surgery, sepsis). One of the ways pts respond poorly is vasodilation,
which can be addressed with both hydrocortisone and IV fluid.

If chronic AI, give hydrocortisone 20–30 mg/d

Chronic AI requires only replacement (<30 mg) rather than stress dose (100 mg).

Determine if it is primary or secondary/tertiary chronic AI

If primary AI, give fludrocortisone (mineralocorticoid replacement) 0.05–1.0 mg/d.

Regardless of type of AI, workup underlying cause and treat

CUSHING SYNDROME

S **Does the pt complain of proximal muscle weakness?**
Pt may report difficulty in rising from a chair or climbing stairs.

Does the pt report weight gain?
Increased cortisol results in distributory weight gain.
   – Moon facies   – Pendulous abdomen   – Cervical Fat Pad

Is there evidence of androgen excess?
   – Hirsutism   – Oligomenorrhea/amenorrhea
   – Acne   – Decreased libido

Does the pt have a history of conditions associated with cortisol excess?
   – Hypertension   – Kidney stones   – Diabetes mellitus   – Osteoporosis

Review medications
Long-term glucocorticoids: Systemic is most common, but topical, inhaled, and intra-
   articular still pose some risk.

O **Examine the VS for signs of excess cortisol**
Hypertension

Perform a complete PE, looking especially for
Gen: central obesity, thin extremities
Skin: thin, dry, ecchymosis, violaceous stria of abdomen or proximal extremities, hir-
   sute, acne, muscle wasting
HEENT: cataracts, moon facies, facial plethora, supraclavicular fullness, buffalo hump
   (cervical fat pad)
Abd: mass

Review basic metabolic panel
The K and Cl will tend to be low, whereas the bicarb and glucose will be high.

Perform a screening test
Overnight dexamethasone suppression test
   • Administer 1 g dexamethasone at 11 PM, then measure cortisol at 8 AM.
   • AM cortisol <5 µg/dL rules out Cushing syndrome.
Consider 24-hr urine collection for cortisol.
   • Increased serum cortisol results in an increased filtered cortisol.
   • Urine cortisol >40 in a woman or >80 µg/dL in a man suggests Cushing syndrome.

Order tests needed to determine etiology
Distinguish between adrenocorticotropic hormone (ACTH)-dependent and
   ACTH-independent.
Check cortisol, ACTH between midnight and 2 AM. If the cortisol is high (>15 µg/dL),
   look at the ACTH:
   • ACTH (<5 pg/mL) suggests adrenal tumor.
   • ACTH 5–24 pg/mL requires CRH stimulation test.
   • ACTH 25–150 pg/mL suggests Cushing disease.
   • ACTH >150 pg/mL (usually ~ 500) suggests ectopic production.

Order appropriate imaging
Consider MRI sella turcica to rule out pituitary adenoma.
Consider MRI of adrenal glands to rule out adrenal tumors, and if it is positive for adre-
   nal tumor, consider measuring 24-hr urine ketosteroids.
   • >30 mg/24 hr indicates carcinoma.
   • Low excretion indicates adenoma.
Consider CT chest/abdomen/pelvis to rule out malignancy.

Consider petrosal venous sinus catheterization and measurement of ACTH
If above imaging is negative, measurement distinguishes pituitary versus ectopic ACTH.

Cushing syndrome

A condition characterized by round facies, cervical fat pad, purple abdominal striae, truncal obesity, and muscle wasting, caused by excess endogenous (from the adrenal cortex) or exogenous glucocorticoids

Cushing disease

The same as the syndrome except that the excess glucocorticoids are caused by excess ACTH from the pituitary. To quickly review, the hypothalamus makes cortisol-releasing hormone (CRH), which stimulates the release of ACTH from the pituitary. ACTH stimulates the release of glucocorticoids from the adrenal cortex.

Differential diagnosis

Pituitary adenoma
Ectopic CRH secretion
Adrenal tumors or hyperplasia
Long-term steroid therapy
Ectopic ACTH production
- Small Cell lung carcinoma
- Pheochromocytoma
- Bronchial carcinoids
- Medullary thyroid carcinoma

Pseudo-Cushing
- Obesity
- Hypothyroidism
- Chronic alcoholism
- Insulinoma

P **Monitor glucose and lipids closely and treat as indicated**

Diabetes and hyperlipidemia are well-recognized effects of glucocorticoid excess.

Recognize and treat osteoporosis with calcium, vitamin D, and bisphosphonate therapy if necessary

Recognize that Cushing places the pt at higher risk for osteoporosis.

Consider starting the pt on a proton pump inhibitor

Pts with Cushing are also at higher risk of peptic ulcer disease.

Treat cushing disease (pituitary adenoma) with surgery, glucocorticoid replacement, and if necessary irradiation

Transsphenoidal resection of microadenoma is curative in more than 80% of pts.
Give replacement glucocorticoids daily for 6–12 months postoperatively.
If no cure after resection, therapy includes pituitary irradiation.
Few pts may need bilateral adrenalectomy for cure.

Treat ectopic ACTH- or CRH-producing tumors with surgery or medical management of symptoms

If possible, resect underlying tumor.

Treat high cortisol with adrenal enzyme inhibitors (ketoconazole or metyrapone)

Treat hypokalemia with spironolactone

Resect adrenal tumors surgically when possible and provide replacement glucocorticoids

Bilateral adrenalectomy (bilateral hyperplasia)
Unilateral adrenalectomy (unilateral adenoma or carcinoma)

OSTEOPOROSIS

S **Does the pt have risk factors for osteoporosis (OP)?**
Any of the following pose a risk for OP:

- Thin (Low body weight)
- Female
- Family history of fractures

- Elderly (age >65)
- Smoking
- Postmenopausal

- Caffeine intake

- Caucasian
- Previous fractures
- Alcohol

- Eating disorder (bulimia, anorexia nervosa)

Does the pt report bone pain?
A bone fracture may be the first presentation of underlying OP.

Does the pt report a loss of height?
Typically, the pt has 2–4 cm loss in height.

Does the pt have a history of prolonged immobilization?
Pts who are paralyzed or bedridden may suffer significant bone loss.

Does the pt have a history of endocrinopathy?
A pt with any of the following disorders is at risk for developing OP:

- Hyperthyroidism
- Cushing syndrome

- Hyperparathyroidism
- Diabetes mellitus

Is there a family history of disorders associated with OP?

- Ehlers-Danlos syndrome
- Marfan syndrome
- Hemochromatosis

Review medications
Any of the following drugs pose a risk for OP:

- Chronic steroid therapy
- Phenytoin
- Selective estrogen modulators

- Benzodiazepines
- High doses of thyroid hormone

- Phenobarbital

O **Review VS and perform a PE**
Measure height and weight and look at habitus.
Look for thyromegaly or thyroid mass.
Look at spine for kyphosis (anterior curvature of thoracic spine).
Palpate ribs for occult fractures, and perform full skeletal exam.

Review the results of the pt's CBC and comprehensive metabolic panel
There are no diagnostic lab abnormalities in OP.
Rarely, alkaline phosphatase and calcium may be increased.

Perform a dual-energy x-ray absorptiometry (DEXA) scan
Indications include:

- All women > age 60

- Hyperparathyroidism
- Long-term steroid therapy

- Postmenopausal women with risk factors
- Abnormal x-ray (osteopenia, fracture)

Diagnostic criteria:

- T-score <−2.5, OP

- T-score <−1.0, increased risk of OP

Pts with suspected secondary causes require further lab tests
Check TSH and, if abnormal, free T4.
Check PTH, increased in hyperparathyroidism, decreased in malignancy.
Check 24-hr urinary calcium excretion.
- Decreased (<50 mg/24 hr) in malabsorption or malnutrition
- Increased (>300 mg/24 hr) in high bone turnover states

Check fasting glucose.
Check free urine cortisol.

Consider spine x-ray
Especially in pt with documented height loss of 1–1.5 in

A Osteoporosis

Weakness of bone resulting from loss of bone mass, causing increased risk of fractures
There are three major types of primary osteoporosis:
- Type I: Usually occurs in >50-year-old postmenopausal women
  o Lack of estrogen causes increased trabecular bone loss.
  o Associated with distal forearm and vertebral body fractures.
- Type II: Men and women >70 y/o
  o Increased loss of both cortical and trabecular bone loss.
  o Associated with fractures of pelvis; and proximal humerus, tibia, and neck.
- Idiopathic: Occurs in younger age groups; likely caused by unidentified secondary cause

Etiologies
- Idiopathic
- Malabsorption (osteomalacia)
- Prolonged use of steroids
- Hyperparathyroidism
- Renal disease/failure
- Cushing syndrome
- Disuse atrophy
- Menopause (without HRT)

Differential diagnosis
- Physical abuse
- Bone tumor
- Paget disease
- Accidental trauma
- Advanced untreated thalassemia
- Secondary causes (see Etiologies)
- Multiple myeloma
- Osteogenesis imperfecta
- Metastases
- Leukemia/lymphoma
- Osteomyelitis

P Identify fractures and consult orthopedics for management

If the pt has a hip or spinal fracture, evaluate for signs of internal blood loss or spinal cord compression. If noted, admit the pt and make consultation emergent.

Obtain a pain score and address/control the pain
In mild cases, analgesics such as NSAIDs should be sufficient, but in cases involving fractures, such as those mentioned above, narcotics will likely be needed.
Calcitonin spray has also been found to be of benefit in some cases.

Educate all pts about how to prevent OP
The key to reducing OP is primary prevention. It is much more effective to prevent OP than to try to treat it when the pt has developed it.

Discuss simple changes the pt can make at home to avoid fractures
- Smoking cessation
- Medication adjustments
- Home safety to prevent falls. Occupational therapist can visit the home.
- Alcohol abstinence
- Weight-bearing exercises

Give supplementation to improve bone strength
Calcium 1,000–1,200 mg per day
Vitamin D (200–600 IU per day)

Consider treatment with medical therapy
- Estrogens
- PTH (teriparatide)
- Monoclonal antibody (denosumab)
- Bisphosphonates (alendronate, risedronate)
- SERMS (raloxifene), or nasal calcitonin

DYSLIPIDEMIA

S **Does the pt have risk factors for coronary artery disease (CAD)?**
Major risk factors include:
- Smoking   – Hypertension   – Diabetes
- Age (men >45 yr, women >55 yr)
- First-degree relative with early CAD (men <55 yr, women <40 yr)

Other risk factors (not considered major) include:
- Obesity   – Physical inactivity

Does the pt have CAD equivalents?
The following are considered equivalent to CAD:
- Peripheral artery disease   – Carotid artery stenosis
- Abdominal aortic aneurysm   – Diabetes mellitus (DM)

Does the pt have medical problems that secondarily cause dyslipidemia?
Any of the following disease states pose a risk for abnormal lipids:
- Hypothyroidism   – DM
- Chronic renal failure   – Long-term steroid use

O **Review VS and perform a PE**
Some findings to note are obesity, earlobe creases, thyromegaly, arcus senilis, and
xanthomas.

What are the results of renal and liver function tests?
Increased BUN/Cr; if chronic suggest secondary cause.
Abnormal LFTs: contraindication for lipid-lowering agents.

Check lipid panel
All pts aged 20 years and older should get a fasting lipid panel every 5 years.
According to ATP III classification:

Low-density lipoprotein

LDL cholesterol		Total cholesterol	
<100	Normal	<200	Desirable
101–129	Near or > optimal	200–239	Borderline
130–159	Borderline high	>240	High
160–190	High	>190	Very high

High-density lipoprotein

HDL cholesterol			
>60	Optimal		
		<40	Low

Look for the metabolic syndrome
Pts with any three of the following criteria have metabolic syndrome:
- Waist circumference >40 inches in men, >35 inches in women
- Fasting triglycerides >150 mg/dL
- HDL cholesterol <40 mg/dL in men, <50 mg/dL in women
- Blood pressure >130/85 mm Hg
- Fasting plasma glucose >110 mg/dL

A **Dyslipidemia**
Abnormal lipoprotein levels: high cholesterol (>200), triglycerides (>150), LDLs (>130),
or low HDLs (<40 in men, <50 in women)

Etiology
Primary (genetic)
Secondary:
- Hypothyroidism   – Obstructive liver   – DM
                                          disease
- Long-term steroid use   – Chronic renal failure

P **Educate the pt about the risks of the disease and importance of lifestyle**

Lifestyle modifications such as exercise, nutrition (low-fat diet), and weight loss are the first-line treatment of dyslipidemias.

In order to be motivated to make such changes, the pt must understand the consequences (stroke, MI, peripheral vascular disease) of the disease.

Optimize treatment of any secondary causes

This not only improves the dyslipidemia but also addresses two problems or risk factors at once. If a diabetic has better glycemic control, it will be easier to control lipids, and both of those things are important improvements.

Count the number of risk factors to determine target goals of medical therapy

Pts with CAD or CAD equivalent (LDL goal <100 mg/dL):
- LDL >130 mg/dL: initiate drug therapy
- LDL 100–129 mg/dL:
  ○ Lifestyle modification for 3 months
  ○ Initiate drug therapy if no improvement after 3 months

Pts with more than two risk factors (LDL goal <130 mg/dL):
- LDL >130 mg/dL:
  ○ Initiate lifestyle modification for 3 months. Repeat lipid panel. In 6 weeks, if not improved, intensify lifestyle changes.
- Initiate drug therapy if >130, after 3 months, and repeat lipid panel in 6 weeks.

Pts with zero to one risk factors (LDL goal <160 mg/dL):
- Initiate lifestyle modification for 3 months. If persist 160–189 mg/dL, then begin drug therapy.

Treatment with lipid-lowering agents

Cholesterol-lowering drugs are listed in Table 7-1, with the more common, easily tolerated drugs at the top and the less used, lesser tolerated drugs at the bottom.

TABLE 7-1   Lipid-Lowering Agents

Drugs	Lower LDL	Lower TG	Increase HDL
Statins	++	+	+
Fibric acids	+	++	+
Nicotinic acids	+	++	++
Bile acid resins	+	––	–

RHEUMATOLOGY

LOW-BACK PAIN

S **Is the pt older than 50 years, a smoker, experiencing weight loss, or having any history of cancer?**
A clinician's greatest concern is to rule out the worst possible diagnoses, in this case, vertebral metastases.

Is there a history of IV drug use or is the pt a diabetic?
Consider osteomyelitis in these pts.

Is there a history of recurrent urinary tract infections or kidney stones?
Pyelonephritis and renal colic can masquerade as low-back pain.

Is there a history of gastroesophageal reflux?
If so, this may represent a perforated ulcer.

Does the pain radiate down the buttock and below the knee?
This is a common presentation of nerve root irritation. Etiologies include the following:
  – Herniated disk   – Sciatica
  – Spinal stenosis   – Sacroiliitis

How does rest affect the pain?
Most degenerative joint diseases of the back improve with rest and worsen with activity.
Pain that is unrelieved by rest or supine position and continues at night is worrisome for malignancy, infection, or cauda equina involvement.
Ankylosing spondylitis (AS) can actually improve with activity and worsen with rest.

Are there any symptoms of a cauda equina process?
  – Multiple nerve root   – Bilateral leg weakness   – Incontinence
    involvement
  – Decreased perineal sensation – Rapidly evolving symptoms

O **Conduct a neurologic examination of the back, hip, and lower extremities**
This will help rule out the more serious diagnoses. Observe for signs of multiple nerve root involvement because this suggests a cauda equina process (tumor, abscess).
Point tenderness over a vertebral body can suggest osteomyelitis or vertebral metastases.
Perform Schober test:
  • Begin by measuring 5 cm and 10 cm above the level of S1, first while standing up straight and then again after bending forward with flexion at the hip.
  • Normally there should be an increase of ≥5 cm between these two points with flexion.
  • If the distance increases only 4 cm or less with flexion, consider AS or another one of the seronegative spondyloarthropathies.
Straight-leg test (pain radiating down the leg with less than 60 degrees of raising) suggests nerve root irritation in L4-L5 or L5-S1.
Decreased sensation over the medial calf, decreased dorsiflexion of the foot, and increased knee tendon jerk are suggestive of L4 nerve root involvement.
Decreased sensation over the medial aspect of the foot and decreased dorsiflexion of the great toe suggests L5 nerve root involvement.
Decreased sensation over the lateral aspect of the foot, decreased eversion of the foot, and increased ankle jerk suggests S1 nerve root involvement.

Look for any other nonrheumatologic causes of low-back pain
Cachexia, breast mass, lymphadenopathy, urinary retention, and enlarged prostate are examples of signs of different malignancies.
Abdominal mass or bruit could signify the presence of an aneurysm.

A **Low-back pain**

The following five diagnoses are the most severe causes of back pain and should be ruled out with the initial examination when possible:

- Cancer: vertebral metastases, cauda equina tumor
- Infection: osteomyelitis, cauda equina abscess
- Fracture
- AS
- Nonrheumatologic conditions: pancreatitis, aortic aneurysm, or perforated ulcer

If you suspect any of these diagnoses, an urgent and aggressive workup is required. With these more serious diagnoses out of the way, the remaining diagnoses can be treated more conservatively:

    – Disk herniation   – Muscle strain   – Sciatica
    – Sacroiliitis   – Degenerative joint disease

These are the most common causes of low-back pain and any one of them can be extremely debilitating for the pt.

P **For pts in whom you suspect one of the first five diagnoses, order a plain radiograph of the lumbar spine immediately**

If you do not suspect these diagnoses, proceed with conservative management for 2–4 weeks because most low-back problems will resolve completely within this time. If after 2–4 weeks symptoms still persist, you should order a plain film at that time.

Order an MRI urgently in any pt who displays cauda equina signs

If the MRI is positive, seek a neurosurgical consultation immediately.

Otherwise, institute conservative measures such as

Reassurance and education (how to properly lift): These are the foundations that the pt needs, particularly because the pain could take as long as 4–6 weeks to resolve.

Bed rest: Many pts want bed rest or feel that it is important. Bed rest should not be continued for more than 2 days.

Physical therapy: After a maximum of 2 days of bed rest, pts should engage in gentle back-mobilizing exercises.

Analgesia: Pain can usually be treated with nonsteroidal anti-inflammatory drugs (NSAIDs) and muscle relaxers. Reserve opioids for severe pain, and even then, for no more than 2 weeks.

Refer to orthopedic surgery if a documented herniation fails to respond to 6 weeks of conservative therapy for consideration of a lumbar discectomy.

POLYARTHRITIS

S **Does the pt report any warmth, swelling, or acute pain at the joint?**
Rule out septic joint because failure to do so may result in permanent disability.
Risk factors for septic joint include IV drug abuse and damaged joints.
Sexually active people (especially women during menses and pregnancy) are at risk for gonococcal infection.

How many joints are involved?
Monoarticular involves one joint (septic arthritis, Lyme disease).
Oligo- or pauciarticular involves two to four joints.
Polyarthritis involves more than five joints (systemic lupus erythematosus [SLE], rheumatoid arthritis [RA]).

When did the symptoms begin?
Acute duration is less than 6 weeks.
Chronic is more than 6 weeks.
The following viruses can cause polyarthritis that subsides in 6 weeks:
  – Rubella – Mumps – Human parvovirus B19 – Enterovirus

What joints are involved?
RA: metacarpophalangeal, PIP, wrists, and MTP
Osteoarthritis (OA): distal interphalangeal (DIP), PIP, and carpometacarpal, weight-bearing joints
Gout: first MTP

Does pt report any morning stiffness?
Helps distinguish inflammatory (RA) from noninflammatory (OA) arthropathy.
Morning stiffness (>1 hour in RA, <1 hour in OA) is an inflammatory symptom.
Swelling, tenderness, warmth, and fever are also inflammatory symptoms.

Is the pain precipitated by motion or weight-bearing and relieved with rest?
These are noninflammatory symptoms associated with OA rather than RA.

Does the pt report fever, chills, or malaise?
If so, consider septic arthritis, SLE, gout, or RA.

Focus the review of systems on a systemic rheumatologic disease
  – Alopecia – Oral ulcers – Dysphagia – Rash—Hematuria
  – Dry mouth/eyes – Myopathy – Photosensitivity – Raynaud syndrome

O **Review VS for signs of systemic illness**
Fever indicates inflammatory arthritis.
Hypotension suggests septic shock from septic joint: address emergently.

Perform a PE
This will give information about joint pain and disability.
Gen: Assess ability to bear weight (wheelchair bound or use of canes, crutches).
HEENT: Uveitis, conjunctivitis, episcleritis
Joint: Feel for warmth, soft tissue edema, and tenderness; test for range of motion.
Skin: Urticaria, purpura, psoriasis, subcutaneous nodules, tophi, Heberden (DIP) and Bouchard (PIP) nodes.

Perform an arthrocentesis for an effusion, and review the results
Can help exclude or differentiate between
  – Septic joint – Gout – Calcium pyrophosphate deposition disease (CPDD)
Contraindications to arthrocentesis include
  – Cellulitis – Bleeding disorders – Uncooperative pt

Check gross appearance, cell count with differential, Gram stain, culture, crystals.
- Noninflammatory: <3,000/µL WBC (white blood cell), <25% PMN
- Inflammatory: >3,000/µL WBC, >50% PMN
- Purulent: >50,000/µL WBC, >90% PMN
- Gout: negatively birefringent crystals
- CPDD: weakly positive birefringent crystals

Review CBC
Leukocytosis, especially with left shift indicative of infection

Review the results of renal and liver function tests and urinalysis
Renal and liver involvements are common with rheumatologic disease.

Check ESR and CRP (nonspecific markers of inflammation)
CRP is a more reliable marker of acute phase response than erythrocyte sedimentation rate (ESR).

Consider further serologic tests
Consider antinuclear antibody if suspect rheumatologic disease.
Check rheumatoid factor (RF), if suspect RA.
- A negative test does not rule out RA, 30% with seronegative RA.
- High titers are more diagnostic and indicate poor prognosis.

Polyarthritis
Inflammation of multiple joints at once

Etiologies
Noninflammatory: OA, trauma
Inflammatory:

– RA	– Gout	– Pseudogout
– SLE	– Scleroderma	– Fungal
– TB	– Reactive arthritis	– Juvenile rheumatoid arthritis

Purulent: Bacterial

Differential diagnosis

– Arthrogryposis	– Osteomalacia	– Crohn disease
– Renal osteodystrophy	– Hemarthrosis	– Vaso-occlusive disease
– Tendonitis	– Fibromyalgia	

Identify septic joint and consult orthopedic surgeon for drainage
Failure to identify septic joint will result in permanent damage.

Panculture and start broad-spectrum antibiotics
Most common organisms are *S. aureus*, strep, gram negative.
If suspect gonococcal arthritis, start ceftriaxone 1 g IV qd.
Lyme *(B burgdorferi)*: doxycycline 100 mg bid or amoxicillin 500 mg tid for 3–4 weeks
Tuberculosis (TB): four anti-TB meds (e.g., INH, rifampin, PZA, and ethambutol).
Candida: fluconazole 200 mg bid

Identify OA and begin treatment with lifestyle changes and anti-inflammatory medications
Weight loss and physical therapy
NSAIDs, glucosamine, capsaicin cream

Gout and pseudogout (see Crystal-Induced Arthropathy, p. 111)

RA (see RA, p. 112)

SLE (see SLE, p. 118)

Scleroderma (see Systemic Sclerosis, p. 122)

GOUT

S

What is the pt's age?
Acute gout is common in men aged 30–60 years.
In women, gout usually occurs after menopause.
Early-age onset (<25 years) suggests a genetic component.

Does the pt report a history of alcohol and/or high-protein foods?
High-protein foods and some alcohols worsen gout by increasing uric acid load.
Alcohol can also worsen gout by inhibiting enzymatic clearance of uric acid.

Is there a family history of arthropathy predisposing disorders?
Lesch-Nyhan syndrome, X-linked
CPDD, AD
Polycystic kidney disease
      – Glycogen storage disease, AR   – Sickle cell   – Leukemia
      – Medullary cystic kidney   – B-thalassemia

How long have symptoms been present?
Acute duration is typically defined by days to a few weeks.

What specific joints are involved?
Gout is commonly monoarticular, metatarsophalangeal of great toe, but also frequently
  in ankle.
CPDD involves knee most commonly but can be seen in all joints.

Does the pt report any precipitating factors?
      – Recent trauma or illness   – Postop   – Alcohol use

Review medications, especially those known to increase uric acid level
      – Thiazide or loop diuretics   – Nicotinic acid
      – Cyclophosphamide (posttransplant)   – Pyrazinamide

Does the pt have a history of kidney stones?
May precede symptoms of gout.

O

Review the VS
Owing to inflammation in gout and CPDD, fever may be present.
Hypertension and obesity are commonly associated with gout.

Perform PE, paying particular attention to the following
Joints: Feel for warmth, tenderness, effusions, and look for erythema
Ext: Valgus knees suggest CPDD
Skin: Tophi (urate crystal deposit), especially on ears

What are the results of the arthrocentesis?
Both CPDD and gout reveal inflammatory fluids.
Send cell count, Gram stain, and cultures because septic arthritis is common.
Look carefully for crystals.
   • Gout (monosodium urate): needle shaped, (–) birefringence
   • CPDD: rhomboid, weakly (+)

What are the results of the CBC, ESR, and comprehensive metabolic panel?
There are no diagnostic abnormalities common to gout or CPDD.
   • Leukocytosis and increased ESR is caused by inflammation.
   • Increased BUN and creatinine may suggest urate-induced nephropathy.

Consider uric acid level
This is not diagnostic and may be normal even in acute gout attack.
The risk of developing kidney stones is more than 50% if levels are >13 mg/dL.

Consider the following laboratory tests if suspect CPDD-associated disorders

– Hypothyroidism (TSH)   – Hemochromatosis (ferritin)
– Hyperparathyroidism (calcium, PTH)   – Amyloidosis (fat biopsy)

Consider x-ray, looking for characteristic findings

CPDD: punctate or linear densities (chondrocalcinosis) in articular cartilage
Gout: varies, may see soft tissue swelling or, in chronic stages, can see atrophic or hypertrophic erosions (overhanging edge)

Consider 24-hour urine collection for uric acid to differentiate overproducers from underexcreters in gout

More than 800 mg/24 hr suggests overproduction.

Crystal-induced arthropathy

Joint inflammation related to overproduction and subsequent crystallization of a molecule such as monosodium urate in the case of gout or CPDD in pseudogout.

Differential diagnosis

– Septic joint   – Gout   – Pseudogout
– Osteoarthritis   – Rheumatoid arthritis – Adult-onset Still disease
– Cellulitis   – Reactive arthritis   – Psoriatic arthritis

Rule out septic joint in acute monoarticular arthropathy by aspirating the joint

Send fluid for both Gram stain and crystals.
If suspicious for septic joint, treat empirically with broad-spectrum antibiotics until results of tap are obtained.

Treat acute gout/CPDD with indomethacin 50 mg po q 8 hours until symptoms resolve

Treatment is aimed at relieving symptoms of arthritis and decreasing inflammation.
Consider also giving colchicine 0.5–0.6 mg po qh until pain relief (max 8 mg/d and adjust dose for renal or liver disease).

If NSAIDs or colchicine are contraindicated, may use steroids

Either systemic or intra-articular steroids may be used.
Transplant pts can be treated with intra-articular steroids.

Do not use allopurinol or febuxostat because this may worsen attack

Allopurinol or febuxostat should not be started for at least 2 weeks after the acute attack.

Educate pts about prevention of gouty attacks

– Weight loss   – Avoid alcohol   – Low-purine diet   – Avoid aspirin

After acute attack, check 24-hour urine and serum uric acid to determine if pts are overproducers or underexcretors

Use allopurinol or febuxostat if pts are overproducers to decrease production or in pts with tophi, nephrolithiasis, and chronic renal insufficiency.
Although some pts are underexcretors of uric acid, these pts should still be treated with allopurinol or febuxostat. This is because uricosuric agents, such as probenecid, require that the pt take in greater than 1,500 mL/d of water and have a creatinine clearance of >60 mL/min. Pts may be unable to meet these expectations.

RHEUMATOID ARTHRITIS

S **How long have the symptoms been present?**
Generally, RA is a chronic disease (symptoms present for more than 6 weeks).
If acute (less than 6 weeks), consider infectious or crystal-induced etiologies.

Does the pt report morning stiffness?
With RA, pts complain of morning stiffness lasting at least 1 hour.
With OA, morning stiffness lasts less than 30 minutes.

What joints are involved?
MTPs may be the first joints involved.
Wrists, MCPs, PIPs, TMJ, and knees are commonly involved.
DIPs, lumbar spine, and SI joints are generally spared in RA.

How many joints are involved?
RA is generally considered polyarticular and symmetrical.

Does the pt report any systemic symptoms?
　－ Fever　　　－ Chills　　　－ Weight loss　　　－ Fatigue　　　－ Anorexia

Does the pt report extra-articular manifestations associated with RA?
Dry eyes, dry mouth (Sjögren syndrome)
Dysphagia or dysphonia (inflammation of cricoarytenoid joint)
Acute paresthesias (mononeuritis multiplex)
Chest pain, shortness of breath, change in exercise tolerance (pleuritis)

O **Review VS**
Fever may be present from inflammation or underlying infection.

Perform a PE
Gen: Assess the pt's functional capacity
HEENT: neck stiffness
 • C1-2 subluxation increases risk of spinal cord compression.
 • Requires further assessment with lateral flexion cervical spine x-rays.
Abd: splenomegaly
 • Recall triad RA, splenomegaly, and neutropenia in Felty syndrome.
Joint:
 • Feel for warmth, tenderness, effusions, and synovial thickening.
 • Look for erythema, edema, and test for range of motion.
 • Look for deformities:
　o Flexion contracture
　o Ulnar deviation at MCP
　o Swan-neck deformities (flexion DIP, hyperextension PIP)
　o Boutonniere deformity (flexion PIP, hyperextension DIP)
Skin: Look for nodules over pressure points like extensor surfaces of upper extremities.
Neuro: Perform Phalen and Tinel tests. (Carpal tunnel syndrome is common in RA.)

Review the result of arthrocentesis if palpable effusion is present
Inflammatory fluid common with WBC >20,000 (mostly PMNs), without crystals

Consider x-rays
Early in disease, x-rays are normal.
Erosions are not present until months or years after disease onset.

Review the results of the CBC, liver, and renal function tests
Obtain baseline values; some medications used to treat RA may be contraindicated.

Check the pt's rheumatoid factor (RF)
RF positive found in 85% of pts with RA.
RF titer correlates with severity; higher values denote worse prognosis, but it is not
　necessary to follow titer once documented to be positive.
RF can also be positive in chronic infectious/inflammatory states (SLE, TB, carcinoma).

Consider erythrocyte sedimentation rate (ESR)

This is a nonspecific inflammatory marker for following the course of disease.

Consider CXR

Findings include interstitial fibrosis, lung nodules (Caplan syndrome-interstitial pneumoconiosis + nodules), pleurisy, and pleural effusions.

Thoracentesis generally reveals very low glucose levels, high lactate dehydrogenase.

Consider ECG

Findings include pericarditis and conduction abnormalities.

Echocardiogram may reveal valvular abnormalities.

Rheumatoid arthritis

Autoimmune inflammation of the articular cartilage of multiple joints for longer than 6 months. Diagnose if at least four of the seven following criteria are met:

1. Morning stiffness (at least 1 hour) for 6 weeks
2. Swelling of hand joints (wrists, MCP, PIP) for 6 weeks
3. Swelling of three or more joints
4. Symmetric joint swelling for 6 weeks
5. Rheumatoid nodules
6. Erosive synovitis on x-ray of the hands
7. RF positive

Differential diagnosis

- Osteoarthritis
- Scleroderma
- Rheumatic fever

- Gout/pseudogout
- Juvenile rheumatoid arthritis
- Polymyalgia rheumatica

- SLE
- Spondyloarthropathies

Diagnosis of rheumatoid arthritis is life changing; discuss disease progression, treatment options, side effects, and prognosis

Pt education is crucial for adherence to therapy and subsequent disease control.

Refer to rheumatologist and physical therapy early in disease

Experience/expertise in RA management makes a significant difference.

Occupational and physical therapy are important for maintenance and preservation of function as the disease progresses.

Treat joint pain and swelling with NSAIDs or COX-2 inhibitors

This will help address the pain and discomfort of the disease.

Use disease-modifying antirheumatic drugs to limit joint damage

Hydroxychloroquine: regular ophthalmology follow-up (retinopathy)

Sulfasalazine: monitor CBC

Methotrexate: monitor CBC, LFT, renal function, folate supplementation

Tumor necrosis factor inhibitors: infliximab, etanercept

T-cell modulator: abatacept

Interleukin-1 receptor antagonist: anakinra

Monoclonal antibody: rituximab, tocilizumab

Low-dose glucocorticoids

Treat refractory extra-articular manifestations with systemic steroids

Steroids will not modify the disease, but they can make the pt feel better.

Surgical referral for joint replacement or carpal tunnel release

SERONEGATIVE SPONDYLOARTHROPATHIES

S **What is the pt's age, racial background, and gender?**

There are associations between type of arthropathy and age, race, and gender:
- AS
  - Presents in late 20s
  - M:F 5:1
  - Native Americans > other
- Reactive arthritis (Reiter's)
  - Young men
  - M:F 9:1
  - White > black

Does the pt have a history of inflammatory bowel disease (IBD)?

Pts with inflammatory bowel disease (IBD) (Crohn disease > ulcerative colitis) are at risk for arthritis.

Does the pt have a history of psoriasis, skin disease, or chronic rash?

Pts with psoriasis are at risk for psoriatic arthritis.

Does the pt report recent illness?

There are various illnesses associated with reactive arthritis:
- Occurs 2–4 weeks after infectious diarrhea: *Salmonella*, *Shigella*, *Campylobacter*, *Clostridium*, *Yersinia*
- Genitourinary infections: *Chlamydia*, *Ureaplasma*
- Respiratory infections: *Chlamydia pneumoniae*

Does the pt report genitourinary symptoms?

Reactive syndrome includes urethritis:
  – Dysuria   – Penile or vaginal discharge

Does the pt have eye symptoms?

Reactive arthritis includes conjunctivitis:
  – Eye pain   – Redness   – Eyelid crusting

AS associated with uveitis
  – Unilateral pain   – Photophobia   – Lacrimation

Ask specifically about joint pain

Asymmetrical oligoarticular pain

LE joint involvement typical for reactive arthritis.

Hand DIP joints suggests psoriatic arthritis.

Back pain, if worse with rest and improved with exercise, is typical for AS.

Buttock pain that radiates into the thigh, worse with rest, suggests sacroiliitis.

O **Review VS and perform a PE**

Skin: rash on palms or soles
- Keratoderma blennorrhagicum associated with reactive arthritis
- Psoriatic arthritis: pitting nails, scaly lesions on elbow, knees

Ext: dactylitis (sausage digits)

Eye: conjunctivitis (reactive arthritis), uveitis (AS)

Heart: listen for murmur (AI suggests aortitis in AS)

Genital: lesions on shaft of penis (circinate balanitis), cervical ulcer

Joint:
- Feel for warmth, tenderness, and edema; test for range of motion.
- Tenderness at tendon sites (enthesitis)
- Press on sacrum while pt is prone (sacroiliitis)

Check urinalysis

A pt suspected of having reactive arthritis must be ruled out for urethritis.

- Sterile pyuria suggests underlying venereal infection.
- Send *Chlamydia* antigen.

Send urethral and cervical cultures for *Chlamydia* and *N. gonorrhea*.

Review the result of arthrocentesis

Pt's synovial fluid most consistent with inflammatory process.

- Send Gram stain, bacterial, and *N. gonococcal* cultures.

Consider x-rays

Order x-rays of the feet for pts with heel pain: May have erosions of calcaneus.
Check a spinal x-ray on pts with AS: Bamboo spine and fusion sacroiliac joint

Consider test for HLA-B27

The incidence of HLA-B27 is common, highest with AS more than 90%.

A ### Seronegative spondyloarthropathy

The seronegative spondyloarthropathies are a rather heterogeneous group of RF-negative conditions involving inflammation of the intervertebral joints.

Etiologies

- AS
- Reactive arthritis (Reiter's)
- Psoriatic arthritis
- IBD associated

P ### Identify and treat septic arthritis

Acute monoarticular arthropathy must be ruled out for septic joint.
Treat pt empirically with broad-spectrum antibiotics until tap results are obtained

Treat AS with conservative measures and pain relief

Physical therapy for proper posture
Regular stretching and spinal exercise
NSAIDs (indomethacin or diclofenac)

Treat reactive arthritis by addressing uveitis, urethritis, and arthritis if culture is positive for chlamydia, give azithromycin 1 g po one time

An alternative is doxycycline 100 mg po bid for 7 days.
Remember to also treat the partner.

Treat arthritis with NSAIDs (indomethacin or diclofenac)

Use COX-2 inhibitors if pt does not tolerate NSAIDs.
Use methotrexate or sulfasalazine in refractory cases.

For psoriatic arthritis, treat the psoriasis and address arthritis

Treatment arthritis with NSAIDs (indomethacin) as above but may also use methotrexate or gold for refractory cases.
Do not use hydroxychloroquine or β-blockers because they can exacerbate skin disease.

Treat IBD-associated arthritis by addressing underlying disease; this is vital because arthritis is related to flares of IBD

INFLAMMATORY MYOPATHIES

S What is the pt's age?
Generally, myositis has a bimodal age distribution: 10–15 years and 50–60 years of age.
Malignancy-associated myositis and inclusion body myositis (IBM) are common
>50 years.

What is the pt's racial background and gender?
African-Americans are affected more than Caucasians.
Women affected more than men (2:1), except with IBM men affected more than women.

Ask about muscle pain
Onset is generally insidious.
Affects symmetrical proximal muscles (neck and proximal extremities). Pt typically
reports difficulty in rising from a chair or washing hair.
IBM is generally asymmetric, with distal muscle weakness.
Facial and ocular muscles are spared.
Dysphagia (especially with initiating swallowing) and dysphonia

Review medications
Many medications cause proximal muscle weakness:
- Steroids
- Colchicine
- Alcohol
- Antiretrovirals
- Statins

O Review the pt's VS and perform a PE
Skin: heliotrope rash, Gottron papules, shawl sign (erythema shoulders and neck), V
sign (chest, neck), mechanic hands
Lung: dry late inspiratory crackles (interstitial fibrosis)

Review CBC, liver, and renal function tests
Myopathies are often associated with occult malignancy.

Look for serologic markers of muscle damage
With myositis, muscle enzymes like CK, aldolase, AST, ALT, and LDH should be
elevated.

Consider checking antibodies to try to further delineate the type of myositis
Anti-Jo-1 Ab presents polymyositis more than dermatomyositis.
- Associated with interstitial lung disease (ILD).
- Associated with antisynthetase syndrome: myopathy, ILD, arthritis, Raynaud phe-
  nomena, and mechanic hands.
Anti-Mi-2 is specific for dermatomyositis.
Anti-SRP (signal recognition particle) implies a poor prognosis. Associated with cardio-
myopathy and distal muscle involvement.

Consider EMG
This is not a diagnostic test because some pts have normal electromyography (EMG), but
common findings include fibrillations, high-frequency discharge, and low amplitude.

Get a CXR
This may be normal, but look for signs of fibrosis.

Get a muscle biopsy
Necrosis and inflammation are seen with polymyositis and dermatomyositis.
Intracellular vacuoles and myeloid bodies are seen with IBM.

A Chronic inflammatory myopathy
A group of idiopathic disorders in which muscle damage is caused by immune system
activity (inflammation)

Etiologies
Polymyositis: proximal muscle weakness, elevated muscle enzymes, characteristic EMG

Dermatomyositis: proximal muscle weakness, heliotrope rash, Gottron papules
IBM: proximal and distal muscle weakness, elevated muscle enzymes, usually over age
  50 years of age

Differential diagnosis

- Myositis associated with malignancy
- Thyroid disease
- Fibromyalgia
- Lupus (SLE)
- Muscular dystrophy
- Guillain-Barré syndrome

- Eaton-Lambert syndrome
- Myasthenia gravis
- Botulism
- Tick paralysis
- Drug-induced myopathy
- Sarcoid/HIV (associated with polymyositis)

P Identify potential life-threatening complications, such as acute respiratory failure caused by respiratory muscle weakness, and admit pt to a monitored bed if indicated

Obtain ABG, if evidence of CO_2 retention, and monitor closely and prepare for intubation.

Screen for underlying malignancy

Dermatomyositis is associated with an increased risk for malignancy.

Educate pt about disease and prognosis

As with any disease, compliance is improved with good pt education.

Refer to physical or occupational therapy

To help with recovery as well as adaptations to muscle weakness

Obtain a swallow evaluation

To monitor for esophageal dysfunction caused by polymyositis

Treat inflammatory myopathies with medications to reduce inflammation

Steroids (prednisone 40–60 mg qd)
Methotrexate or azathioprine can be used if the pt does not respond to steroids.

Monitor disease activity by changes in serum muscle enzymes

See above.

SYSTEMIC LUPUS ERYTHEMATOSUS

S

What is the pt's racial background and gender?
Women, especially in their reproductive years, are affected more than men (9:1).
African-Americans and Hispanics are at increased risk.

Does the pt have a family history of systemic lupus erythematosus (SLE)?
High frequency is seen among first-degree relatives.
Commonly associated with HLA-DR2, HLA-DR3

Does the pt have coexisting autoimmune diseases?
Previous/current autoimmune disease is higher risk for another.
- Autoimmune thyroiditis
- Autoimmune hemolytic anemia
- ITP
- Sjögren syndrome

Has the pt had recurrent spontaneous abortions or thrombosis?
There is an association between antiphospholipid syndrome and SLE.

Review medications for those associated with a lupus-like syndrome
- Procainamide
- Quinidine
- INH
- Hydralazine

Does the pt have any constitutional symptoms common in SLE?
- Fever
- Malaise
- Weight loss

Is there evidence that multiple organ systems are involved?
Mucocutaneous:
- Alopecia (patchy)
- Rash (malar or discoid)
- Oral ulcers
- Photosensitivity
- Dry eyes/mouth (Sjögren syndrome)

Joints: Symmetric polyarticular distribution (proximal interphalangeal, metacarpopha-
langeal, wrists, knees) as in RA.
- Pain
- Stiffness
- Swelling

Pulmonary: hemoptysis, pleuritic chest pain, shortness of breath
Cardiac: pleuritic chest pain that changes with position (pericarditis)
Central nervous system (CNS): mood changes, anxiety, memory loss, headache, change
in vision
Raynaud phenomena: changes in skin on exposure to cold or stress

O

Review the VS
Fever is common and may indicate an underlying infection or active disease.
High blood pressure suggests underlying renal disease.
Hypotension (with distant heart sounds and jugular venous distention) indicates cardiac
tamponade.

Perform a PE
Skin:
- Discoid (raised patch with overlying scale on face, scalp, ears, neck)
  - Alopecia
  - Malar rash (spares nasolabial folds)
  - Palpable purpura
HEENT: oral ulcers
Joint: Look for erythema; feel for warmth, edema, effusions, tenderness
Heart: Listen for murmurs, pericardial friction rub
Lung: decreased air entry; decreased tactile fremitus

Review CBC
- Leukopenia
- Anemia
- Thrombocytopenia

Check urinalysis
The presence of proteinuria and red blood cell (RBC) casts suggest lupus nephritis.
- Consider 24-hour urine collection for protein and creatinine.
- Consider a renal ultrasound to assess kidney size.
- Renal biopsy is indicated if it will change the management course.

Check an antinuclear antibody (ANA)
Found in up to 95% of pts with SLE, but poor specificity.

Check anti-dsDNA and anti-Smith
Unique to SLE (100% specific, low sensitivity).
Anti-dsDNA is important for following renal involvement.

Check anti-Ro/La
Anti-Ro has a strong association with neonatal lupus and subacute cutaneous lupus.
Approximately 10%–30% of mothers with anti-Ro will deliver babies with congenital heart block.

Check complement levels and erythrocyte sedimentation rate
Serologic markers for disease activity and inflammation

A Systemic lupus erythematosus

Diagnosis requires 4 of the following 11 criteria:
1. **M**alar rash
2. **D**iscoid rash

3. **N**euro (Sz, Psychosis)
4. **O**ral ulcers
5. **P**hotosensitivity
6. **A**rthritis (>2 joints)

7. **R**enal disorder (proteinuria, cellular casts)
8. **I**mmunologic markers (anti-dsDNA, anti-Sm, or antiphospholipid Ab)
9. **S**erositis (pleuritis or pericarditis)
10. **H**eme (anemia/leukopenia/thrombocytopenia)
11. **ANA** (+)

A brief mnemonic is "MD NO PARISH ANA."

Differential diagnosis
Vasculitis: polyarteritis nodosa (PAN), microscopic polyangiitis (MPA), Wegener granulomatosis
Infectious: HIV, syphilis, Epstein-Barr virus, brucellosis, Lyme disease
Rheumatic: RA, mixed connective tissue disease, Crohn
Neoplasm: perineoplastic syndrome, leukemia, lymphoma

P Identify any life-threatening illness in an SLE pt
CV: myocardial infarction, cardiac tamponade, pulmonary embolism, serositis
CNS: vasculitis, stroke
Infectious: subacute bacterial endocarditis, bacteremia, myocarditis, pericarditis, meningitis, septic arthritis
Rheumatologic: thrombotic thrombocytopenic purpura, ITP

Identify and remove precipitating factors such as medications (see above) that cause lupus-like syndrome
Removal of some medicines, like quinidine, result in resolution of the symptoms.

Treat coexisting autoimmune disorders
Remember that these pts are at increased risk for multiple autoimmune disorders, so pay attention to signs of other problems in the pt.

Treat SLE with anti-inflammatory/immunosuppressive agents
– NSAIDs, COX-2 inhibitors
– Hydroxychloroquine
– Cyclophosphamide
– Steroids (oral, topical, or intra-articular)
– Azathioprine
– Methotrexate

VASCULITIS

 Does the pt complain of malaise, fever, weight loss, or night sweats?
Vasculitis commonly presents with nonspecific complaints such as these.

Does the pt complain of headaches or changes in vision?
If so, consider giant cell arteritis (GCA), especially in pts older than 60 years with
– Throbbing pain – Painless loss of vision (amaurosis fugax)

Does the pt report GI symptoms?
GCA: dysphagia, trismus, jaw claudication with chewing
PAN, MPA, Henoch-Schönlein purpura (HSP): periumbilical pain, especially after eating, classical for mesenteric ischemia
PAN: cholecystitis and appendicitis
HSP: nausea/vomiting
PAN/HSP: GI blood loss

Does the pt report pulmonary symptoms?
Wegener/MPA/HSP: hemoptysis may be seen with pulmonary capillaritis
Wegener: recurrent sinus, ear, or upper respiratory infections
Churg-Strauss: asthma or allergic rhinitis

Does the pt report skin changes?
HSP: palpable purpura involving buttocks and lower extremities
Cryoglobulinemia: recurrent palpable purpura of lower extremities

Does the pt report joint or muscle pain?
HSP: arthritis of knees and ankles
Polymyalgia rheumatica (PMR): symmetric pain/stiffness in the hips/shoulders
PAN: myalgias involving calves

Ask the pt about neuropathy
PAN: mononeuritis multiplex

Ask about risk factors for hepatitis B or C
Up to 30% of PAN is associated with hepatitis B or C.
Cryoglobulinemia is common with hepatitis C.

 Review VS
– Fever – Hypertension (renin-mediated in PAN)

Perform a PE
HEENT: tender or nodular temporal artery, scalp tenderness (GCA); nasal mucosal lesions or saddle nose deformity (Wegener)
Neuro: foot drop (PAN, MPA)
Skin: livedo reticularis, ulcers (PAN), palpable purpura (MPA, HSP, cryoglobulinemia)

Check CBC
Eosinophilia (PAN, Churg-Strauss)

Check renal and liver function tests

Check erythrocyte sedimentation rate (ESR)

Check U/A
Look for hematuria, RBC casts, proteinuria (PAN, MPA, HSP).

Check ANCA

Order a CXR

Perform a renal biopsy

A **Vasculitis**

Inflammation of blood vessels, usually causing multisystem disease

- Large vessel (>150 μm)
  - GCA/temporal arteritis: Inflammation of the large arteries of the head and neck can lead to blindness.
  - Polymyalgia rheumatica (PMR): hip/shoulder stiffness
  - Takayasu arteritis (pulseless disease): inflammation of the aortic arch leading to arm claudication, amaurosis fugax, headache
- Medium vessel (diameter 50–150 μm)
  - PAN: Involves nearly all tissues but the lungs for an extremely variable presentation.
  - Buerger disease: Thrombophlebitis and eventually ischemia in the distal extremities. Exacerbated by smoking. Rarely involves internal organs.
- Small vessel (<50 μm)
  - HSP: Lower extremity palpable purpura, abdominal pain, and variable kidney involvement. Due to deposition of IgA.
  - Cryoglobulinemia: Recurrent palpable purpura with darkening of skin on resolution of lesions. Associated with hepatitis C.
  - Wegener syndrome: Involves the respiratory tract and kidneys, leading to nosebleeds and renal failure. Associated with C-ANCA.
  - MPA: Causes a pulmonary renal presentation similar to Wegener and Goodpasture syndromes, P-ANCA
  - Churg-Strauss syndrome: asthma, eosinophilia, and P-ANCA

Differential diagnosis

If a pt presents with complaints from multiple organ systems, consider vasculitis along with the other great imitators.

Infectious: HIV, syphilis, Epstein-Barr virus

Neoplastic: perineoplastic syndromes

Autoimmune: SLE, mixed connective tissue disorder, Crohn disease, celiac disease

P **Identify life-threatening complications of vasculitis and treat appropriately**

    – Ischemic bowel or perforation   – Sepsis/infections

    – Capillaritis or glomerulonephritis   – Thrombosis

Verify diagnosis with blood tests and biopsy if necessary. Consider consulting rheumatology for more direction takayasu and GCA can be treated with steroids

Treat vision loss immediately with high-dose steroids to prevent blindness.

Treat stable pts with oral steroids.

Treat PMR with NSAIDs or low-dose steroids

Treat PAN with high-dose steroids

Use bactrim for PCP prophylaxis.

HSP is generally self-limited, but symptoms can be treated with

NSAIDs for arthralgias

Cryoglobulinemia can be treated with INF alpha +/−ribavirin

Wegener syndrome can be treated with high-dose steroids and cyclophosphamide

MPA can be treated with cyclophosphamide and steroids

Churg-Strauss can be treated with steroids

SYSTEMIC SCLEROSIS

S What is the pt's racial background and gender?

The following groups are at risk for systemic sclerosis (SS):
- Females are affected more often than men (7:1).
- Native Americans are at highest risk.

Does the pt report environmental exposures?

There is a questionable association with some environmental toxins:
- Silica dust   – Organic solvents

Secondary scleroderma is reported with the following:
- Bleomycin   – Benzene   – Vinyl chloride

Does the pt have pruritus?

Pruritus can be the initial manifestation seen with skin involvement and is self-limited.

Does the pt have other organ system involvement?

Skin changes: thickening or tightness

Pulmonary symptoms: shortness of breath, dyspnea on exertion, cough
- Pts with SS are at risk for interstitial fibrosis and pulmonary hypertension.
- This is the number one cause of mortality!

Cardiac symptoms: chest pain, palpitations

GI symptoms: dysphagia, malabsorption, constipation

Raynaud phenomenon: changes in skin color on exposure to cold or stress

Musculoskeletal: arthralgias, myalgias

O Review VS

Accelerated hypertension suggests renal crisis (see below).

Perform a PE

Skin:
- Telangiectasia (face, hands, mouth)   – Small mouth (tight, pursed lip)
- Subcutaneous calcinosis   – Sclerodactyly
- Nailfold capillaries, digital ulceration – Hyper/hypopigmentation

Heart: jugular venous distention, loud P2; parasternal heave (pulmonary hypertension).

Joint: warmth, edema, tenderness; listen for tendon friction rubs.

Consider checking antinuclear antibody, anti-centromere, anti-SCL-70

There are no antibodies found in every pt with SS.
- Anticentromere antibody is found in 80% of CREST.
- Anti-SCL-70 (antitopoisomerase) is found in 20% of SS.

Consider CXR and hand x-rays

There is a risk of developing pulmonary disease, so check a baseline CXR.

Common abnormalities on hand films include joint calcinosis or osteolysis of fingertips

Consider an ECG

Pts are at risk for conduction abnormalities.

Consider pulmonary function tests

Pts typically have
- Restrictive lung pattern   – Decreased DLCO   – Lung volumes

Consider an echocardiogram

Pts are at risk for
- Pulmonary hypertension   – Increased pulmonary artery pressure
- Diastolic dysfunction   – >35 mm Hg

A **Systemic sclerosis**

A connective tissue disease characterized by thickening and fibrosis of the skin and some internal organs

SS is further divided into

- CREST:
  - **C**alcinosis
  - **E**sophageal dysmotility
  - **R**aynaud phenomena
  - **S**clerodactyly
  - **T**elangiectasia

Also associated with isolated pulmonary hypertension.

- Diffuse SS
  - Skin thickening involves both extremities and trunk.
  - Rapid onset after Raynaud phenomena
  - Pulmonary fibrosis common

P **Identify life-threatening complications of SS**

- Congestive heart failure (CHF)
- Cardiac tamponade
- Pulmonary embolism
- Arrhythmias
- Pericarditis

Treat ischemic digits with IV prostaglandins (prostacyclin)

It is important to address this problem emergently to avoid or reduce the loss of digits.

Identify pts with renal crisis and treat with ACE inhibitors/ARBs

Renal crisis is defined as acute oliguric renal failure with malignant hypertension.

Risk factors include pregnancy, steroid use, and diffuse disease.

Educate pt early in disease about close monitoring of blood pressure and prophylactic use of ACE inhibitors or ARBs to avoid renal crisis.

Educate all pts about disease progression and prognosis

Immunizations such as influenzae and pneumococcal

Treat symptoms of SS

Treatment aimed at symptom relief:

- Skin moisturizers for dryness
- BP control with ACE inhibitors
- Anti-inflammatories like NSAIDs and COX-2 inhibitors for arthritis
- Calcium channel blockers (nifedipine) for Raynaud's
- Smoking cessation and avoidance of cold temperatures
- Antihistamines for pruritus
- Proton pump inhibitor for reflux

Treat pulmonary hypertension with home oxygen and IV epoprostenol

Management of CHF is also an important component of therapy.

IV epoprostenol (improves exercise capacity).

Consider use of anticoagulation.

TOXICOLOGY

ALCOHOL INTOXICATION AND WITHDRAWAL

S **How much does the pt normally drink? When was the pt's last drink?**

This information can aid in anticipation and management of withdrawal symptoms.

The alcohol-intoxicated patient (pt generally may be unable to give a clear history.

Family members, friends, and close contacts should be called to obtain information focusing on any coexisting medical problems, any history of trauma, last known drink, etc.

O **Note vital signs and assess level of consciousness**

Tachycardia and fever can be signs of onset of delirium tremens.

A Glasgow Coma Score of less than 8 is an indication that intubation may be necessary.

Examine for signs of advanced or chronic liver disease

– Spider angiomata	– Caput medusae	– Palmar Erythema
– Ascites	– Hepatomegaly	– Umbilical hernia
– Testicular atrophy	– Bilateral parotid swelling	– Peripheral neuropathy
– Prolonged PT, PTT	– Hypoalbuminemia	

Examine for evidence of GI bleeding

Hypotension, tachycardia, orthostatic blood pressures (BPs) and pulse, decreasing hemoglobin and hematocrit on serial CBCs, and heme-positive stool

Check a serum alcohol level

A low level may indicate withdrawal or that another substance is responsible for the intoxication.

A serum alcohol level of greater than 400 mg/dL (0.4 g%) is a risk of death and may require urgent hemodialysis.

Examine for possibility of other drug intoxication

Check urine and serum toxicology screen for any evidence of coexisting drugs.

Examine for evidence of other neurologic disorders

Seizure disorder, meningitis, head injury

Examine for glucose or electrolyte abnormalities

Pt is at increased risk for hypoglycemia if malnourished.

Low Mg, K, phosphorus are also common.

An anion gap acidosis or an elevated serum osmolality may indicate intoxication with methanol, ethylene glycol, or isopropanol. Ingestion of any of these substances may be fatal.

- Alcohol dehydrogenase in the liver converts ethanol to acetaldehyde. When this same chemical operation is performed on methanol, it is converted to formaldehyde.
- If ingestion of any of these substances is suspected, levels must be checked directly.

A **Alcohol intoxication**

Alcohol is a central nervous system (CNS) depressant. Early effects include depression of inhibitions and later effects impair motor function, consciousness, and, at maximal concentrations, respiratory drive.

Differential diagnosis

Intoxication by CNS-depressant drugs such as barbiturates, benzodiazepines, or opioids

Pts may be intoxicated by more than one substance at once.

Consider intoxication with methanol, isopropyl alcohol, or ethylene glycol because chronic alcoholics may ingest these substances to attempt intoxication.

Also consider infectious, neurologic, or psychiatric etiologies.

P **Monitor mental status**

Take aspiration precautions in case pt develops withdrawal seizures. Consider intubation to protect airway.

Consider head CT for mental status changes or appearance of focal examination findings neurologic deficits

Optimize nutritional status by replacing magnesium, potassium, phosphorus, thiamine, and folate with an IV preparation known as a "banana bag"

Chronic alcohol abusers tend to be deficient in all of the above electrolytes and vitamins.

Chronic thiamine (vitamin B_1) deficiency can result in either Wernicke or Korsakoff encephalopathy.

- Wernicke encephalopathy is a triad of ophthalmoplegia, broad-based gait, and global confusion.
- Korsakoff pts are demented to the point of confabulating.

Be sure to give thiamine before glucose to avoid precipitating Wernicke encephalopathy.

If ingestion of ethylene glycol or methanol is suspected

Perform gastric lavage.

Give IV sodium bicarbonate to counteract the acid effects and alkalinize the urine to enhance elimination.

For ethylene glycol, activated charcoal may be given.

IV ethanol can be given to compete with these drugs for enzyme metabolism.

For potential isopropanol ingestion

Gastric lavage may be performed.

Charcoal and ethanol will be ineffective.

Consider hemodialysis.

Observe for and treat any signs of withdrawal

Changes in vital signs (fever, tachycardia, hypertension, tachypnea)

Anxiety

Tremor

Hallucinations: 48–72 hours

Seizure activity: within 48 hours of last drink

Delirium tremens: 48 hours up to 2 weeks

- Treat with a short-acting benzodiazepine such as diazepam, lorazepam, or chlordiazepoxide. Chlordiazepoxide is the drug of choice for alcohol withdrawal provided that pts have normal liver function. If not, choose lorazepam.

Contact social services for appropriate rehabilitation referral

COCAINE INTOXICATION AND WITHDRAWAL

S **Does the pt give a history of drug use?**

If the pt is coherent, obtain the following information:
- Previous hospitalizations
- Length of drug abuse
- Drugs used and method of using them (e.g., smoking, snorting, intravenous)

Avoid aggravating an acutely intoxicated pt.

Contact family members or friends

Pts typically present altered and are unable to give a clear history.
The following information is important to obtain:

- Palpitations
- Headache
- History of suicide attempts
- Chest pain
- Trauma
- Recent illness
- Shortness of breath
- Seizure activity
- Change in mentation

O **Does the pt have VS suggestive of intoxication?**

- Tachycardia
- Hypertension
- Fever

Perform a thorough PE, with specific attention to the following

Gen: level of consciousness, anxiety, diaphoresis
HEENT: dilated pupils, dry mucous membranes, nasal septal perforation
Lungs: If the pt has used smokable crack-cocaine, look for pneumothorax.
Neuro: myoclonus, tremor, focal deficit, seizure
Skin: evidence of trauma

Review the results of the CBC with differential

Leukocytosis with left shift: consider infection. If seen, investigate the source.

Review urinalysis for signs of rhabdomyolysis

Look for moderate blood on dip with minimal red blood cells (RBCs) on microscopy.
If suggestive, check CK level, electrolytes, phos and calcium, look for
- Increased CK, BUN, creatinine, potassium, anion gap, and phosphorus
- Decreased calcium

Check serum and urine toxicology screen

Cocaine metabolites can be detected for up to 48 hours or longer in chronic users.
Look for other stimulants (like amphetamines) or depressants (like alcohol). Their use
increases the risk of cocaine toxicity.

Does the pt have an abnormal ECG?

Pt is at risk for ventricular arrhythmias or ischemia caused by cocaine-induced vasospasm. Consider checking troponin I or CK levels.

Consider taking a CXR

Pt is at risk for dissecting aortic aneurysm (chest pain radiating to back with widened
mediastinum on CXR), cardiomegaly, or bilateral infiltrates.

Consider taking a head CT scan

Cocaine use is associated with acute cerebrovascular accidents.

A **Cocaine intoxication**

Cocaine is derived from the coca plant. It is an alkaloid that can be taken orally, nasally,
intravenously, or smoked. It is a stimulant producing a wide range of symptoms, such
as euphoria, tremor, agitation, headache, nausea, fever, and hypertension.

Cocaine overdose produces all of the above symptoms plus lethargy, hyperactive deep
tendon reflexes (DTRs), seizures, hyperthermia, and incontinence. It also causes severe
vasoconstriction, which can cause vascular events like myocardial infarction (MI) and
stroke. More severe manifestations are coma, loss of DTRs, flaccid paralysis, pulmonary edema, and sudden death from arrhythmia, stroke, MI, etc.

Chronic cocaine use can produce addiction, paranoia, and hallucinations.

Cocaine withdrawal can occur as soon as 15 minutes after last use and manifests as an inability to stay awake, excessive hunger, and paranoia.

Differential diagnosis

First consider coingestion of cocaine with other drugs, which is common: alcohol, heroin (speedball), amphetamines, marijuana, etc.

Also consider other intoxications:

    – Lysergic acid diethylamide   – Ecstasy   – Methamphetamines

A differential diagnosis depends on the manifestations your pt has, ranging from altered mental status to chest pain to anxiety and paranoia.

– Schizophrenia	– Anxiety disorder	– Bipolar disorder	– Delirium
– Dementia	– Meningitis	– Encephalitis	– Uremia
– Lupus cerebritis	– Diabetic	– Head trauma	– Stroke
– Neurosyphilis	ketoacidosis		

P **Identify potentially life-threatening complications Admit pt to a monitored bed and give supportive care**

Cocaine overdose is a medical emergency, and interventions such as intubation may be necessary and the need for them should be monitored closely.

If pt is having an acute seizure, give a benzodiazepine IV

IV diazepam, approximately 2–10 mg/dose

If the seizure persists (>10 minutes), give phenobarbital or phenytoin

Seizures lasting longer than 10 minutes should be treated as status epilepticus (see Seizure, p. 424).

If MI occurs, treat appropriately but avoid β-blockers

(See Myocardial Infarction, p. 362 and Unstable Angina, p. 368.)

β-blockers are avoided because cocaine causes sympathetic stimulation including alpha (vasoconstrictive) effects, which will be unopposed with β blockade, leading to worse infarction as a result of vasospasm.

If arrhythmia occurs, identify and treat appropriately

If intracranial hemorrhage (cerebrovascular accident or subacute hemorrhage) occurs, transfer pt to the ICU and notify Neurosurgery

(See Cerebrovascular accident, p. 430)

Look for rhabdomyolysis and treat with fluid resuscitation

Check electrolytes and correct any abnormalities.

Consider renal consultation if renal function does not improve.

If pt is hyperthermic, consider neuroleptic malignant syndrome

Consider cooling measures, supportive care, bromocriptine, and dantrolene.

Chronic cocaine abuse requires a multidisciplinary approach

A social worker, psychiatrist, and a primary internist may all be needed for rehabilitation.

There are no medications effective for detoxification.

Cocaine withdrawal requires supportive care

Agitation may be controlled with IV or po benzodiazepines.

II
PEDIATRICS

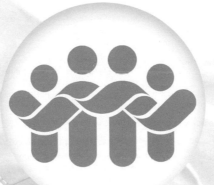

NEWBORN NURSERY

NEWBORN EXAM

S **Obtain a maternal Hx**

Important for determining safety of the neonate

- Maternal sexually transmitted infections (STIs: GC, CT, HSV, syphilis, HBV, HIV)
- Mother's occupation
- Previous children
- Maternal illicit drug use
- Where the baby will live
- ABO blood type/Rh type
- Past pregnancies including congenital anomalies, still births, genetic syndromes

Has the mother had prenatal care and labs? Has she been taking any medications?

Between the mother and her chart, record whether she has the following risk factors:

- Urine culture positive for Group B strep
- Diabetes mellitus
- TB
- HIV
- Hepatitis
- Preeclampsia, hypertension

Medications that can have an adverse effect on the baby include:

- Antiepileptics
- Antibiotics
- Antidepressants/mood stabilizers, hormones, anticoagulants
- Narcotics
- Antihypertensives

O **Examine the baby under a radiant warmer. Review vital signs**

Additions to a general physical exam include observation of general appearance, body position, color, respiratory effort

Measurements: Length, weight, and head circumference.

Head: Size and shape of head, scalp defects. Palpate scalp, anterior and posterior fontanelle; check to make sure the sutures move.

Eyes: Look for a red reflex with an ophthalmoscope. Check for spacing for eyes and symmetry.

Palate: Check for cleft (sometimes a finger may need to be inserted into the mouth for this).

Ears: Look for tags, and make sure the superior attachment is level with the eye. If it is not, the ears are low-set, a possible sign of a genetic disorder.

Hands and feet: Look for extra digits, polydactyly/syndactyly.

Musculoskeletal: Look for clavicular fractures, sacral spine for pits, dimples, or hair tufts.

Abdomen: Palpate both the kidneys. Unusual masses should also be palpable.

Pulses: Place one finger on a femoral pulse and the other on the right brachial pulse. They should be equal and occur at the same time, without delay.

Hips: Perform **O**rtolani (**O**ut) and **B**arlow (**B**ack) maneuvers (feeling for clunks).

- Ortolani maneuver is performed by grasping the proximal thighs with the index finger on the greater trochanter and the thumb on the lesser trochanter and abducting the hips 180 degrees. If a clunk is felt, you have reduced a dislocated hip.
- Barlow maneuver is performed by using the same grasp on adducted hips and pushing down toward the table. If a clunk is felt, you have dislocated the hip.

Infant neuro exam:

- *Moro:* Support the head and make the baby feel as if he/she is falling back. The arms should go out symmetrically, fingers splayed, with a small shake.
- *Gallant:* Place the baby's face down in the palm of your hand, stroke back on L or R, baby's bottom moves to side stroked.
- Palmar and plantar grasp, baby's tone, suck, jitteriness, and for tolerance of feeds.

- Stepping reflex: Holding infant in vertical position with feet in contact with flat surface. It initiates alternate stepping action of flexion and extension of legs.

Skin: Look for any normal or abnormal lesions or jaundice (see Benign Skin Lesions, p. 134 and Jaundice, p. 155).

Genitalia: Confirming gender of newborn. Examine penis, testicles, and scrotum in males. In female infants, size and location of labia, clitoris, and vaginal opening should be assessed.

Ballard exam (a neurologic and physical maturity scale) is used to estimate gestational age.

A **Normal newborn: Decide if the neonate requires a workup for sepsis**

Maternal risk factors:

    – Membranes ruptured >18 hr   – Group B strep (+)   – Uterine tenderness
    – Fever at delivery (>100.4 F)   – Chorioamnionitis
    – Foul-smelling lochia

Neonatal risk factors to suggest sepsis workup:

    – <37 wks' gestation   – Fetal tachycardia   – Grunting

The initial sepsis workup consists of a CBC with differential, CRP, and blood culture. If results are abnormal, transfer the baby to the neonatal intensive care unit (NICU) for presumed sepsis. Sepsis workup also includes lumbar puncture if the infant is clinically stable enough to tolerate the procedure.

Consider transfer to the NICU if

Baby's weight is less than 2,250 g or more than 4,500 g.

Mother is diabetic using insulin.

Gestational age of the baby by Ballard or dates is less than 35 weeks.

Baby has symptoms of distress:

    – Accessory respiratory   – Grunting   – Temperature instability, irritability,
      muscle use   – Cyanosis   poor feeding, vomiting, abdominal
    – Nasal flaring   distension

P **Consider all things that may endanger the neonate before discharge at 48–72 hours**

Rule out subgaleal hemorrhage. Follow CBCs and vital signs if suspected

Subgaleal hemorrhage: If scalp bogginess extends to the back of the neck, observe carefully because a baby can lose its entire blood volume into this space.

For an abnormal red reflex, refer to Ophthalmology

Red reflex abnormalities can mean cataracts, strabismus, or retinoblastoma.

Order an echocardiogram if the cardiovascular exam is abnormal

Murmurs may be congenital heart lesions. Pulse differentials can be a coarcted aorta.

If the hip exam is abnormal, refer for U/S of the hips and then to orthopedics

Hip clunks on the Ortolani and Barlow can be signs of developmental dysplasia of the hip. If the problem is not corrected in early infancy, the child may never walk.

For an abnormal infant neuro exam, consult a pediatric neurologist

Also, if the exam is asymmetric, consider birth trauma, such as a brachial plexus injury.

Check a total bilirubin on the second day of life. Consider NICU transfer if >25

A neonate sent home with a rapidly climbing bilirubin is at risk for kernicterus.

Explain normal and abnormal skin findings to the parents

See Benign Skin Lesions, p. 134.

Use the Ballard exam estimate for gestational age only if it is more than 2 weeks different from the prebirth-estimated gestational age

This is a predetermined pediatric scale.

Vaccinate for hepatitis B. If mom is HBsAg (+) or status is unknown, give HBV IgG

BIRTH TRAUMA

S **Were there any complications in the delivery?**
Trauma risks include:
- Breech presentation
- Scalp electrode
- Vacuum extraction
- Cesarean section
  (scalpel lacerations)
- Forceps extraction

What are the physical characteristics of the mother?
Trauma risks include:
- Primiparity
- Maternal short stature
- Small vaginal canal
- Pelvic anomalies
- Maternal obesity, operative vaginal delivery (use of forceps or a vacuum)
- C-section

How long was the labor?
Prolonged or rapid labor may also be risk factors to the neonate.

What are the physical characteristics of the neonate or amniotic sac?
Oligohydramnios (less than normal amount of amniotic fluid surrounding the baby) increases risk of trauma to baby because of less fluid protecting it from the initial uterine contractions.
A baby with a large head (e.g., hydrocephalus) or shoulders (e.g., macrosomic) may have difficulty passing through the birth canal.

O **Trauma is most commonly seen in the following areas**

Head (the largest and most common presenting part of the fetus)
Caput succedaneum (most common and benign type of extracranial hemorrhage): Occurs when serosanguineous fluid collects in the subcutaneous area between the galea aponeurotica and the skin. It is boggy in texture with poorly defined margins and crosses suture lines.
Cephalohematoma: A subperiosteal collection of blood caused by rupture of a blood vessel on the surface of the bone presenting as a firm, discrete mass that does not cross suture lines. Underlying skull fracture is sometimes present. Rarely associated with significant hemorrhage.
Subgaleal hemorrhage (most dangerous and least common extracranial hemorrhage): Caused by bleeding between the periosteum and the galea aponeurotica. It is a large space, extending from the orbital ridge over the entire skull to the ears and back of the neck, into which the neonate's entire blood volume can be lost. Examine carefully for bogginess, fluctuance, or pitting edema in this entire region.

Exam of the neck and shoulders
Torticollis: The head is held tilted to one side with a palpable sternocleidomastoid mass possibly resulting from birth trauma or intrauterine positioning.
Clavicular fracture (most common neonatal orthopedic injury): Crepitus (crunchy/crackling) or bony irregularity along the clavicle. Often occurs during delivery of the shoulders or shoulder dystocia.

Exam of the arms
Erb palsy: Injury of the fifth and sixth cervical spinal roots, causing the arm to be adducted, internally rotated, with the elbow extended, forearm prone, and wrist flexed. Because the fingers are not involved, palmar grasp reflex is present, but Moro is absent.
Klumpke palsy (rare): Traction of the seventh and eighth cervical nerves, and first thoracic nerve, causing flexed elbow, supinated forearm, extended wrist, and hyperextension of the MCP joints. Grasp is absent. Moro is present.
Entire plexus injury causes an entirely flaccid arm.

Exam of the skin

Petechiae (common): Nonblanching red spots caused by subcutaneous capillary bleeding.

Ecchymosis (bruise): Larger nonblanching areas of subcutaneous bleeding.

Lacerations (common): Cuts in the skin from scalpels, forceps, or other trauma.

Subcutaneous fat necrosis (usually occurs a day or two after birth): Presents as irregularly shaped reddish purple subcutaneous nodules, which are hard to the touch. Often resulting from instrumentation, such as forceps, on the cheek of the baby.

Sucking blisters: Bullae or ulcerations on the wrist, finger, foot, etc. caused by sucking in utero.

Birth trauma. A small DDx includes

Excessive petechiae or subcutaneous bleeding should be ruled out for sepsis and bleeding diathesis such as hemophilia or platelet disorders.

Extensive fractures should be ruled out for osteogenesis imperfecta or other bone disorders.

Mongolian spots (see Benign Skin Lesions, p. 134) can be mistaken for ecchymoses.

Always keep the parents well-informed

This will prevent panic if they find trauma incidentally.

Note and record all injuries in the chart

This should prevent legal action against the obstetrician or pediatrician.

For caput succedaneum and cephalohematoma, confirm that they are not evolving subgaleal hemorrhages. Check CBCs and T bili levels. Take a skull x-ray if skull fracture is suspected

Blood breakdown in these injuries can elevate total bilirubin and lead to jaundice.

If subgaleal hemorrhage is suspected, monitor for signs of volume loss, such as tachycardia and hypotension. Check CBCs. Replace blood and fluids as needed

This should be sufficient to prevent hypovolemic shock in these high-risk neonates.

For torticollis, observe, massage, perform gentle stretching, and place a pillow on the affected side to hold the head away from the shoulders while sleeping

This therapy has been shown to correct torticollis in a matter of weeks to months.

If clavicular fractures are suspected, perform an x-ray to confirm the diagnosis

Nothing else needs to be done except to follow up with x-rays to verify callus formation and normal healing.

For brachial plexus injuries, nothing needs to be done

These usually resolve in 1–2 weeks. The pt should have neurologic follow-up. No improvement by 6 months indicates a poor prognosis.

Suture all wide or deep lacerations

BENIGN SKIN LESIONS

S **Are there any genetic disorders in the family that may present with skin lesions?**

Neurofibromatosis (von Recklinghausen disease): Can present with multiple, large café au lait spots, axillary freckling. In the neonate, more than three spots or any one spot larger than 3 cm should make you suspicious for this disease.

Tuberous sclerosis: Multiple fibromas, ash-leaf spots, Shagreen patch, Lisch nodules.

Waardenburg syndrome: Presents with piebaldism, partial areas of hypopigmentation.

Peutz-Jeghers syndrome: Presents in the neonatal period with multiple, scattered hyperpigmented macules usually found on the nose, mouth, fingers, hands, and mucous membranes of the mouth. Usually associated with intestinal polyps.

Albright syndrome: In adults, it has bony lesions and endocrine abnormalities. In neonates, it presents with a single, large (up to 12 cm), ragged, irregular hyperpigmented lesion.

O **Lesions can be red, brown, white, or blue and can be raised or flat**

Raised red lesions

Erythema toxicum: One of the most common findings on the skin of the neonate. It usually looks like small red marks on the skin, with tiny papules arising from the center of each red macule. It can occur anywhere on the body. It is far more common in healthy, term neonates.

Staphylococcal skin infections: Be sure to differentiate them from erythema toxicum. The pustules are usually grouped periumbilically, in the axillae, or in the groin.

Superficial hemangioma: The old term for this kind of lesion is strawberry hemangioma, and this is highly descriptive. It would be rare in the nursery to have a fully recognizable strawberry hemangioma, but, if present, it would appear as a raised, red nodule, or it may appear as a pale macule with some blood vessels appearing within it.

Flat red lesions

Nevus simplex (salmon patch, stork bite): Usually pink, not red. It is approximately ½–1 cm in size. The most common location is on the nape of the neck, but it may also be found on the forehead, eyelid, or bridge of the nose. It is extremely common.

Port-wine stain (nevus flammeus): Usually unilateral, reddish purple, and commonly found on the face. If it involves the area of the ophthalmic branch of the trigeminal nerve, this is known as Sturge-Weber syndrome.

Raised brown lesions

Nevi: These form when groups of melanocytes are grouped together. Junctional nevi are small and benign. Compound nevi are similar, but they may be hairy and slightly larger. The most obvious is the giant hairy nevus, which may cover 20%–30% of the total body surface area.

Flat brown lesions

Transient pustular melanosis: Difficult to categorize because it may have red raised lesions and brown flat lesions at both extremes. More common in African-American babies. Noninfectious pustules rupture to form raised, then flat brown spots on the skin, and then resolve.

Raised blue lesions

Deep hemangioma: The new term for cavernous hemangioma. Like superficial hemangioma, this is a vascular malformation. It is deep in the skin but tends to cause a raised blue lesion. If it is large, it can sequester blood and platelets (Kasabach-Merritt syndrome).

Flat blue lesions

Mongolian spots: More common in babies of African or Asian descent. Usually disappear by the age of 3 years. Tend to appear blue, like bruising. They can be small or large and occur anywhere, although the lumbosacral region is most common. It is important to note them because they fade slowly and later may make someone suspicious for child abuse.

Raised white lesions

Milia (common): Epidermal cysts appear as tiny white papules on the nose, forehead, and chin.

Sebaceous gland hyperplasia: Like milia, but the papules are smaller and grouped together.

Flat white lesions

Piebaldism and ash-leaf spots as noted above are the main hypopigmented lesions.

It is important to note that there is also a lesion of absent skin

Cutis aplasia: Occurs when the skin does not form. This usually occurs over the midline of the posterior scalp. It looks like a punched-out area (with no hair), 1–2 cm in diameter.

Often you will find more than one lesion in the same pt

A   **Benign skin lesions. DDx includes**

Child abuse: Consider in the case of Mongolian spots and cutis aplasia. However, it is unlikely to occur in the hospital.

Heat rash: May appear similar to erythema toxicum.

P   **All of these lesions are initially benign. Some may require later intervention**

Lesions that require no intervention and will self-resolve

- Transient neonatal pustular melanosis
- Mongolian spots
- Milia
- Superficial hemangioma
- Small deep hemangioma
- Erythema toxicum
- Junctional nevi
- Nevus simplex
- Sebaceous gland hyperplasia

Giant hairy nevi and compound nevi have the potential to become malignant in the future (3- to 20-fold higher risk of developing melanoma) and should be surgically removed

Refer to surgery or dermatology clinic

Port-wine stains are cosmetically undesirable and require pulse-dye laser therapy

Obtain an MRI of the brain for suspected Sturge-Weber pts

An MRI is needed because Sturge-Webber pts can have underlying brain lesions.

Large deep hemangiomas may require surgical resection

If large enough, they can cause anemia, thrombocytopenia, and high-output heart failure.

Place a surgical dressing over cutis aplasia

This will prevent injury or infection.

PEDIATRIC CLINIC

WELL-CHILD CARE: INFANT

S **Ask developmental questions appropriate for age for each visit**

1 week: Visually fixes

1 month: Raises head slightly from prone, tight grasp, alerts to sound, regards face

2 months: Raises chest off table, tries to steady head briefly when held, social smile (6 weeks), recognizes parents, relaxes grasp

4 months: Rolls front to back, coos/laughs, explores visually, hands midline, no head lag

6 months: Rolls back to front/sits, raking grasp, recognizes stranger, babbles

9 months: Says "mama/dada"/gestures, pincer grasp, holds bottle/throws, cruises, imitates sounds

12 months: Says "mama/dada" (specific), walks, comes when called, three-word vocabulary

What is the baby eating? How often is the mother feeding?

Exclusively breastfeeding q 2–3 hours is best for the baby until about 6 months, then start baby food and water. Breastfeeding may be continued as long as the mother feels comfortable.

For bottle/formula feeding, from 1 week–6 months should take up to 3 ounces every 3 hours. At 6–12 months, give no more than 4 ounces every 3 hours to allow for adequate intake of solid foods.

How many diapers per day? How many with stool?

Stool: Initially occurs after every feed (q 2–3 hours for breastfeeding and q 3–4 hours for bottle-feeding). As the infant approaches 1 year, stooling will become less frequent (about 1/d).

Urine: About 8 wet diapers per day. If significantly less, consider dehydration or urinary tract infection.

How is the baby sleeping?

Newborns sleep about 15 hours per day, sleeping only a few hours at a time.

By about 4 months, they should be able to sleep through the night (about 5 hours at a time).

By 12 months, they should sleep about 14 hours a day (10 hr/night and two naps during the day).

O **Perform a PE, making sure to include the following**

Growth parameters: Weight, height, and head circumference should be plotted on a growth curve so as to not miss malnutrition, failure to thrive, or poor brain growth.

Vital signs: Temperature, respiratory rate, heart rate

Fontanelles: Posterior closes at about 2 months, anterior closes at about 18 months.

Eyes: Looking for leukocoria (white instead of red reflex). Differential diagnosis: retinoblastoma or cataracts.

Infant neuro exam:
- Tone: Hypertonic (CP), normal, or hypotonic (CP, botulism, metabolic disorder)
- Primitive reflexes: Palmar/plantar grasp, Moro, Gallant = birth to 3–6 months
- ATNR (asymmetrical tonic neck reflex) = birth to 4 months
- Postural reactions: Head righting and Landau by 3 months, derotational righting by 5 months, parachute by 6 months, Ant/Lat/Post Propping by 5, 6, and 7 months, respectively.

Hip clunks: **O**rtolani (**O**ut) and **B**arlow (**B**ack) (see Newborn Exam, p. 130).

Umbilical cord: Should have fallen off by 1 month. If not, consider leukocyte/neutrophil defect.

Testes down bilaterally: Abdominal testes have increased risk of testicular cancer.

A **Well infant, age**

Assess development

Some diagnoses to consider while assessing developmental delay are cerebral palsy, hearing deficit (poor language development), and autism (poor social and language development).

Assess appropriateness of growth

Term infants may lose up to 10% of their body weight in the first few days and then regain birth weight by 10–14 days of age. Infants double their birth weight by 4 months of age and triple their birth weight by 1 year. Plot the height, weight, and head circumference. If any of them is below the 5th percentile or the current plot is not following the expected growth curve, this should be investigated further.

P **Give anticipatory guidance. Recommend contacting the doctor if there is**

Runny nose/congestion that interferes with breathing
Prolonged fatigue or irritability
Vomiting and decreased oral intake
Audible wheezing
Diarrhea and dehydration
Fever in an infant younger than 1 month

Offer appropriate anticipatory guidance related to the safety of the infant's environment

- No unlocked guns in the home
- All possible poisons out of reach
- Electric outlet protectors
- Infants should not be left in the bath alone (they can drown and die in as little as 1 in of water)
- Smoke detectors
- Prevent falls
- Reset water heater to 120°F

Give appropriate vaccinations

Because the regimens change regularly, and many combination vaccines with different administration schedules are available, it is best to find the most recent version of the vaccination schedule at www.cispimmunize.org.

Recommend exclusive breastfeeding (bottle-feeding as a second choice) until about 6 months

Endorse breastfeeding because there is no better food for the baby.
Introduce solids at 6 months of age. Feeding earlier increases risk of food allergies.

At 6 months, recommend introducing baby food and the cup

Infant cereals (rice cereal) and pureed meats be offered first as they provide zinc and iron. Once these foods are accepted, strained or pureed fruits and vegetables may be added.
Fruit juice generally should not be offered to infants younger than 12 months.
Highly allergenic foods such as eggs, fish, peanuts/peanut butter, tree nuts may be introduced at 6 months of age.
With the cup, the bottle should be phased out.

At 8–10 months, recommend starting things in small pieces such as

Cereal, pasta, banana, crackers, cooked chicken, and vegetables

Discuss foods to avoid before 1 year of age

Honey because of the risk of infant botulism, cow's milk, plant-based milks, fruit juice
Foods that the baby can choke on, such as nuts, seeds, popcorn, chips, grapes, raisins, raw vegetables
Sugar-sweetened beverages should be avoided during infancy

Check CBC and lead level at the 1-year visit to rule out anemia or lead ingestion

WELL-CHILD CARE: TODDLER

S **During a well-child visit, you should always start off by asking how the child is doing**

In addition to any complaints, be sure to assess eating, sleeping, stooling, and voiding.

Obtain a developmental history

For developmental assessment use developmental screening tools recommended by American Academy of Pediatrics such as Ages and Stages Questionnaires (ASQ), Child Development Inventory (CDI), Denver-II Developmental Screening Test, M-CHAT, etc. (brightfutures.aap.org).

Failure to reach developmental milestones appropriately is a red flag.

Screen for exposure to lead, smoking, domestic violence, and guns in the home (Table 11-1)

TABLE 11-1 Developmental Assessment

	18 mo	24 mo	36 mo
Gross motor	Walks fast; runs; walks up stairs; throws a ball	Runs well; walks down stairs; kicks a ball	Walks up stairs on toes; uses tricycle (3 yr = 3 wheels); hops on 1 foot
Fine motor	Builds a tower of 4 cubes; scribbles spontaneously; copies a vertical line	Builds a tower of 6–7 cubes; copies a horizontal line; uses a spoon with less spilling	Builds a tower of 9–10 cubes; draws a head; copies a circle
Social/emotional	Takes off clothes; feeds self (spills); hugs a doll	Refers to self by name; says when needs the toilet; plays in parallel	Shows concern for others; plays cooperatively; dresses with help
Language	Follows two-step commands; looks at book; names one object; says 10–20 words	Uses 2- to 3-word phrases; 150- to 200-word vocabulary; uses "I" "me" "you"; 25%–50% intelligible	75% intelligible; 4- to 5-word phrases; tells stories
Intellectual	Understands cause and effect; points to named body parts; understands object permanence	Solve by trial and error; understands time	Asks "why?"; recites rhymes; follows daily routine

O **Check the toddler's height, weight, and head circumference**

Height should increase by 12.5 cm over the second year of life and 6.25 cm over the third. Children gain 2 kg per year (4.4 lb) between 2 years of age and puberty.

Head circumference should continue to be followed until age 36 months.

Plot on growth curve. If not in normal range or growth rate decreasing, investigate.

Perform a PE

Usually, a child younger than 3 years continues to experience stranger anxiety.

Examine the chest first so that you may be able to auscultate before the child begins to cry.

Then examine the abdomen, extremities, and genitalia. The abdomen softens and can be palpated when the child inhales to cry.

The exam of the head, ears, eyes, nose, and throat should be done with the child seated on mother's lap. Mother should hold both of the child's hands in one hand, and use her other hand to hold the head, which prevents sudden movements during the exam.

If the child bites down on the tongue blade, slide it slowly and gently forward. When the gag reflex is triggered, the child will open the mouth and you may examine the throat.

A Well toddler, age: _____

Consider the following possible complicating diagnoses, which may present in this period

Gross/fine motor abnormalities: Cerebral palsy, hypothyroidism, muscular dystrophy.

Social/emotional/language failures: Autism, hearing impairment, mental retardation

Intellectual failures: Consider mental retardation

Obesity: Calculate the BMI = (weight in kg)/(height in m)^2; plot it on the BMI curve; and if pt is obese or at risk of obesity, address this issue with the family. Be aggressive because obesity will significantly shorten children's lives.

Failure to thrive: If the child is not gaining weight, this should be investigated as well. Both social and medical causes should be considered.

Evaluate for medical conditions related to the complaint of the parents or child.

P Give anticipatory guidance. Advise the parents on the following safety issues

Climbing risks, falling risks, ingestion risks (both chemical and foreign body).

Pool should be gated (if there is one).

Lock up cleaning supplies or place them in unreachable areas.

Lock up all guns with ammunition locked away separately.

Adult supervision is needed while the child is near or crossing the street (driveways, ice cream trucks, exiting car).

Discuss AAP-recommended car seat guidelines with parents.

Advise the parents on toilet training techniques, including

Positive reward systems, a special potty chair, and to avoid making it a struggle, which usually ends in constipation

Advise the parents on discipline for temper tantrums, especially the time-out method

Studies have shown that time-outs are more effective at decreasing tantrums than corporal punishment. Spanking, although tolerated, is no longer advised (see WCC: Child, p. 140).

Advise decreased bottle use and minimized juice intake

The bottle is bad for the toddler's teeth. Juice has little nutritional value and leads to obesity.

Vaccinate for DTaP at 15 months and two dose series of hep a between 12 and 23 months. Check lead level (for toxicity), CBC (for anemia), if none in last 2 years

Anemia is very common and is usually secondary to increased milk intake. Advise no more than 20 oz of milk per day in children aged 1–5.

For milestone failures, follow-up in 3 months to check for milestone attainment

Screen the hearing for all language failures. If failure persists, refer to a child developmental specialist or your local Social Services center for support.

WELL-CHILD CARE: CHILD

S **Begin with a typical open-ended question about whether there are any problems, and then move to developmental questions that are appropriate for the child's age**

4 years: Balances on one foot for 3 seconds, alternates feet going down steps, uses all utensils (except knife), can name colors, understands concept of past, speech 100% intelligible, speaks in paragraphs, can draw a plus sign, buttons

5 years: Balances on one foot for 10 seconds, can jump over low obstacles, ties shoes, spreads with knife, competitive play, asks for definitions, can draw a square

6 years: Counts to ten, knows right from left, can draw a triangle

8 years: Sounds out words, can print name, can draw a diamond

10 years: Tells time, does chores, does well in school

What is the child eating?

Explain that it is the parent's job to offer a balanced diet (limit junk food) and the child's job to select from among the options. It is very common for parents to think that their children don't eat enough. As long as the child is growing normally (confirm by plotting the child's growth curve), everything will be fine.

If the child is obese, this question will help you learn what foods may be easy to eliminate.

Ask how things are going at home, school, and in the child's outside activities

Problems in one or all of these areas will give you reason to investigate things such as domestic violence, discipline, and learning disabilities.

Ask questions related to the safety of the home environment

Ask specifically about smoke alarms (and whether there are functioning batteries), and if there are guns, violence, drugs, or tobacco in the home.

O **Review and plot growth parameters on a growth chart**

It is important to plot not only height and weight but also to calculate body mass index (BMI: weight in kg/[height in m]²) because many children are obese, and it is important to recognize its severity when you see it. A child with BMI <5th percentile for age and sex is underweight, BMI between 5th and <85th percentile is normal. A child with BMI between 85th percentile and <95th percentile is overweight, and a child with BMI of 95th percentile and higher is obese.

Watch how the child and parents interact

You may see clues to make you consider discipline problems, ADHD, or even child abuse.

Perform a PE. Order appropriate tests as necessary

If you assess delayed development or school problems, a hearing and vision screen would be an appropriate first step.

If you pick up scoliosis on PE, you should check an x-ray of the spine.

A **Well-child, age**

Assess the development of child

If you assess delay, check hearing and vision and consider conditions such as autism and ADHD.

Assess the safety of the home environment

If any of the answers to the questions you asked above indicate an unsafe environment, such as guns, violence, drugs, or lack of smoke detectors in the home, give appropriate anticipatory guidance.

Assess whether the pt is obese

As described above, this is becoming a very common problem. In the United States, prevalence of obesity among school-aged children increased between 1976–1980 and 2013–2014 from 6.5%–19.6 %.

P Give anticipatory guidance

Car seat guidelines:

- Infants and toddlers: Rear-facing only or rear facing convertible until 2 years of age or until they reach the maximum height and weight for their seat.
- Toddlers and preschoolers: Convertible or forward facing with harness for as long as possible, up to the highest weight or height allowed by their car safety seat manufacturer.
- School-aged children: Use belt positioning booster seat until the vehicle seat belt fits properly, typically when they have reached 4 ft 9 in and are 8 through 12 years of age.
- All children younger than 13 years should ride in the back seat.

Safety helmets for bikes, roller-blades, skates, scooters, etc.

Crossing the street safely is very important because pedestrians versus automobiles is a common reason for admission. All children should be supervised by an adult while crossing the street.

Water safety: There should always be a fence around pools and an adult supervising.

Recommend exercise or some sort of physical activity

Limit junk food, desserts, sodas, and chips to prevent obesity.

Limit TV time to prevent inactivity, snacking, obesity, and improve interaction with the family.

Brush twice a day and floss nightly and visit a dentist to prevent tooth decay.

Discuss why hitting children for punishment is wrong

It sends the wrong message that hitting and being hit is okay. A more effective method is the time-out. When the child misbehaves, say "Time-out, hitting" or whatever short phrase that is applicable and calmly remove the child from the environment, isolating him or her (facing a wall, corner, or any other uninteresting place) until the time has been completed. Because of the limited attention span of children, the time-out should last about 1 minute for each year of life. Time-outs can be used repeatedly without any harm to the child.

Discuss sex education

It is always better for the parents to address this issue in the prepubertal age before any of the child's friends who think they are experts on the subject get to them first.

Puberty/menarche: Prepubertal girls should know what menses is before it happens.

Discuss the use of money

Children in this age group should be given supervised opportunities to use money.

Discuss school readiness

If a learning, hearing, or vision problem is detected, it should be addressed before it interferes with school.

Discuss drugs, tobacco, and alcohol and the dangers of using them

As with sex education, it is best to demystify this topic in the doctor's office rather than on the school playground.

Give appropriate vaccinations

DTaP, IPV, varicella, and MMR should be given at 4 years of age, before starting school.

WELL-CHILD CARE: ADOLESCENT

S **If the parent is present, begin the interview with the parent and adolescent together. After discussing the parent's concerns, ask her or him to wait in the waiting room**

Talk to adolescents alone so they can talk about things they do not want their parents to hear.

Explain that confidentiality is broken only to prevent serious harm to someone.

Remember to use open-ended questions and the mnemonic HEADDSS:

H **(home): How are things at home?**
Ask about: Live with parents, friends, homeless; physical, sexual, verbal abuse; discipline

E **(education): How is school?**
Ask about: Grade level, performance, goals; detention, truancy, expulsion; learning difficulties

A **(activities): What do you do when you're not in school?**
Ask about: Jobs, what they do for money; sports, hobbies, clubs; gangs, arrests

D **(diet): What do you normally eat?**
Ask about: Number of meals per day, junk food; using laxatives, vomiting

D **(drugs): Do you use any drugs?**
Ask about: Alcohol (how much, what kind); smoking (packs per day, how many years); illicit drugs

S **(sex): Are you having sex?**
Ask about: Age at first intercourse; age and sex of partner; use of contraception; type of sex (vaginal, rectal, oral); number of partners; condom, dental dams; STDs, discharge, genital lesions; sex for money, housing, or food; unwanted sex

S **(suicide): Do you feel depressed? Do you ever feel like hurting yourself?**
A good mnemonic for depression is SIG E CAPS:
- *S*leep (insomnia or oversleeping)
- *I*nterest (less for normal activities)
- *G*uilt
- *E*nergy (lack of)
- *C*oncentration (lack of)
- *A*ttention (lack of)
- *P*sychomotor agitation (nervous activity)
  -*S*uicidal thoughts

   If they have thought of hurting themselves, ask about SLAP (Suicidal, Lethality, Attempts/ Access, Plan):
- *S*uicidal thoughts currently
- *A*ccess to lethal means
- *L*ethality of plan
- *P*lan about how to do it
- Previous Attempts

   Do they have thoughts of hurting or killing someone else? If so, do they have current plans?

O **Perform a general PE**
This can be done with the parent present or absent, depending on the adolescent's choice.

Check growth and development
Note rapid increases in weight or decreases in height velocity.
Assess sexual development (breast, pubic hair, genital) by Tanner Sexual Maturity Rating:
- I: No breast development or pubic hair, prepubertal testes
- II: Breast bud diameter < areolar, sparse thin pubic hair
- III: Breast bud diameter > areolar, sparse coarse pubic hair, penis lengthens.
  Menarche for girls usually occurs after Tanner Stage III

- IV: Mounding of areola, coarse hair confined to mons, penis grows in width
- V: Adult breast development, pubic hair extending to thigh, adult testes

If breast enlargement (gynecomastia) found in males, reassure that it's normal and will resolve.

Screen for sexually transmitted infections (STIs) in those who are at high risk

Screen for HIV in all adolescents aged 13 and above

Adolescents should also be assessed for

Pubertal delay or short stature: If there are no signs of sexual development by age 14, investigate chromosomal or endocrine causes

Home problems: From abuse to homelessness

School problems: From learning difficulties to behavior problems

Eating disorders: Anorexia, bulimia, or obesity

Risk-taking behaviors: Such as substance abuse, reckless driving, unprotected sex, homelessness

Suicidal ideation: Caused by problems at home, abuse, or clinical depression

Scoliosis and any other general medical problems

Anticipatory guidance and counseling

It is extremely helpful for the teen to hear advice from a nonparental authority figure.

Home problems: Investigate abuse and take appropriate measures depending on severity

Learning problems: Offer a referral to the appropriate school services assessment

Behavior problems: Identify the source of the problem, such as abuse or influence of friends.

If you suspect apathetic effort, try to counsel on the importance of education.

Counsel the teen regarding dangerous activities, such as gangs, that may lead to arrest.

Diet: Counsel regarding problems with obesity, anorexia, or bulimia

All will significantly shorten the adolescent's life.

Drugs: AAP/Bright Futures Guidelines recommend using CRAFT screen (car, relax, alone, forget, friends, trouble) to identify substance use

Assess for alcohol, smoking, and drug use. Offer a referral to programs such as Alcoholics Anonymous or other rehabilitative programs. Counsel on the dangers of the following

Alcohol: Cirrhosis, varices

Smoking: Cancer, chronic obstructive pulmonary disease

Drugs: Overdose, HIV, hepatitis

Sex: Assess for high-risk behaviors and counsel on the risk of pregnancy, dangers of STIs (HIV, herpes, etc.), and offer testing, treatment, barrier methods, and contraception

Give Tdap and meningococcal vaccine at 11–12 years of age. HPV vaccine at 11–12 years

Return to clinic in 1 year, or sooner if indicated by above possible social problems.

HYPERACTIVE AND SCHOOL-RELATED COMPLAINTS—ADHD

S **What symptoms does your child have?**

Hyperactivity: Leaving his or her seat in class, running or climbing at inappropriate times, fidgeting, squirming, talking excessively

Attention deficit: Frequent careless errors, not listening when spoken to directly, not finishing schoolwork or chores, losing things necessary for tasks (like schoolwork), obvious distraction by extraneous stimuli

Impulsivity: Blurting out answers before questions are asked, not waiting his or her turn, interrupting others

What is the child's sex?

Attention deficit hyperactivity disorder (ADHD) is far more common in male than female children in up to a 4:1 ratio.

How old is the child?

The child should be school age. Toddlers who act in the aforementioned manner are acting age appropriately. Just because the parents are exasperated does not mean the child has ADHD.

Teens with onset of these symptoms may be using mind-altering drugs that might be responsible for their behavior. They may also be developing an oppositional disorder. If symptoms were not present by age 7 years, the child is unlikely to have ADHD.

Does the child have symptoms in more than one setting?

Hyperactivity just at school or just at home does not count as ADHD.

ADHD must be pervasive in more than one setting.

How long have the symptoms been going on?

In order to diagnose ADHD, symptoms have to have been present for at least 6 months.

Obtain a birth history

Risk factors for ADHD include:

- Maternal substance abuse
- Low APGAR scores
- Prematurity

Does the child take any medicines?

The following medications can cause symptoms that mimic ADHD:

- Beta-agonists
- Theophylline
- Phenobarbital

Is there a family history of ADHD, learning disability, tics, obsessive compulsive disorder, or Tourette syndrome?

The gene loci for these problems are very close, and 70%–80% of the problems that cause ADHD are genetic. An example is Fragile X syndrome, a common genetic cause of ADHD.

O **Observe the child in the clinic while you are obtaining the history**

As noted above, symptoms of hyperactivity or impulsiveness should be present in more than one setting. That may include the clinic.

Perform a general PE including a detailed neurologic exam

The child may be excessively clumsy and do poorly on the neuro exam. This includes poor finger-to-nose, sliding heel on shin, rapid alternating movements, and an inability to walk heel to toe. These are neurologic "soft signs," but in this case they are extremely significant.

Also check the child's kinesthetic sense: ability to recognize a paper clip by touch or telling the difference in size between a penny and a quarter.

On the PE, be sure to check for physical signs of a genetic disorder. Fragile X presents with long facies, prominent ears, and large testicles.

Perform the test of attention preferred by your hospital or facility

Multiple tests of attention exist, including the TOVA, the IVA, the Stroop Color Word Test, and the Wisconsin Card Sort Test.

Refer for an EEG

There may be fairly nonspecific abnormalities in ADHD; however, this will be diagnostic if you suspect your pt has absence seizures. These pts exhibit a three-per-second spike and wave pattern on the EEG. This is characteristic of absence or petit mal seizures.

A **Rule out ADHD**

Per the DSM-5 (the psychiatric reference manual), pts may either have the predominantly inattentive presentation, the predominantly hyperactive/impulsive presentation, or the combined presentation.

Studies show that ADHD may actually result from deficiencies of dopamine in the prefrontal cortex or caudate nucleus, or deficiencies of norepinephrine in the locus ceruleus.

Therefore, treatment attempting to increase these normally activating neurotransmitters should actually correct the problem.

Differential diagnosis

- Absence seizures   – Medication side effect   – Developmental delay
- Street drug effect   – Autism

P **Use a behavior rating scale to make the diagnosis and monitoring of ADHD**

These are usually surveys filled out by the parent, the teacher, and the pt.

Scales include the Connor's, Behavior Assessment System for Children (BASC), ADHD Rating Scale, Vanderbilt Assessment Scales. You should use whichever instrument your institution is most familiar with.

Have the parents return with all three completed forms in 1–2 months. If the scores are appropriate, the diagnosis of ADHD can be made and treatment can begin.

Begin treatment with methylphenidate (Ritalin or Concerta) or atomoxetine (Strattera)

These are the first-line agents for ADHD.

Concerta is longer-acting than Ritalin but has the same mechanism of action. Start 2.5 mg orally twice daily and during the course of 1 week; increase the dose as necessary up to 7.5 mg three times per day.

Adderall and Dexedrine can be also be started as first-line therapy for ADHD in children.

If your first choice has been ineffective at treating symptoms, you may switch to the other.

In follow-up visits, monitor for side effects such as irritability, anorexia, nausea, weight loss, insomnia, depression, or growth impairment. Change meds or adjust the dose as needed

CHRONIC COUGH AND WHEEZE—ASTHMA

S **Has the child had shortness of breath caused by cough, wheeze, or chest tightness?**

The response to this question can help you diagnose asthma as the problem. Many asthmatics have a chronic nighttime cough, which goes unrecognized. As a result, they are inappropriately treated with cough medicine or antibiotics instead of albuterol and inhaled corticosteroids.

How often do these symptoms occur at night? How often do they occur during the day?

The response helps categorize the asthma (see Table 11-2).
The categorization is important because it directs treatment.

What makes the asthma symptoms worse or better? What triggers the asthma?

It is important to identify what triggers the child's asthma. Common triggers include:
- Weather changes   – Exercise   – Pollens
- Dust   – Mold   – Cockroaches

If the pt already uses albuterol (or other asthma medications), how often is it used?

If pts report mild symptoms but they use their medicine five nights a week, this could suggest a more severe asthma that is not adequately controlled.

How many times has the child been intubated, hospitalized, or brought to the ER with asthma?

These are important indicators of the severity of the asthma and how aggressively to treat (Table 11-2).

TABLE 11-2 Asthma Categorizations

Category	Symptoms	Nighttime Symptoms
Mild intermittent	<2×/wk	<2×/mo
Mild persistent	>2×/wk	3–4×/mo
Moderate persistent	Daily	>1×/wk
Severe persistent	Throughout the day	7×/wk

O **Look at the pts overall and assess whether they are in respiratory distress based on the following symptoms**
- Unable to speak in full   – Accessory respiratory   Tripod posture
  sentences   muscle usage
- Tachypnea   – Tachycardia
- Straining facial   – Low O_2 saturation
  expression

Look closely at the chest wall and abdomen for signs of increased work of breathing

Sometimes the pt will look fairly comfortable until you take off the shirt and look closely at the chest wall and abdomen to see signs of respiratory distress. These include:
- Subcostal retractions   – Accessory muscle use   – Abdominal breathing

Listen to the chest wall for breath sounds

Listen for wheezing (a high-pitched sound during expiration), prolonged expiratory phase, and poor air movement. Examine the lungs carefully, auscultating and percussing the lung fields for signs of other lung pathology such as pneumonia.

Always recheck the breath sounds after a breathing treatment

Often, after a treatment, you may be better able to hear wheezing because there is better air movement.

If breath sounds are unchanged, airways may not be reactive. Other diagnoses should be considered.

Asthma

Asthma is the most common chronic inflammatory disease of the airways. It is a complex pathologic state in which chronic airway inflammation leads to increased mucus production and bronchoconstriction. Bronchoconstriction causes lower airway obstruction, which is intermittent and reversible with bronchodilators.

Differential diagnosis

     – Aspirated foreign body   – Vocal cord dysfunction   – Pulmonary infection
     – Heart disease   – Cystic fibrosis

Assess severity of disease

Classify the asthma as mild intermittent, mild persistent, moderate persistent, or severe persistent, based on the system noted in Table 11-2.

If the exacerbations occur more than once a day or last several days or are particularly severe (requiring intubation), then the classification should be upgraded.

Explain to the pt how, when, and why to use the asthma medications

Demonstrate and explain the correct use of the medicine and then observe the pt doing it correctly. Put the spacer on the inhaler and put the other end of the spacer in the mouth. Press down on the inhaler and breathe in slowly for 5 seconds. Hold breath for 10 seconds and then repeat.

Explain the need for spacers

Ensures that the medicine is small enough particles to reach the lungs.

Without the spacer, much of the medicine deposits in the throat and not the lungs.

Without the spacer, you get more of the side effects and less of the benefits of the medicine.

Explain the difference between relievers/rescue inhaler and controllers

Relievers are rescue medicines such as albuterol that are used to stop an exacerbation.

Controllers are medications such as inhaled corticosteroids, leukotriene antagonists, and a long-acting beta-2-agonist that are used daily regardless of how the pt feels.

Prescribe the appropriate medications based on the severity of the asthma

Mild intermittent: Albuterol as needed

Mild persistent: Add a low-dose inhaled corticosteroid twice daily

Moderate persistent: Increase the dose of corticosteroids to medium, or add a long-acting beta-2-agonist. A leukotriene antagonist or theophylline may substitute for the long-acting beta-2-agonist daily.

Severe persistent: High-dose inhaled corticosteroids and a long-acting beta-2-agonist twice daily. Add oral corticosteroids as needed. Attempts should be made to reduce corticosteroid dosages at every visit during which symptoms are well controlled.

If the asthma is difficult to control, look for signs of associated diseases and treat them

The following diseases are often found in association with asthma, and many difficult-to-control asthmatics improve when these specific comorbidities are addressed and treated:

     – Allergic rhinitis   – Sinusitis   – Gastric reflux

CHRONIC RUNNY, STUFFY NOSE—ALLERGIC RHINITIS

S **Does the child have a cough at night or a stuffy nose? If so, how often?**
Often this will not be mentioned by the parents and will only come up randomly in one
of the routine visits. This question is a good way of screening for allergic rhinitis and
other respiratory problems such as asthma. If the parents answer yes, then you should
probably follow up with more questions about the actual chronicity and frequency of
the problem.

Has the child had his or her tonsils and adenoids removed?
Hypertrophy of the lymphatic tissues that form the Waldeyer ring (including the tonsils
and the adenoids) can be responsible for these symptoms.

What other symptoms does the child have?
Runny nose (rhinorrhea)
Red or itchy eyes
Dry, itchy skin
Rashes may imply atopic dermatitis, which is often linked with chronic nasal symptoms
A chronic cough can be from postnasal drip, asthma, or gastroesophageal reflux disease

What is the seasonal variation in the child's symptoms?
Discovering a seasonal variation may help uncover an allergy.
- Winter: Cold temperatures can cause tissue swelling. Also, it is the most common
  time of year for viral infections.
- Spring: Pollen is a very common allergen.
- Summer: Cut grass is another common allergen.
- Fall: Leaf cutting and leaf blowing can lead to these symptoms.

**If the child has year-round symptoms, ask about some common household
antigens**
    – Pets   – Smoking   – Cockroaches   – Dust

**Does anyone else in the family have similar problems with allergies, asthma,
or snoring?**
Family history in the parents, siblings, or other family members can help suggest a
diagnosis.

 Examine the ears
Serous effusion: Clear fluid behind the tympanic membrane suggests swelling, obstructing passage of air through the Eustachian tube.

Examine the nose
Look for edema of the nasal mucosa that is narrowing the passages. Erythema suggests
an infection, whereas a boggy, blue color suggests allergy. Also check for polyps (pink,
round, fluid-filled structures, protruding down), which suggest that you should start a
workup for cystic fibrosis.

Look at the eyes
Allergic conjunctivitis: Mild erythema or increased vessels in the conjunctiva bilaterally
Allergic shiners: Blue-tinged ring under the eyes

Have the child open his or her mouth in order to view the oropharynx
Cobblestoning: Oropharyngeal bumps resembling a cobblestone road suggest postnasal
drip.
Tonsilar hypertrophy: Tonsils visibly enlarged, touching, or almost touching but not red
or purulent in nature. If the tonsil crosses the midline it is 4+, midline is 3+, 1+ is just
visible.

Gently press on the child's face over each eyebrow and on each cheekbone
Pain on this exam suggests the possibility of sinusitis.

Listen to the lungs

Air should move freely in all areas. Listen for wheezing (a high-pitched noise on expiration); have the pt blow out long and hard to flesh out a wheeze (highly suggestive of asthma).

Examine the skin

Atopic dermatitis: Dry, scaly, nonerythematous rash, especially in the antecubital fossae

Allergic rhinitis

Allergic rhinitis is a chronic inflammatory disease of the nasal mucosae that affects the sinuses, ears, and throat. It can be exacerbated by a variety of allergens, which are likely to be different in different pts.

Differential diagnosis

Viral upper respiratory infection: Likely to be associated with fever, be less itchy, and be more acute in nature

Nasal foreign body: Unilateral, discrete time of onset, less itchy

Comorbid conditions

As noted above, on exam you may find evidence of:

– Chronic sinusitis   – Tonsillar hypertrophy   – Asthma
– Atopic dermatitis   – Allergic conjunctivitis   – Cystic fibrosis

If you have a difficult time controlling allergic rhinitis, consider that there may be a component of one of these conditions and either investigate the possibility further or just treat empirically.

Recommend avoidance of any known allergen

If the parent or pt can identify a clear exacerbating factor such as dust, cockroaches, or mold, the best thing is to limit contact with these things. Allergy testing may also be helpful.

Start inhaled nasal steroids, once a day

These have minimal systemic absorption, so side effects are uncommon. They are highly effective at decreasing the immune response and inflammation, but pts must be aware that they must be used daily, not prn (as needed) for them to work. They do not acutely alleviate symptoms.

Consider a systemic nonsedating antihistamine as the next step in treatment

Cetirizine, fexofenadine, or loratadine are useful alternatives.

Consider obtaining a sleep study for tonsillar hypertrophy. If (+) for apnea, refer to an ear, nose, and throat (ENT) specialist

Sleep apnea should not be allowed to continue because it can cause many problems for the pt. The ENT will likely remove the pt's tonsils and adenoids.

If chronic sinusitis is suspected, start amoxicillin 80 mg/kg/d divided into three doses for 21 days

This should be effective treatment, but if symptoms persist, second-line therapy is Augmentin. If that is still not effective, third-line treatment is clindamycin.

Refer to Chronic Cough (see p. 146) for a detailed discussion on the treatment of asthma

Start lubricating eye drops such as artificial tears for eye symptoms.
Recommend applying moisturizing creams for suspected atopic dermatitis

If, after all of the above treatments, your pt does not improve, refer to an allergist.

HEART MURMUR

S **Have parents ever been told the child has a murmur? Are there any symptoms of heart failure, chest pain, exercise intolerance, cyanosis, or syncope?**

Symptoms of heart failure: Tachypnea, poor exercise tolerance, sweating with feeds, poor weight gain, pallor, periorbital edema, cool extremities.

If there is chest pain, ask specifically about location, radiation, frequency, duration, exacerbating or relieving factors, palpitations, dizziness, syncope.

If cyanosis is intermittent, ask about precipitating factors such as breath-holding or eating.

If there is exercise intolerance, ask about normal activity, comparison with peers, relation to fatigue.

For pts with syncope, see Syncope, p. 366.

Has the child had rheumatic fever (RF) or any of its signs or symptoms?

The Jones major criteria for RF (a good mnemonic is J ♥ NES):
- *J*oints (arthritis)
- ♥ (carditis)
- *N*odes
- *E*rythema marginatum
- *S*ydenham chorea

Were any drugs or medications taken during pregnancy (most likely heart lesion in parentheses)?

Hydantoin (ventricular septal defect [VSD], pulmonary stenosis, aortic stenosis [AS], patent ductus arteriosus [PDA], coarctation)

Valproate (atrial septal defect [ASD], VSD)

Lithium (Ebstein anomaly)

Alcohol (ASD, PDA, VSD, ToF)

Retinoic acid (aortic and conotruncal abnormalities)

Are there any congenital abnormalities or a family history of heart disease?

Trisomy 13, 18, and 21 (VSD)

DiGeorge (ToF, truncus arteriosus)

Williams (supravalvular aortic stenosis, peripheral pulmonary stenosis)

Turner (coarctation, bicuspid aortic valve)

Ehlers-Danlos (mitral valve prolapse [MVP], tricuspid valve prolapse, aortic dilation)

Marfan (MVP, aortic dilation/dissection)

Family history of congenital heart disease, sudden death, or myocardial infarction (MI) in <50-year-old, diabetes mellitus, or hypertension

O **Look at the general appearance**

Consider syndromes such as VACTERL, DiGeorge, Turner, Williams, and Marfan.

Is there a murmur and, if so, is it systolic or diastolic?

To assess whether a murmur is systolic or diastolic, listen very carefully for S_1 and S_2. S_1 should coincide with the pulse and S_2 should split with inspiration. Systole comes after S_1, diastole after S_2.

Where is the murmur best heard?

Aortic sounds: second intercostal space, right upper sternal border

Pulmonic sounds: second intercostal space, left upper sternal border

Tricuspid sounds, VSD: fourth intercostal space, left lower sternal border

Mitral sounds: fourth to fifth intercostal space, midclavicular line with axillary radiation

What does the murmur sound like?

In general, stenosis murmurs are crescendo-decrescendo, and regurgitant murmurs have a uniform sound, with onset coinciding with the valve closure.

What is the grade of the murmur?

Grade I (very hard to hear), II (easy to hear), III (loud/no thrill), IV (loud/thrill), V (loud with stethoscope near chest), VI (no stethoscope needed)

After examining the heart, perform a focused PE

Feel for a hyperdynamic or displaced precordium, thrills, pulses, and organomegaly. Listen carefully to the lungs for rales or wheezes.
Check for clubbing, cyanosis, retractions, and chest surgery scars.

 Heart murmur

Murmurs and bruits, which can be auscultated and sometimes palpated, are created whenever there is turbulent blood flow. The more turbulent the flow, the louder a murmur.

Differential diagnosis

Innocent murmurs:

- *Still murmur*: By far the most common. A systolic vibratory or twanging sound that can be heard at the left lower sternal border and over the mitral valve. Most common in children 4–6 years old but can be in any age.
- *Venous hum*: A continuous murmur (not associated with heart sounds) that can only be heard in the sitting-up position. Usually heard just under the clavicles bilaterally, it is the sound of venous blood returning from the head to the heart. It sounds like a cascading waterfall.
- *Flow murmur*: Can be aortic or pulmonic; occasionally Grade III but usually less; they are whispering midsystolic sounds. They do not sound harsh like stenosis murmurs.
- *Mammary soufflé*: The pulsing sound of increased arterial blood flow to the breast; it only occurs in pregnant women.

If the murmur is not one of these, it is likely pathologic. The most common include:

- *Ventricular septal defect (VSD)*: A regurgitant murmur at the left lower sternal border. It may last throughout systole or may terminate midsystole if the defect closes as the septum contracts. The murmur is louder as the defect becomes smaller.
- *Aortic stenosis (AS)*: A loud, harsh systolic murmur, soft at the end of S_1, loud in midsystole, and soft before S_2 over the aortic area. Note that in the case of congenital bicuspid aortic valve, this murmur is associated with an early systolic click over the mitral valve area.
- *Patent ductus arteriosus (PDA)*: Usually a continuous murmur with a "washing machine"–type quality. It is best heard in the left midclavicular line at the second intercostal space.
- *Mitral stenosis*: Rarely occurs in pts who have not had rheumatic fever; it presents as a low-pitched, diastolic rumble after an opening snap that radiates to the left axilla.
- *Mitral valve prolapse (MVP)*: No sound is heard after S_1 and then a midsystolic click or pop can be heard, followed by a soft blowing sound over the mitral area, which lasts until S_2. It is more common in women and pts with Marfan syndrome.
- *Atrial septal defect (ASD)*: Doesn't cause a murmur per se, but it causes a fixed split to the S_2 (which should normally only be split during inspiration) and, in later years, can mimic tricuspid stenosis as increased right-sided blood volume pours over a size-restricted tricuspid valve.

 Get an echocardiogram, ECG, chest x-ray, and consult cardiology if a pathologic murmur is suspected

All of the above pathologic murmurs can cause serious problems for the pt in the future. ECG and chest x-ray will be helpful, but the echocardiogram will definitively characterize the lesion and the cardiologist will have to evaluate it.

HARD STOOL OR NO STOOL—CONSTIPATION

S **What are the symptoms of constipation in this pt?**
Constipation occurs when the lower colon does not completely evacuate. Symptoms include:
- Involuntary soiling (encopresis)
- Decreasing stool frequency
- Pain with defecation
- Hard stools

Occasional painful defecation and decreased stool frequency alone do not constitute constipation. A child who has only two stools per week is not constipated if these stools are large and soft, and the child is fully evacuated when finished.

At what age did the child become constipated?
Functional constipation: Onset is with a transition in feeding or stooling pattern:
- Breast milk to formula
- Baby food to table food
- Starting cow's milk
- New toilets (preschool)
- Toilet training

Hirschsprung disease: Onset is at birth. Usually the child was kept in the hospital for a delayed first bowel movement.

Does the child soil his or her underwear?
Encopresis (fecal incontinence) represents severe constipation. The colon continues to absorb water from the impacted or retained stool. Soon a large, dry mass plugs up the distal colon and rectum. New liquid stool leaks around the hard mass and is deposited in the underwear.

What are the stools like?
History of small, hard ball–like stools implies incomplete evacuation of any kind.
Rare passage of large, voluminous stools indicates functional stool retention.
Pencil-thin stools and a lack of encopresis are more indicative of Hirschsprung disease.

Is there a family history of constipation or of a constipating disease?
- Hirschsprung disease
- Cystic fibrosis
- Hypothyroidism
- Neurofibromatosis
- Myopathies

O **Check the growth curves for height and weight**
Failure to grow correctly is a red flag for the aforementioned genetic or metabolic diseases.

Perform a complete neurologic exam, including normal sensation of the perineum
An occult myelomeningocele (a disorder where a portion of the spinal cord protrudes through a partially fused spine) can present with mild lower extremity weakness or no more than saddle anesthesia and constipation with encopresis.

Examine the abdomen
Listen for normal bowel sounds.
Palpate the abdomen. Make sure that it is soft and feel for balls of retained stool. Mild tenderness diffusely is consistent with chronic constipation.

Examine the anus externally
Look for fissures or signs of local infection that may produce pain on defecation.

A rectal exam is necessary if you have reason to suspect Hirschsprung disease
Use a lubricated, gloved finger. A normal anal canal will be tight initially, but will relax within moments. A canal that remains tight should lead you to consider Hirschsprung disease or some other cause of distal rectal obstruction.

A plain x-ray of the abdomen may be necessary if the history and PE are inconclusive
Impacted stool will be very clear on KUB.

If you continue to suspect Hirschsprung disease, send the pt for a barium enema

The rectum should be the largest structure; in Hirschsprung disease, it is smaller than the sigmoid.

 ## Constipation

Infantile rectal confusion: Infants cannot voluntarily retain stool, but they can develop an inability to coordinate their Valsalva maneuver with pelvic floor relaxation.

Stool holding or functional constipation (most common): Begins when the child is faced with a situation when he or she feels the urge to defecate, but for some reason wishes to prevent it. This causes little problem in the short-term, but over long periods, the distal colon and rectum begin to become distended. The child resists passing the large, hard stool for as long as possible because of the expected pain. When the stool passes, their expectations are fulfilled. For a few days, their symptoms are relieved, but the cycle continues.

Hirschsprung disease: A defect of the rectum beginning at the anus involving a variable distance of rectum and even colon. The involved large bowel fails to develop normal innervation, so when stool arrives it fails to dilate. The proximal normal bowel distends until it is noticed and corrected surgically.

Differential diagnosis

Lack of stool: Infantile botulism, irritable bowel syndrome, intestinal atresia/stenosis

Encopresis: Crohn disease, ulcerative colitis, bloody diarrhea (colitis), cystic fibrosis, malabsorptive syndromes

Pain on defecation: Rectal fissures/fistulas, herpes

Blood in stool: Colitis, fissure/hemorrhoids, rarely cancer

 ### Educate the parents regarding the threefold treatment of functional constipation

Increased dietary fiber is ineffective until muscle tone is restored. Treatment failure is common and usually results from weaning medications too quickly. Even with proper treatment, up to 50% recur.

Start with total evacuation, the first phase of treatment

Mineral oil followed by enemas. Polyethylene glycol orally for 2–5 days.

Next recommend diet changes, behavior modification, and medications to maintain evacuation

Place the pt on a low-dairy, low-fiber diet, and give oral mineral oil, milk of magnesia, or lactulose.

Encourage the child to use the toilet with positive rewards and a daily star chart.

If evacuation is sustained after 3–12 months, slowly wean the medication

Decrease by one dose each month until the medication is stopped.

May use a bisacodyl suppository if the child goes 3 days without stooling.

If the barium enema indicates Hirschsprung disease, refer to a surgeon for a biopsy looking for aganglionic bowel

SHORT STATURE

S **Has the child always been small or has he or she just recently stopped growing?**
A child who has always been small may have genetic short stature. The parents may not be very tall, or the child may have a genetic syndrome.

Was the child small at birth?
A child with intrauterine growth restriction may have a genetic reason to be small.

What are the parents' expectations for the child's height?
Occasionally, short parents have unrealistic expectations of their child's height.

Obtain the height of both parents and whether either had a delayed growth spurt
Using this information a mid-parental height can be calculated to see if the family has delayed growth.

Does the child have any chronic illnesses that the parents know of?
All of the following can cause short stature:

- Inflammatory bowel disease
- Chronic anemias
- Celiac disease
- Treatment with steroids
- Renal disease
- Diabetes
- Cystic fibrosis
- Congenital heart disease
- Liver disease
- Asthma

How is the child eating?
Malnutrition can be a cause of short stature (e.g., a picky eater who consumes no protein).

O **Plot the child's growth on a standardized growth chart**
The child's height may fall within the normal range for age.
It is very common for the parent to think that the child is short when he or she is actually normal.
If the child is below the 5th percentile for height, it is important to recheck to make sure that the measurement was done accurately.

- Three heights should be measured with a stadiometer and then averaged.
- Make sure the child has his or her head, shoulders, and bottom against the wall.

If this is not the pt's first visit to the clinic, there should be other data available on the growth chart. Check a growth velocity. Normal growth is as follows:

- Toddlers grow 7.5–13 cm in the second year of life.
- From 3 years to puberty, children should grow at about 5–6.5 cm per year.
- Adolescents have a variable growth rate, but increased growth follows the onset of puberty. Girls generally begin puberty at age 10 years, whereas boys start later, at about age 12.5 years. If a girl reaches age 13 or a boy 15 with no signs of puberty, this should be investigated.

A child who is below the fifth percentile but has normal growth velocity is probably normal.
If the growth velocity is less than normal, it should be worked up.

Plot a mid-parental height on the growth chart
For girls it is [(the father's height − 13 cm) + the mother's height]/2.
For boys it is [(the mother's height + 13 cm) + the father's height]/2.
A child's target height is the mid-parental height ± two standard deviations (about 10 cm).
Therefore, a child's current percentile spot should track to the mid-parental height ± 10 cm. If it does, then the child's height is appropriate, even if the child is less than the fifth percentile.

Now plot the child's weight

Weight should track to a similar percentile as height.

If the child is obese compared with the current height, and the child is tracking to below the mid-parental height, consider an endocrinopathy such as:

- Hypothyroidism
- Cushing syndrome
- Growth hormone deficiency

If the child's weight percentile is below where the height is plotted, and the child is tracking to below the mid-parental height, consider a chronic disease such as:

- Renal failure
- Cystic fibrosis
- Celiac disease
- Inflammatory bowel disease

Perform a generalized PE, looking for signs of chronic disease

A child with hypothyroidism may have coarse skin, hair loss, and eyebrow thinning.

Cushing syndrome may present with centripetal obesity, muscle wasting, and striae.

Hepatosplenomegaly and jaundice are consistent with chronic liver disease.

Abnormal features may indicate a genetic or chromosomal anomaly. Webbed neck, shield chest, and widely spaced nipples may indicate Noonan or Turner syndromes.

If the pt does not track to near the mid-parental height, check a CBC, an erythrocyte sedimentation rate (ESR), a chem 7, a thyroid-stimulating hormone, and order a radiographic bone age

These labs will help you rapidly rule out renal failure, inflammatory disorders (if the ESR is normal), and hypothyroidism.

A Familial short stature versus constitutional growth delay

Familial short stature: The pt is less than fifth percentile for height, has a normal growth velocity, and tracks to the appropriate mid-parental height. The pt is genetically short.

Constitutional growth delay: These pts are less than fifth percentile, have a normal growth velocity, and a delayed bone age. Labs are normal. The pt will be a "late-bloomer," have a growth spurt later on, and catch up to where he or she needs to be.

Differential diagnosis of abnormal growth velocity and delayed bone age

- Renal disease
- GI disease
- Hypothyroidism
- Cushing syndrome
- Genetic syndrome
- Growth hormone deficiency
- Cerebral palsy
- Cystic fibrosis
- Any chronic condition

Abnormal growth velocity with advanced bone age

Precocious puberty

P If the child has familial short stature or constitutional growth delay, give reassurance

In the case of constitutional growth delay, the child will grow normally and will achieve the expected mid-parental height. In the case of familial short stature, the child will not be tall but is appropriate. No treatment is needed.

For suspected endocrinopathies or chronic diseases, refer to an endocrinologist for possible growth hormone therapy

NOSEBLEEDS

 How often does the child have nosebleeds?

Chronicity may imply an ongoing problem such as:

- Nose-picking   – Dry environment
- Telangiectasia   – Bleeding diathesis

How long do the nosebleeds last?

If the nosebleed is treated appropriately, it should not last more than a few minutes.

What is the child doing to stop the bleeding when it occurs?

Stopping a nosebleed requires tight pressure applied just anterior to the bony part of the nose for about 2–5 minutes without checking to see if it is still bleeding.

If the child is holding the pressure up on the bone instead of in front of it or leaning over a bowl with ice on the forehead and not holding the nose, bleeding may last longer than expected.

Which side of the nose bleeds?

Nosebleeds tend to occur from only one nostril.

When the pt has bleeding from both nostrils at once, this should make you concerned regarding a problem with clotting (see Easy Bruising or Mucosal Bleeding, p. 188).

Ask the child "Which finger do you use to pick your nose?"

Trauma from nose-picking is far and away the most common reason for recurrent nose-bleeds, and this question has a way of surprising the answer out of children.

Does the child have cold symptoms such as cough, runny nose, and stuffy nose?

Although it would be rare for the parents to leave this information out of the history, upper respiratory infections are associated with nosebleeds.

Nasal congestion may lead to the parent using a topical decongestant spray. These tend to irritate the nasal mucosa and may cause bleeding.

Is the child coughing up or spitting up blood?

This is a symptom of inappropriate therapy. It is often worrisome for the parents, who will usually bring it up on their own.

Implies the head is being held back to stop the bleeding and blood is dripping into the throat.

Does the child put foreign bodies (tissue, marbles, etc.) in his or her nose?

Foreign bodies can cause nosebleeds from irritation and erosion of the mucosa.

O **Is the child actively bleeding at this time?**

If the child is actively bleeding, stop the bleeding using the technique described above.

How does the child appear?

Other than slightly frightened over the nosebleed, the child should appear well with a normal energy level and entirely interactive with the parent and you. Check for any pallor or jaundice.

Using an otoscope with a speculum, examine the inside of the nose

If the child has been bleeding recently, you may see dried blood in one nare.

The mucosa should appear pink and healthy.

Make note of any clusters of capillaries (telangiectasias) on the mucosa.

Mucosa that has been exposed to chronic decongestant use may appear red and swollen, leaving little room for the passage of air.

Blue, boggy mucosa may be irritated because of allergies.

If you live in a dry climate, or it has been dry recently, the mucosa may appear dry.

A foreign body should be apparent if it is present.

In an older child or adolescent, rarely the mucosa will appear black. This may be a sign of a necrotizing lesion. The differential diagnosis is small:

- Cocaine usage can cause necrosis of the septum and nosebleeds.
- In diabetics or neutropenics, a fungal infection called *Mucor* can have this appearance. It is an emergency referral to otolaryngology (ENT).
- Wegener granulomatosis

Complete a rapid PE

A blowing heart murmur or an S_3 may represent high-output heart failure secondary to extreme blood loss or anemia.

Note any hepatosplenomegaly or other abdominal masses.

A petechial rash (small red spots that do not blanch when you press on them) represents bleeding under the skin. Together with nosebleeds, this is a sure sign that the child has a bleeding diathesis such as idiopathic thrombocytopenic purpura (ITP).

Blood dripping down into the oropharynx represents a posterior nasal cavity bleed.

A Epistaxis (nosebleed)

Epistaxis is commonly associated with a set of blood vessels known as Kiesselbach plexus. This plexus may bleed spontaneously, although picking is the most likely cause.

Differential diagnosis

Bleeding diathesis: von Willebrand disease, hemophilia, leukemia, ITP

Other processes: Wegener granulomatosis, nasal steroids, mucormycosis, vitamin C deficiency, vitamin K deficiency, taking aspirin, being on heparin, nasal cocaine

P First, stop the bleeding as indicated above. Educate the parents on how to do the same

Parental education should also include the benign nature of the disease and that nosepicking may be the cause. Parents also need to understand that nasal decongestants cannot be used chronically without serious side effects on the nasal mucosa.

If bleeding cannot be stopped, or there is reason to suspect a bleeding disorder, check a CBC with differential, PT, PTT, and a chem panel

This should help rule in or rule out a chronic disease.

If the bleeding still cannot be stopped, call ENT for packing or cautery

Remember that adolescent males may have a benign tumor of the sinuses called an angiofibroma. It may cause recurrent bleeding and will require ENT evaluation as well.

ACNE

S **What is the pt doing about his or her acne?**

This is a way of bringing up the topic. Many times, acne is not the chief complaint. It will not even be mentioned as a problem until you bring it up, but when you do, you will usually see the pt respond with relief and interest that you addressed the issue.

It is also important to know what medications have been used in the past or are currently being used to attempt to treat the acne so therapy can be tailored appropriately.

What medications are being used?

It is important to obtain a drug history. Those medications for other conditions that may worsen acne include:

– Corticosteroids	– Lithium	– Isoniazid
– Rifampin	– Hydantoin	

Oral contraceptive pills may worsen or improve acne.

What hair or cosmetic products are being used?

Makeup with lanolin or oil or any grease used in the hair can worsen acne.

How many times a day does the pt wash his or her face?

It is important that the pt understand that frequent washing with harsh soaps can actually make acne worse. Adolescents should only wash once or twice a day with a mild soap.

What type of activities is the pt involved in at school or after school?

Activities such as football, with helmets, shoulder pads, etc., can worsen acne.

If the teen is involved in working out at the gym, you may want to ask if he or she is using anabolic steroids. These are certain to increase acne.

When was the pt's last menstrual period, and have they been regular?

Oligomenorrhea may suggest other comorbid conditions that worsen acne (see below). However, it is worth noting that adolescents in the first 2 years of their menstrual cycle commonly have irregular and infrequent periods.

Ask if the pt is sexually active

Some of the acne medications, including isotretinoin (Accutane) and tetracycline can be extremely teratogenic. Using two forms of contraception simultaneously is advised.

O **Observe the lesions and describe what you see**

Acne lesions can be broken down into three groups:

- *Obstructive lesions*: Comedones are small; white (closed comedones) or black (open comedones) papules that may or may not be surrounded by an area of erythema. These are the "whiteheads" and "blackheads," respectively.
- *Inflammatory lesions*: Erythematous papules, pustules, or nodules. Pts with nodules are more likely to develop cysts and scars, so they should be treated aggressively.
- *Cysts and scars*: Cysts are nodular lesions without overlying erythema, and scars have the appearance of pits. These are often irreversible changes, so these pts should be treated aggressively.

Carefully examine the face, chest, and back and be careful to document the numbers of each type of acne lesion in each area so an assessment of improvement can be made at the next visit.

A **Acne (see below for classification)**

Acne occurs when the sebaceous glands that make the oil that coats the skin become clogged. This becomes extremely common with the hormonal changes seen in adolescence. Open comedones are black because environmental dirt colors them. Inflammatory lesions have become infected with *Propionibacterium acnes*, an anaerobic organism that is ubiquitous on the skin.

Differential diagnosis
Acne has a fairly typical appearance that is not usually confused with other entities, but
    you should consider the following:

- Tuberous sclerosis syndrome
- Congenital adrenal hyperplasia
- Obesity
- Polycystic ovarian disease
- Cushing syndrome
- Pregnancy

You may also see acne-like lesions in babies. This is neonatal acne or neonatal pustular
    melanosis, neither of which requires treatment.

Consider activities or products that may be contributing to the acne
Activities such as football or working in greasy environments such as fast-food restau-
    rants can exacerbate acne and, in severe cases with nodules or scaring, pts should
    consider avoiding these activities.

Hair care products and make-up are good examples of things that can be changed or
    removed from the daily routine to improve the acne.

Assess the severity of the acne (Table 11-3)
The more lesions and locations and the more scars or nodules that are seen, the more
    aggressively you should treat the acne.

TABLE 11-3   Acne Classification

Type of Acne	Total Lesions	Comedones	Inflammatory	Cysts
Mild	<30	<20	<15	0
Moderate	30–125	20–100	15–50	<5
Severe	>125	>100	>50	>5

P Recommend washing with gentle soap at most twice a day
Clarify that acne is not improved and can actually be made worse with frequent
    washing.

Point out that the make-up or hair products they are using may be worsening their acne.

For mild acne, start with 5% benzoyl peroxide gel once a day

For pts with moderate acne, start with 5% benzoyl peroxide gel plus (depending on type)
For comedonal acne: Tretinoin 0.025% cream nightly (to avoid the side effect of sun
    sensitivity)

For inflammatory acne: Clindamycin 1% cream twice a day

For pts with severe acne, use benzoyl peroxide, tretinoin, and oral erythromycin or tetracycline

Consider referral to Dermatology to limit or prevent permanent scar formation
The dermatologist may wish to start the pt on Accutane.

PEDIATRIC EMERGENCY ROOM
ANAPHYLAXIS

S **Is there a constellation of symptoms suggestive of anaphylaxis?**

General: sudden behavior change, irritability, cessation of play
Neuro: Feelings of doom, mouth tingling, tightness in the chest
Resp: Shortness of breath
CV: Dizziness, palpitations
FEN/GI: Stomach pain, nausea/vomiting, diarrhea
Ob/Gyn: Menstrual cramping
Derm: Hives, itching

Ask about previous episodes or history of allergies or anaphylaxis

A history of allergic reactions or anaphylaxis in the past to things such as peanuts, sea-
food, antibiotics, or insect stings will increase your clinical suspicion.

Ask specifically about exposure to medicines, food, and insects or recent exercise

Drugs: Sulfonamides, penicillins, antiepileptics, contrast
Foods: Peanuts, tree nuts, crustaceans, eggs
Stings: Hymenoptera venom (i.e., bee, wasp, fire ants)
Other less common but well-known causes of anaphylaxis include latex, vaccines,
hormones, aspirin, and exercise
Latex allergies commonly cross-react with stone fruits such as avocado, plum, peach, or
cherry

What was the time course of the reaction?

Most anaphylaxis occurs within 30 minutes of exposure (although it can be longer with
ingestions), and in some cases there may be a recurrence 1–8 hours later. The more
rapidly the anaphylaxis occurs and progresses, the more likely the reaction is to be
severe and life-threatening.

O **Examine the pt**

Vital signs: Hypotension and tachycardia are extremely common. Tachypnea would also
be expected.
Neuro: The pt may have altered mental status, a late sign of shock.
Eyes: Periorbital swelling, erythema, injected conjunctiva.
Oropharynx: Tongue and pharyngeal swelling (causing muffling of the voice) can both
occur as hallmark symptoms of angioedema.
Lungs: Wheeze and stridor are both common in anaphylaxis.
Skin: Sweating is common, but the most common finding is of urticaria (erythematous,
raised lesions on the skin that may change location), commonly known as hives. The
pt may be scratching them.
Urticaria and angioedema are the most common symptoms of anaphylaxis (>90%).
The next most common manifestations are respiratory difficulty, then dizziness, syncope, and GI symptoms.

Labs

β-Tryptase level can be drawn to confirm the diagnosis in retrospect. A level above
10 ng/mL indicates mast cell activation.

A **Anaphylaxis or, at its worst, anaphylactic shock**

Anaphylaxis occurs when the immune system is exposed to an allergen, recognized by
an immunoglobulin E (IgE) antibody bound to the surface of a mast cell. If the allergen
is present in sufficient number as to cause cross-linking of IgE on the mast cell surface,
the mast cell is stimulated to degranulate. Its inflammatory cytokines, especially histamine, induce multiple changes, including massive vasodilation and capillary leak.

Differential diagnosis

– Hypovolemic shock	– Septic shock	– Cardiogenic shock
– Panic disorder	– Foreign body aspiration	– Acute intoxication
– Pulmonary embolus	– Seizure	– Vasovagal reaction

Vasovagal reaction will present with bradycardia, whereas anaphylaxis presents with tachycardia.

Rarely will any of the above diagnoses be concurrent with urticaria.

Quickly check responsiveness, assess ABCs, and then place an oxygen delivery system (nasal cannula, or face mask), secure an IV, and attach a monitor

Shock is a medical emergency and should be dealt with as such. Assessing the ABCs is always a good place to start.

Place the pt supine with the feet higher than the head

This will allow for adequate blood return to the heart (and thus to the brain) by gravity.

Administer epinephrine, 1:1,000 (1 mg/mL) at a dose of 0.01 mL/kg (max 0.3 mL in children and 0.5 mL in adults). Repeat Epi as needed every 15 minutes

The number-one drug for treating anaphylaxis is epinephrine.

It can be given intravenously or via an intraosseous line. If no access has been secured, it can even be given down the endotracheal tube.

Consider endotracheal intubation if necessary for laryngeal edema or respiratory failure

Signs of this include worsening stridor or hypoxia over time.

If hypotensive, give boluses of NS 10–20 cc/kg and consider pressors such as dopamine

This may be necessary to counteract the massive vasodilation.

If lower airway obstruction, consider β_2-agonist nebulizer

This may be necessary to open up airway.

If source is insect bite, consider placing tourniquet above reaction site. Be sure to release the tourniquet about every 3 minutes

This will prevent further circulation of the toxin.

Also administer

Diphenhydramine **or** hydroxyzine (H_1 blocker)
Famotidine, ranitidine, **or** cimetidine (H_2 blocker)
Albuterol
Hydrocortisone

If the pt is not improving on these medications or has required intubation, admit to the pediatric intensive care unit. Otherwise, give discharge instructions and a prescription for a home epinephrine delivery system

Tell the pt to avoid the allergen and to return to the ER if the symptoms recur.

Educate on the proper use and storage of home epinephrine.

If this is a recurrent event, and the allergen is unknown, refer to an allergist for testing

SEIZURE

S **When did the seizure start?**

Status epilepticus is defined as more than 30 minutes of continuous seizure activity or two or more sequential seizures without full recovery of consciousness between seizures.

The longer the seizure lasts, the more refractory it becomes to treatment.

Treat seizures lasting longer than 10 minutes as if they are status epilepticus.

Also specify how many seizures in the past 24 hours and length of postictal period.

What did the seizure look like?

Generalized tonic-clonic seizures: Characterized by whole body stiffening, then shaking

Partial seizures: Demonstrate one specific body part twitching or shaking

Absence seizures: Brief spells of staring

What was the child doing before the seizure started?

More specifically, was there head trauma, prolonged fast, or a new medicine before the seizure?

Has the child had a seizure before?

A first-time seizure or new seizure pattern prompts more of an investigation (head CT scan or MRI and EEG) than another seizure in a pt with a known seizure disorder.

Does the child have a known brain disorder?

Cerebral palsy, autism, and many genetic lesions are associated with seizure. Even if the child has never had a seizure before, these conditions would suggest the onset of a seizure disorder.

Did the child have a fever?

If seizure occurs at the time of a fever, consider two things: meningitis and febrile seizure.

Any focal aspects?

I.e., unilateral movements, eye deviation, head turning in one side.

O **Is the pt stable?**

Look at the pulse oximeter and vital signs. If they are not stable, go back to the ABCs (i.e., airway, breathing, circulation) of pediatric advanced life support and consider intubation if a gag reflex is absent.

Is the pt still having a seizure?

Neuro exam: Responsiveness, pupillary reaction, reflexes, posture, tone

Seizure stopped: Responsive and verbally follows commands (if age appropriate)

Seizure ongoing: Tachycardia, eye deviation, increased tone, and/or clonic movements

If febrile and between the ages of 6 months and 6 years, look for a source of infection

This especially pertains to the ears, throat, and urine. Identifying a source of fever may save this child from having a lumbar puncture if you suspect febrile seizure.

Check some stat labs to rule out some of the common/easily modifiable causes of seizures

Glucose: Hypoglycemia can precipitate a seizure. May check quickly by fingerstick.

Electrolytes: If the seizure is ongoing. Hypo/hypernatremia can both cause seizures.

Consider a blood and urine toxicology screen (see Chemical Ingestions, p. 182).

Antiepileptic medication levels: Check for low levels, indicating a need for either increased dose or increased adherence to therapy.

Seizure

Seizures represent massive neuronal discharge in the brain, producing physical symptoms.

Differential diagnosis

Generalized tonic-clonic (GTC) or *grand mal:* Stiffening, then shaking of the entire body.

Absence (petit mal): Generalized seizure with loss of consciousness (LOC). Subtle movements (blinking/lip-smacking). Lasts seconds. EEG shows 3-Hz spike and wave pattern.

Complex partial: Starts with abnormal movements restricted to one part of the body. Consciousness is lost. Commonly, secondary generalization occurs.

Simple partial: This rare seizure type involves abnormal movements of only one body part. The "simple" designates the fact that there is no LOC.

West syndrome (infantile spasm) (poor prognosis): Neurodegenerative disorder that presents at about 3–6 months of age with a unique seizure where the infant bends at the waist and throws arms out to the sides.

Psychogenic: This is a nonepileptic seizure with high frequency movements, negative EEG, eyes are usually closed during event, and associated with sobbing, moaning, or coughing usually when other people are around. History of childhood trauma or physical/sexual abuse is usually involved.

Febrile seizure versus meningitis

Febrile seizures: Are usually GTC and last <15 minutes. Postictal period tends to be short and mild. Rarely occur in children before 6 months of age and never after 6 years. They are completely benign (no damage to the brain) and are extremely unlikely to recur.

Meningitis: If the seizure was focal, lasted >15 minutes, the pt had >1 seizure, is <6 months or >6 years, or is obtunded, then rule out meningitis. Check CT, LP, and admission for observation.

For pts with known seizure disorder, fever lowers the seizure threshold.

 If there is no resolution within 10 minutes, give IV lorazepam 0.1 mg/kg or rectal diazepam 0.4 mg/kg. Repeat lorazepam if there is no resolution in 5 minutes

Benzodiazepines are central nervous system (CNS) depressants that are safe and effective at stopping seizures.

If the seizure continues, give fosphenytoin 20 mg phenytoin equivalents/kg IV q 15 minutes up to two times. Then begin a maintenance dose of 4–8 mg PE/kg q 12 hours if the seizure stops

Phenytoin (Dilantin) stabilizes sodium channels and is highly effective at stopping a seizure. Fosphenytoin is a preparation that runs faster in an IV and causes less local tissue damage.

If the seizure continues, intubate and give phenobarbital 20 mg/kg loading dose and then 5 mg/kg/dose q 15 minutes until seizure controlled

Barbiturates, like benzodiazepines, are effective CNS depressants.

Consider a Versed or propofol drip for further active seizure activity

Admit

Intubated pts who are still having a seizure to the ICU

New-onset seizures (unless they are febrile or absence) for workup

All suspected meningitides for treatment

Discharge

Suspected febrile seizure pts home with parental reassurance.

Pts with known seizure disorders whose seizures have stopped. Be sure to redose their medications.

Suspected absence seizures with an outpatient EEG and neurology clinic follow-up.

SYNCOPE

S **Have the parent and child (if old enough) and any witnesses available to describe the event**

Often the parent will tell you that the child appeared pale, diaphoretic, and nonresponsive.

Rarely, you will hear of involuntary, "seizure-like" movements and urinary incontinence. This history does not necessarily indicate a seizure.

Pt's symptomatic prodrome often includes:
- Lightheadedness
- Darkening visual field
- Auditory changes
- Headache
- Nausea

Unconsciousness should not last more than a minute or two.

What was the child doing before loss of consciousness (LOC)?

Syncope during exercise: Represents cardiac pathology until proven otherwise.

Vasovagal reaction: Caused by activities that increase intrathoracic pressure, such as coughing, urinating, defecating, and even strong emotions such as fear or surprise.

Prolonged upright posture: Especially in a warm environment with knees locked, can lead to blood pooling in the lower extremities and poor venous return.

Breath-holding: A benign syncope in infants and toddlers in which the child gets so worked up during a temper tantrum that he or she does not breathe.

Hyperventilation: Reduces serum carbon dioxide levels. When this happens, cerebral blood flow decreases and unconsciousness may ensue.

Has this ever occurred before?

Benign reflex syncope (vasovagal response) often recurs for 1–2 years and then resolves.

History of previous syncope with exercise raises suspicion of cardiac disease.

Ask about other possible symptoms of cardiac syncope

Palpitations or chest pains before LOC

Lack of warning signs, especially if there was an injury with the associated fall (a pt with a vasovagal response is likely to gently slump to the ground or try to lie down)

Has the pt had a recent history of increasing fatigue or decreasing exercise tolerance?

This may be another sign of a worsening cardiac lesion.

Is there a family history of syncope, early-unexplained death, or any other heart problem?

All of these should once again prompt a cardiac evaluation.

O **Begin by checking the pt's vital signs**

Tachyarrhythmias and bradycardia can both be causes of syncope.

Carefully check orthostatic blood pressure

Have the pt lay supine for 2 minutes. Record the heart rate and BP.

Have the pt sit up for 3 minutes. Record the heart rate and BP again.

Have the pt stand for 5 minutes. This gives the final heart rate and BP.

If the heart rate increases by more than 15 bpm or the systolic blood pressure drops by more than 20 mm Hg on any change of position or between lying down and standing, the pt is said to be orthostatic.

This may indicate a low circulating blood volume or that the autonomic nervous system is not compensating well for postural changes.

Perform a thorough cardiac exam and auscultate in both the supine and upright positions

Record all murmurs and rhythm irregularities. Checking in both positions is important because some pathologic murmurs can be positional. Hypertrophic obstructive cardiomyopathy (HOCM) is a common cause of LOC and sudden cardiac death in these pts. The murmur is systolic and harsh and decreases with passive leg raise.

Obtain an ECG

Arrhythmias: Ventricular tachycardia, supraventricular tachycardia, heart block.

Electrical disturbances:

- *Wolff-Parkinson-White (WPW) anomaly:* An accessory pathway carries electrical signals around the AV node. Shortened PR interval and slurred QRS upstroke (delta wave).
- *Prolonged QT syndrome:* Characterized by a QT interval corrected for rate (QTc) greater than 450 ms. At that rate, a new QRS complex can occur before T wave repolarization has finished, causing an R on T phenomenon, and ventricular tachycardia can result.

A   Benign reflex syncope (a.k.a. vasovagal response)

The pt develops an increased vagal tone, causing bradycardia and hypotension, which resolves when the pt is horizontal and gravity allows redistribution of blood to the brain.

Must rule out neurologic and cardiac causes to make this diagnosis.

Although up to one-quarter of the pediatric population (including adolescents) will develop syncope at some point in their lives, significant pathology is found in <10% of pts.

Differential diagnosis

Breath-holding spell: Benign LOC usually occurs in a crying infant/toddler.

ALTE: See Infant Who Stops Breathing or Changes Color.

Seizures: Involuntarily shaking, convulsion, staring, blinking, or lip-smacking. May not have a prodrome. Lightheadedness and slumping to the ground are uncommon. Pts tend to have minor injuries, including tongue biting. Injury is more common in seizure than syncope.

Cardiac abnormality: WPW, HOCM, long QT syndrome, anomalous coronary artery.

P   If you suspect a cardiac cause, admit the pt and obtain an echocardiogram and cardiology consult

Because of risk of sudden death, monitor the pt until pathology is ruled out or corrected.

For vasovagal responses, encourage increased hydration and increased dietary salt intake

Explain that the child is normal, and although this may recur, it is entirely benign.

If benign syncope is recurrent, you may refer your pt for a tilt-table test

In this test, the pt is strapped to a table that is rotated to a 90-degree position and held there for 10–60 minutes. This may aid in the diagnosis of an etiology for recurrent syncope.

SHORTNESS OF BREATH, WHEEZE, COUGH—ASTHMA

S **Does the child have a history of asthma?**
Previously diagnosed asthma in the pt may make the diagnosis more likely, but be sure to consider alternative diagnoses if the presentation is not typical.

Has the child been to the ER with this problem before?
Multiple previous ER visits may suggest a more severe or poorly controlled asthma.

Has the child been intubated or in the ICU before?
History of previous intubations or ICU admissions for asthma warrants more aggressive treatment to prevent reintubation and risk of death.

Does the child have a history of intubation in the NICU?
This suggests possible lung disease such as laryngo- or tracheomalacia or broncho-pulmonary dysplasia. Clinical course can be more severe as a result of less ability to compensate.

Does the child have frequent nighttime cough?
This may indicate a previously undiagnosed asthma.

Does anyone else in the family have asthma, eczema, or allergic rhinitis?
A family history of allergic disease makes the diagnosis of asthma more likely.

Review other risk factors
More than two admissions in the past year, more than three ER visits in the past year, More than two SABA refills in the past month.

O **Check a pulse oximetry reading and perform a quick, focused PE**
Quickly assess the pt's level of respiratory distress:

– Unable to speak in full sentences
– Accessory respiratory muscle usage
– Tachypnea
– Tachycardia
– Low O_2 saturation
– Nasal flaring
– Tripod posture
– Subcostal retractions
– Abdominal breathing
– Suprasternal retractions

To see most of these symptoms, you must expose the pt's chest wall. A common mistake is the failure to do exactly this. The pt may look very comfortable until you take the shirt off and see retractions and abdominal breathing.

Listen carefully to the lungs
Pts with reactive airway disease will typically have:
• *Wheezing:* A high-pitched sound on expiration; indicates lower airway obstruction.
• *Poor air movement* (a worrisome sign): Lack of sound with visible chest wall excursion.

After treatments, the lungs may actually sound worse, with more wheezing, crackles, and rhonchi because more of the airways have opened up and are subsequently making noise.

Obtain a chest x-ray (CXR)
– Hyperinflated lung fields
– Flattened diaphragms
– Lack of infiltrates
– Atelectasis
– Peribronchial cuffing
– Lobar infiltrates or unilateral pathology suggests other illnesses

If pts can cooperate, have them blow as hard as they can into a peak flow meter
Peak flow will help assess the severity of an acute asthma exacerbation.

Asthma (a.k.a. reactive airway disease), acute exacerbation

Asthma is the most common chronic inflammatory disease of the airways. It is a complex pathologic state in which chronic airway inflammation leads to increased mucus production and bronchoconstriction. Bronchoconstriction causes lower airway obstruction, which is intermittent and reversible with bronchodilators.

Differential diagnosis

Foreign body in the airway if not easily seen on CXR may appear as unilateral hyperinflation of a lung caused by air trapping. The right lung is the more common because the left mainstem bronchus takes off at more of an angle than the right.

Respiratory syncytial virus/viral bronchiolitis: Usually presents with fever and is unlikely to improve with breathing treatments.

Laryngotracheomalacia or bronchopulmonary dysplasia is usually accompanied by a history of a prolonged NICU course with intubation.

Vascular rings and slings are congenital malformations of the aortic arch, which constrict the airway and may lead to wheezing or stridor.

Assess severity of an exacerbation

If the peak flow is less than 30% of the predicted value, this indicates a severe attack. More than 60% is considered a mild attack. Treat severe attacks more aggressively.

Provide supplemental oxygen

Until the pt is no longer hypoxic. Maintain oxygen saturation >94%.

Give a short-acting β_2 agonist, such as albuterol

Begin with a handheld nebulized β_2 agonist (2.5 mg in infants/toddlers [<15 kg], 5 mg in older children/adolescents [>15 kg]) in addition to the supplemental oxygen. If the pt improves significantly, repeat as needed. If not, continue with the treatment until improvement occurs.

Give ipratropium

0.5 mg neb if moderate to severe distress

Give corticosteroids

Equivalent of 2 mg/kg prednisone per day for 5 days should reduce the inflammation. If you are only treating for 5 days, there is no need to taper the dose.

Admit for

Only mild improvement with ongoing respiratory distress or hypoxia. The pt will need albuterol q4h with a respiratory check every 2 hours. If the pt needs continuous albuterol, assess carefully whether pt should be on the regular ward versus in a more monitored setting.

If pt fails to respond or worsens, prepare to transfer to the PICU and consider intubation.

Discharge if

The pt responds well to treatment with complete resolution of hypoxia, retractions, and other signs of respiratory distress. Prescribe a 5-day course of corticosteroids with β_2 agonist as needed. Give clear instructions to the pt's caregivers to return to the ER if symptoms return or if relief medicine (β_2 agonist) is being used regularly without improvement and for patient to follow up with PCP. Ensure that you give an asthma action plan on discharge.

Try to assess whether this is intermittent or persistent asthma

If you assess the pt as persistent, be sure to prescribe a controller medication such as an inhaled corticosteroid for daily use. Give clear instructions to the pt (if old enough) and pt's caregivers on proper use of the spacer and inhaler and be sure to provide a clear asthma action plan (see Chronic Cough/Wheeze, p. 146).

INFANT WHO STOPS BREATHING (BRIEF RESOLVED UNEXPLAINED EVENT—BRUE)

S **Begin by calming the parent(s) and asking them to describe what happened**

Parents may run into the ER with a well-appearing baby in a panic because their baby stopped breathing at home.

Typical stories depict an infant whom the parent observes to be suddenly not breathing, grunting, or straining. There will often be a history of facial (especially perioral) color change to pale or blue.

How long did the event last?

It is important to discern for how long the baby seemed not to be breathing. BRUE refers to events lasting <1 minute in an infant <1 year that is associated with greater than or equal to one of the following: absent, decreased, or irregular breathing; cyanosis or pallor; altered level of responsiveness; or marked change in muscle tone (hypertonia or hypotonia).

How did recovery occur?

One should find out if an attempt was made at CPR, or if other attempts at stimulation were made (shaking or backslapping), or if the infant simply recovered spontaneously.

Has anything like this ever occurred before or since?

To get a general idea of whether this baby has a chronic condition, you would want to know a history of similar events. Recent recurrence, on the other hand, would give an indication of an acute process the child is currently undergoing.

Is the baby premature?

Premature infants have underdeveloped respiratory drive centers and poorly developed lungs. Apneas are more common.

Was the child crying forcefully immediately before the episode?

If so, consider a breath-holding spell, a benign syncope in infants and toddlers in which children get so worked up that they literally stop breathing. Loss of consciousness can result. It can be followed by jerking movements and circumoral pallor or cyanosis but always resolves spontaneously.

O **Place the infant on a monitor to check the vitals and oxygen saturation levels**

Oxygen saturation should be 100%. The infant should be afebrile, heart rate in the 120s–160s with a respiratory rate in the 30s–40s.

Check the growth parameters

Weight or length less than the 5th percentile might indicate failure to thrive.

Head circumference less than the 5th percentile indicates microcephaly. These infants may have underdeveloped brains, which may lead to apneas.

Large infants (greater than 95th percentile) may have been born to diabetic mothers. They are typically immature for their size and may have apneas.

Is there any evidence that the infant is in distress?

– Accessory respiratory muscle usage	– Tachypnea	– Tachycardia
	– Nasal flaring	– Suprasternal retractions
– Low O_2 saturation	– Grunting	– Gasping
– Subcostal retractions		

Perform a full PE, starting with the heart and lungs, proceeding to check capillary refill time and complete the rest of the regular exam

Lungs: Should sound clear without wheezes, rhonchi, or rales.

Heart: There should be no heart murmurs.

Capillary refill: Should be 1–2 seconds.

Facial features: Dysmorphism may indicate a syndromic child.

Anterior fontanelle: Should be flat and soft.

Nares: Should be patent with no mucosal congestion.

Labs

Check CBC and blood cultures to rule out sepsis or other infections.

If in the winter, consider a nasopharyngeal swab to test for respiratory syncytial virus.

 ### Brief resolved unexplained event, a.k.a. BRUE

In the past this event was termed "apparent life-threatening event" but now BRUE is used to describe whenever the event is transient and remains unexplained after an appropriate medical evaluation.

Considered low risk if the patient has ALL of the following: age >60 days, gestational age ≥32 weeks and postconceptional age ≥45 weeks, occurrence of only one BRUE, duration of BRUE <1 minute, no CPR needed, No concerning historical features or physical examination findings.

Because there is no test to prove that it was a simple benign choking episode caused by a momentary lapse in swallow coordination, the only way to be safe is to rule out more dangerous causes such as seizure, decreased respiratory drive caused by a central nervous system (CNS) abnormality, aspiration, etc.

Differential diagnosis of etiologies of a BRUE

Infections: RSV, sepsis, meningitis

Gastroesophageal reflux: Causes laryngeal chemoreceptor stimulation

Neurologic disorders: Seizures; CNS anomalies; breath-holding spells

Idiopathic

 ### Admit most BRUEs for workup and monitoring

Low-risk BRUEs need continuous pulse oximetry, and consider ECG to look at QT interval. In patients with cough, consider testing for pertussis. There is no need for evaluating for systemic infection, blood testing, urine analysis, or imaging. Parents need education and training in CPR and 24 hour with PCP should be recommended.

High-risk BRUEs need a thorough workup including complete blood count, urinalysis, metabolic profile, CXR, and ECG. In addition, if the patient has had change in sensorium, evaluation should include history and laboratory testing to detect accidental ingestion of poison or medications. GERD, neurologic problems, and respiratory infections account for the greatest number of episodes, but it is not enough to rule these in and say this was the cause without ruling out other possibilities.

If the history is highly suggestive of a breath-holding spell, this would be a case where admission and workup are not necessary. Educate the parent

Instruct the parent that the next time the child seems to be crying hard enough to lose consciousness, to quickly blow air in the child's face. This usually averts an episode.

CHEST PAIN

S Ask the child, "Where does it hurt most?"
Have the child point with one finger to the place where it hurts most.

Does the pain radiate, travel, go anywhere else?
Radiation to the jaw or left arm is more consistent with myocardial ischemia (angina).
Radiation to the back is more consistent with pancreatitis or dissecting aorta.
It is unlikely that the child will have any of these problems.

Obtain a good description of the timing of the pain: onset, duration, and frequency
Cardiac chest pain tends to be of sudden onset, lasts minutes, and recurs with exertion.
Noncardiac pain lasts only seconds or is chronic, with gradual onset and variable recurrence.

What number would you use to describe the pain on a scale of 0 to l 0?
Pain scores give an idea of the severity of the pain from the pt's perspective. Keep this in mind if the child appears comfortable, without tachycardia, and says the pain is a l0 out of 10.

How would you describe the pain (sharp, dull, burning, etc.)?
Cardiac pain is usually dull, pressure-like. Sharp, stabbing, or burning pain is less worrisome.

Ask what makes the pain worse or better
Angina: Pain that is worse with eating or exertion.
Pericarditis: Pain that is worse with lying down and improved with leaning forward.
Musculoskeletal: Pain with chest wall palpation and not associated with exertion.
Pain that wakes a child up from sleep is always a worrisome sign.

Are any other symptoms associated with the pain?
Possible cardiac symptoms (all can occur with anxiety as well): Sweating, nausea, paresthesias in the left arm, palpitations, dizziness, syncope, dyspnea
Respiratory symptoms: Dyspnea, cough, wheeze

Ask if the child has ever had this pain before
It is always useful to know if this has ever happened in the past, and if so, what became of it.

Ask a pertinent past medical history. Red flags include
- Malignancy
- Cardiac disease or surgery
- Sickle cell
- Infections (tuberculosis, HIV)
- Previous aortic dissection or conditions such as Marfan, type IV Ehlers-Danlos, or Turner syndrome
- Risk factors for pulmonary embolism
- Rheumatic fever
- Kawasaki disease

Has anyone in the family had a history of heart problems? Red flags include
- Cardiomyopathy
- Inherited hypercoagulable state (factor V Leiden, protein C or S deficiency)
- Sudden death in <50 yr of age
- Syncope

O Perform a physical exam, specifically including
Look for any features suggestive of genetic syndromes associated with a cardiac anomaly.
Look for vital signs consistent with pain (tachycardia or isolated systolic hypertension).
Look for fever (associated with pericarditis, myocarditis or pneumonia).
Look for tachypnea (seen in spontaneous pneumothorax, asthma, pneumonia, pulmonary embolism, hyperventilation syndrome).

Be aware for hypotension (concerning for serious cardiac, pulmonary, or infectious cause of chest pain).

Watch out for narrow pulse pressure or pulsus paradoxus >10 mm Hg (present in patients with large pericardial effusion associated with cardiac tamponade).

Palpate and auscultate the chest wall for tenderness, thrill, displaced point of maximal impulse, or murmur.

Obtain an ECG

This will rule out any major cardiac causes and make the pt and parent feel better.

Check other studies to rule out pathology if indicated by the H&P

Chest x-ray to look at lung fields, heart size, and great arteries

Echocardiogram to check origin of coronary arteries, heart and aortic size, and ventricular function

Exercise stress test to look for arrhythmia or ischemia

 Chest pain

Pain can occur for a variety of different reasons, but because myocardial infarction (MI) is the number-one killer of adults in the United States, we are often overly concerned about this rare possibility in pediatrics. Having said this, keep in mind that in rare situations, such as anomalous coronary artery or ectasias caused by Kawasaki disease, pediatric MIs are still possible.

Differential diagnosis

Benign adolescent chest pain: 8–16 years old, symptoms for months, sharp knife-like pain, variable severity, occurs at rest, brief paroxysmal episodes, normal PE and ECG

Chest wall (35%): Trauma, herpes zoster, costochondritis, slipping rib, muscle strain

Pulmonary (10%): Asthma, pneumothorax, pulmonary embolus, pneumonia

GI (5%): GERD, odynophagia, esophageal spasm, pancreatitis, biliary colic

Psychogenic (10%–30%): Hyperventilation syndrome, anxiety attack, stress

Unknown (10%)

Check the ECG for ST segment elevations corresponding to different coronary arteries (Table 12-1)

If you see ST segment elevations in any of the above patterns, strongly consider MI. If the ST segment elevation is in all leads, consider pericarditis.

Evaluate the ECG for ventricular hypertrophy, long QT (>0.45 second), or arrhythmia.

A normal ECG does not rule out a cardiac etiology, but it does make it less likely.

TABLE 12-1   ECG Results

I	H	aVR	X	V1	S	V4	A
II	I	aVL	H	V2	S	V5	L
III	I	aVF	I	V3	A	V6	L

High Lateral corresponds to I and aVL = left circumflex
Inferior corresponds to II, III, and aVF = right coronary artery
Septal corresponds to V1 and V2 = left anterior descending septal branch
Anterior corresponds to V3 and V4 = LAD diagonal branch
Lateral corresponds to V5 and V6 = left circumflex

 If you suspect noncardiac pain, perform tests to diagnose and treat causes appropriately. If the pain is psychogenic, give reassurance and refer to psychiatry

More than 99% of chest pain pts will be like this. Reassure and send them home.

If the pain is cardiac, monitor the pt carefully and consult Cardiology for intervention

If you suspect MI, give supplemental O$_2$, sublingual nitroglycerine, aspirin, and if necessary, morphine to control the pain. Check a serum troponin level

A good mnemonic to remember this is **MONA**.

   Troponin is a cardiac enzyme. It is present if there is myocardial injury.

ABDOMINAL PAIN—RULE OUT APPENDICITIS

S **When did the symptoms start, and where is the pain located?**

If the pain is long-standing, consider constipation, irritable bowel syndrome (IBS), or possibly inflammatory bowel disease (IBD). For more acute processes, the location is very important:

Generalized: Small bowel obstruction (SBO), Henoch-Schönlein purpura, constipation, IBS, IBD, colitis, gas

RUQ: Hepatitis, cholecystitis, choledocholithiasis, liver abscess

LUQ: Peptic ulcer disease, gastritis, pancreatitis

Periumbilical: Pancreatitis, appendicitis, Meckel diverticulum

Flank: Pyelonephritis, kidney stone

RLQ: Appendicitis, Meckel diverticulum, colitis/IBD

LLQ: Meckel diverticulum, constipation, colitis/IBD

Suprapubic: Urinary tract infection (UTI)

Pelvic: In adolescent females, is associated with a wide differential, including:

– Pelvic inflammatory disease (PID)   – Ovarian torsion

– Endometriosis   – Mittelschmerz

What are the associated symptoms?

Fever, vomiting, and/or diarrhea: Appendicitis, cholecystitis, Henoch-Schönlein purpura, pyelonephritis, hepatitis, liver abscess, UTI, PID

Bilious (dark green) emesis: SBO or ileus

Bloody emesis: Peptic ulcer disease

Bloody stool: Colitis/IBD, Meckel diverticulum, intussusception

When was the pt's last normal bowel movement (BM)?

Important for generating the differential diagnosis. No BMs versus diarrhea suggests different entities.

O **How old is the pt and is he or she the appropriate size?**

Age is also an important factor in making diagnoses such as pyloric stenosis more or less likely.

Pts with chronic inflammatory processes are usually small for age.

Perform a PE

Some illnesses that can mimic abdominal complaints include:

• *Group A strep pharyngitis:* Causes a mesenteric adenitis, mimicking an appendicitis

• *Pneumonia:* Can cause RUQ or LUQ pain

• *Testicular torsions:* Radiate to the lower quadrants

Does the pt have a surgical or nonsurgical abdomen?

Surgical abdomens (suggesting diseases that will require surgery) imply peritonitis:

• *Guarding:* The abdominal musculature will contract on palpation of the area with pain.

• *Rebound:* Pain occurring when you abruptly remove your fingers after palpating deeply.

• *Percussion tenderness:* Significant pain with tapping abdominal wall.

• *Pain with movement:* Pts with peritoneal inflammation hold very still. If the pt is writhing in pain, it is less likely to be a surgical abdomen. If you are uncertain, have the pt jump up and down (if it is a child) or have the mother bounce the pt on her knee (if it is a toddler). If this is tolerated without pain, surgical abdomen is unlikely.

Although the entire abdomen may be tender, there is usually a point of maximal tenderness:

• *RLQ:* Appendicitis

• *Epigastrium:* Perforated peptic ulcer disease

• *RUQ:* Cholecystitis

• *Periumbilical area:* SBO, pancreatitis (pancreatitis will rarely require surgery)

Perform specific tests for appendicitis, if it is suspected

Rovsing sign: Palpation anywhere in the abdomen causes pain in the RLQ.

Psoas sign: Hyperextending the right leg at the hip causes pain.

Obturator sign: With the right leg flexed at the knee and hip, abducting the hip worsens pain.

Rectal: Palpation of the right rectal wall is exquisitely tender.

Perform an abdominal x-ray (kidney-ureter-bladder, KUB)

This will not always give you the diagnosis, but it may show an RLQ fecalith in the case of appendicitis, calcifications in the case of kidney stones, or distended loops of bowel in an SBO.

If highly suspecting appendicitis, obtain an ultrasound and/or CT scan.

Rule out appendicitis

Appendicitis can occur at any age but is most common near adolescence.

Most common cause of abdominal pain requiring surgery in children.

Results from an obstructed, infected appendix with pus and pressure.

Presentation is variable, but it commonly begins with periumbilical pain and then vomiting and loss of appetite. In several hours, the pain moves to the RLQ and the pt will hold still so as to not exacerbate the pain. If left untreated, the pain worsens, comes to a climax, and then improves as the appendix perforates. If still left untreated, pain will again worsen and the pt may become septic. If an abscess cannot be walled off, death may follow.

Differential diagnosis

As can be implied from the subjective portion of this SOAP, the differential diagnosis is massive. If the pt has an H&P consistent with appendicitis, consider:

- Constipation   – Mittelschmerz   – Ovarian torsion
- Colitis   – PID

P   **If the abdomen is surgical, call the surgery team immediately to evaluate it. These pts should be admitted. If the abdomen is nonsurgical, further diagnostic tests include**

Blood for CBC, chemistry panel (Na, K, Cl, HCO_3, BUN, Cr, glucose; especially if the pt has been vomiting), liver panel, amylase, and lipase (elevated in the case of pancreatitis).

Elevated WBC count, neutrophilia, and bandemia on CBC are all consistent with an inflammatory process but are very nonspecific.

Check a U/A

Leukocyte esterase and nitrites positive suggest a UTI.

Blood could indicate a stone or Henoch-Schönlein purpura.

Perform an U/S and/or CT of the abdomen and pelvis if still unsure of the diagnosis

Appendicitis is sometimes seen. Other diagnoses may also be made this way.

INFANT WITH PROJECTILE VOMITING—PYLORIC STENOSIS

S **How old is the child? How long has this been going on?**
Pyloric stenosis usually occurs at about 2–4 weeks of age but may be seen up to
   3 months of age.
Emesis will usually start around the second to third week of life and progressively
   worsen.

How long after feeding does the child vomit? How many times per day?
Vomiting should occur within about half an hour of every, or nearly every, feed.

Is the vomiting truly projectile?
The vomiting should be described as traveling some distance, possibly across the room.

What is the color of the emesis?
Emesis should look like the recently consumed milk. It should not be dark yellow or
   green. This would imply the presence of bile in the emesis, which would suggest
   another diagnosis.

Is the pt a boy or a girl, and is there a family history of pyloric stenosis?
For some reason, boys are more likely (4:1) than girls to have pyloric stenosis.
There is also often a parent or close family member with a history of surgery in infancy.

O **Examine the child carefully. Look for the peristaltic wave and the olive**
Observe the feeding and subsequent vomiting if you are able to. The baby should appear
   hungry during the feeding but forcefully vomit the feed within about half an hour.
Look at the child's abdomen and watch the epigastrium for the peristaltic wave.
Examine the abdomen for the olive by holding the infant's knees up toward its chest.
   Palpate in the epigastrium for a discrete, mobile mass about the size and shape of an
   olive.

Look for signs of dehydration and assess degree of dehydration
See Dehydration, p. 228. A dehydrated baby is consistent with the diagnosis.

Check an abdominal plain film x-ray
A gas-filled stomach with little gas elsewhere supports the diagnosis of pyloric stenosis.

Obtain an U/S of the abdomen
U/S is the best modality with which to look for pyloric hypertrophy. The pylorus
   thickness should be ≥4 mm, pylorus diameter should be ≥10 mm, and pylorus length
   ≥15 mm long to be consistent with pyloric stenosis.

**Check a stat chem 7 and a U/A. Consider CBC, amylase, lipase, liver
aminotransferases**
Hypochloremic alkalosis: Frequent emesis causes a loss of electrolytes produced in the
   stomach, mainly chloride and hydrogen, increasing serum bicarbonate and potassium.
Hypokalemia: In the presence of low intravascular volume, aldosterone increases the
   renal uptake of sodium and wastes potassium and hydrogen. As a result, serum K+ is
   usually low.
Paradoxical aciduria: Despite the apparent metabolic alkalosis (elevated serum bicarbonate), the urine pH will be low. Aldosterone increases H+ excretion to preserve
   intravascular volume.

A **Pyloric stenosis**
This phenomenon occurs in infants at the end of their neonatal period in which the
   pyloric musculature becomes hypertrophied and ingestions cannot pass. More
   common in males. Approximately 30 percent of cases occur in firstborn children. It is
   usually idiopathic, and the natural history is that it would resolve in 1–2 months if left
   alone. Unfortunately, it would be difficult for the infant to survive that long untreated.
   Surgery is the better option.

Differential diagnosis

Gastroesophageal reflux: Must differentiate between true vomiting and spitting up.

Metabolic disorder: Poor weight gain and emesis.

Malrotation/volvulus: Can happen at any age, but is common in this age group. It is differentiated from pyloric stenosis by its bilious emesis and intermittent symptoms. If it is missed, midgut volvulus can compromise blood flow, causing necrotic bowel. Death follows.

Appendicitis: Rarely diagnosed clinically in pts younger than 1 year but has an extremely atypical and serious presentation in this age group because of the inability of the child to talk and the lack of a well-developed omentum to localize the infection.

Duodenal atresia/stenosis: Will generally present with bilious emesis in the NICU.

Necrotizing enterocolitis: Mostly premature babies in the NICU with vomiting, feeding intolerance, heme-positive stools, and radiographic findings.

Hernia or adhesions: Any hernia that becomes incarcerated or adhesions after abdominal surgery can cause a small bowel obstruction, which is associated with bilious vomiting resulting from the dilated proximal small bowel.

Enteritis: Causes large, voluminous, watery stools often resulting from viruses (such as rotavirus and the noroviruses) and bacteria (such as *Escherichia coli* [not O_{157} H_7], *Vibrio cholerae*, and *Salmonella*). The vomiting is caused by distention of the small bowel with the voluminous diarrhea. There may be an associated fever (see Vomiting and Diarrhea, p. 176).

UTI: Many infants with urinary tract infections will vomit, likely secondary to the ileus caused by bowel touching the inflamed bladder or kidney. Fever should be present.

Meningitis: Central vomiting can occur with meningitis caused by any infectious agent but is especially prevalent in viral meningitis. Again, one should see fever.

P **Admit this pt. Assess the degree of dehydration and correct it intravenously**

See Dehydration and Intravenous Fluid Management, p. 228. Maintenance fluids can be started when the dehydration improves.

Make the child NPO, place a nasogastric tube to gravity, and consult a surgeon

After a variable time, decompressing the stomach and getting it to relax some from all of its recent activity, the surgeons will perform a pylorotomy.

Pylorotomy: Involves cutting along the pylorus transversely and sewing it up horizontally, relieving some of the stenosis. The surgery is usually curative, and the child will slowly begin to eat over the next few days and then completely recover with usually no residual sequelae.

VOMITING AND DIARRHEA—ENTERITIS

S **How long has the child been vomiting? Having diarrhea? How many times per day?**

When the pt presents with what may be enteritis, it is important to differentiate it from other possible causes of vomiting and diarrhea.

The time course is important; it is almost always vomiting before diarrhea. Consider alternative diagnoses if:
- *Vomiting follows diarrhea:* Colitis with sepsis, hemolytic uremic syndrome (HUS)
- *Diarrhea never appears:* Pyelonephritis, meningitis, appendicitis

The number of times of each episode per day indicates the severity of the disease.

Is the child's urine output decreased?

A decrease in the average number of wet diapers or voids suggests dehydration.

What is the color of the emesis/diarrhea? Is there blood or bile present in the emesis or blood present in the stool?

Bloody emesis: Suggests an upper gastrointestinal bleed. This may be a component of enteritis, but it can also suggest something more serious.

Bilious emesis: Suggests an intestinal obstruction, often associated with decreased stooling, not diarrhea.

Diarrhea can be many different colors, but frank blood suggests a lower GI bleed, possibly colitis (see Bloody Diarrhea, p. 178). Mucus in the stool also suggests colitis.

Black stool: Suggests an occult upper GI bleed.

Is the child keeping any oral intake down?

This is the most important question; if all of the other questions are missed, this must be asked. All therapy is based on hydrating the child.

O **What are the vital signs?**

Tachycardia indicates a volume-depleted infant. Children can have a normal BP until shortly before cardiovascular collapse. Fever may be present but is less common than with colitis.

How does the child look?

General appearance: A happy, playful child, or a child actively resisting the doctor is likely to be better hydrated than a weak-appearing child with poor coloring.

Hydration: Palpate the fontanelle (if less than 1 year old), assess tear production, assess lips and buccal mucosa for moisture, and capillary refill time.
- Anterior fontanelles may be sunken with dehydration.
- Dehydrated children do not produce tears. This sign is unreliable in infants younger than 3 months.
- The lips and oral mucosa should appear moist and not tacky.
- Push down over the child's heel or great toe and release. Count the number of seconds until the pink color returns. Less than 2 seconds is normal.

Send the blood for electrolytes and BUN and creatinine

If the pt has been vomiting and having a lot of diarrhea, he or she could easily have electrolyte abnormalities or acute renal failure.

Send the stool for viral and bacterial culture

Rotavirus can be tested for using an enzyme-linked immunoassay of the stool.

The only reasons to send stool for ova and parasites are if the pt is immunocompromised or if you suspect *Giardia* or *Entamoeba*.

Enteritis

If the pt has large, voluminous, watery diarrhea, it is likely to be enteritis. The next step is to consider what organism is causing it:

Viral (viruses are usually the cause of enteritis):

- *Rotavirus:* Increased incidence in winter and in children 6 months to 3 years old. Vomiting usually precedes diarrhea, and there may be mild AST/ALT elevation.
- *Norovirus:* Used to be classified as Norwalk viruses, but this is a whole family of viruses that cause enteritis. This form of enteritis is not seasonal and has the same attack rate in all ages. Often associated with outbreaks at gatherings such as picnics or on cruise ships.
- *Adenovirus:* Although they are rarer, adenoviruses can cause enteritis, but they are more commonly associated with upper respiratory tract infections.

Bacteria:

- *Salmonella:* Need more than 5,000 organisms to cause infection. Often associated with raw eggs, ice cream, and people with pet turtles or salamanders. The diarrhea can be bloody.
- *E. coli:* Not $O_{157}H_7$ (causes colitis and HUS) but rather ETEC (enterotoxogenic *E. coli*).
- *V. cholerae:* Massive, up to 10 L per day! Nonexistent outside of the third world.

Protozoa: Giardia actually causes a duodenitis, which leads to large, smelly, fatty stools with bloating, cramping, and gas. It would rarely be confused with enteritis.

Differential diagnosis

 – Colitis – Appendicitis – UTI – HUS – Meningitis

Assess degree of dehydration

See Dehydration and Intravenous Fluid Management, p. 228.

If the child tolerates oral liquid at home and the PE reveals a well-hydrated or 5% dehydrated child, reassure the parents

The child will do well as long as he or she continues to take liquids. Solids will return in time.

If the parents state that the child keeps no oral liquid down, begin oral liquids 1 teaspoon at a time

If the child takes oral liquid in the ER, he or she may be sent home with instructions on slow hydration.

For 10%–15% dehydration, or if the pt fails the oral liquid trial (emesis within 30 minutes), start 20 cc/kg normal saline IV bolus. Draw stat electrolytes while the IV is being placed

Continue IV normal saline until the child makes urine and the appearance improves.

For 15% dehydration and a lethargic child, obtain emergent venous access via an intraosseous line (tibia) bolus NS as above

A child in this state is on the verge of cardiovascular collapse.

Admit for

Failure to tolerate oral liquid, >5% dehydration, or continuing to appear ill after receiving IV fluids.

BLOODY DIARRHEA—COLITIS

S **When did the diarrhea start? How many times per day? Large or small amount? Is there any blood or mucus in the stool? Is there any vomiting?**

Gastroenteritis, as it is commonly called, is actually a misnomer because there is no stomach inflammation associated with the vomiting. In reality, there are two clinical entities:

- *Enteritis:* Few, voluminous, watery, nonbloody stools without mucus, preceded by vomiting. It is more common and more benign.
- *Colitis:* Small, frequent, bloody stools with mucus, rarely with vomiting. These questions will help you distinguish the two.

Is there abdominal pain?

Colitis is often associated with crampy belly pain and tenesmus.

Did the child eat anything out of the ordinary recently?

Because food poisoning is a possible cause of this condition, eating food from street vendors, a restaurant, or just something questionably old from the refrigerator are all useful clues.

Has the child traveled anywhere recently?

Travel increases the risk for an exotic parasitic or bacterial infection.

Is anyone else sick at home?

If other people, both children and adults, are also suffering from this same problem, it is another suggestion that this may be infectious diarrhea.

Is the child's urine output normal or decreased?

This question is a quick way to assess the hydration status of the child.

O **Perform a PE and review of the vital signs**

Vital signs: Tachycardia indicates a volume-depleted infant. Children can have a normal BP until shortly before cardiovascular collapse. Fever is common.

General appearance: A happy, playful child, or a child actively resisting the doctor is likely to be better hydrated than a weak, pale-appearing child.

Hydration: Palpate the fontanelle (if less than 1 year old), assess tear production, assess lips and buccal mucosa for moisture, and capillary refill time.

- Anterior fontanelles may be sunken with dehydration.
- Lack of tears suggests dehydration unless the patient is <3 month old.
- The lips and oral mucosa should appear moist and not tacky.
- Push down over the child's heel or great toe and release. Count the number of seconds until the pink color returns. Less than 2 seconds is normal.

Order appropriate lab tests

Check a CBC. It rarely makes a diagnosis but may help in the following areas:

- WBC count is more likely to be elevated with colitis than enteritis.
- Anemia may suggest prolonged bleeding (iron deficiency) or chronic inflammation. Both can be signs of colonic inflammation.
- Eosinophilia can suggest a parasitic infection.

An erythrocyte sedimentation rate is helpful if autoimmune colitis is suspected.

Check stool for WBCs and occult blood. A guaiac may be performed in the ER to check the latter. Both can be signs of colonic inflammation.

A stool bacterial culture is always a must if colitis is even suspected. If there is still a possibility that this could be enteritis, rotavirus studies may be sent. If the pt is immunocompromised, add a cytomegalovirus (CMV) viral culture as well.

If you suspect parasitic infection, check the stool for ova and parasites (O&P).

Check the stool for *Clostridium difficile* toxin if the patient has been on antibiotics.

Colitis

Bacterial causes:

- *Shigella:* Only infects humans, does not enter bloodstream (septicemia), and is associated with seizures caused by shiga toxin. WBC is mildly elevated with significant left shift (bandemia). Treat with ceftriaxone or azithromycin to reduce the carrier-state in symptomatic children.
- *Salmonella:* Can infect animals such as chickens and turtles and can enter the bloodstream and cause septicemia, especially *Salmonella typhi.* If enteric or typhoid fever is present, it may be without diarrhea with a low (<4,000) WBC. Antibiotics may increase the carrier-state.
- *Campylobacter:* Number-one cause of colitis. It is associated with Guillain-Barré syndrome. Treat with macrolide antibiotics.
- *E. coli* $O_{157}H_7$: Associated with hemolytic uremic syndrome (HUS), which is intravascular hemolysis (schistocytes on peripheral smear), acute renal failure, and thrombocytopenia. Do not give antibiotics because this increases the chances and severity of HUS.
- *Yersinia enterocolitica:* Presentation can mimic appendicitis.
- *C. difficile:* Antibiotics kill the usually protective commensurate organisms in the bowel. The clostridia then grow and secrete a toxin that creates a pseudomembrane over the normal mucosa. Hence the name pseudomembranous colitis.

Parasitic causes:

- *Entamoeba histolytica:* The only reason to check O&P if your host is immunocompetent.
- Infectious worms can cause disease, but unless your patient has traveled to an endemic area, these should be thought of as rare causes.

Immunosuppressed patient: Think of cryptosporidia, microsporidia, isospora, cryptococcus, mycobacterium-avium complex, and CMV.

Inflammatory bowel disease (IBD) such as Crohn disease or ulcerative colitis is the main noninfectious cause of colitis.

Differential diagnosis

- Appendicitis   – Meckel diverticulum   – Intussusception
- Milk protein allergy   – Enteritis

P **Treat hypovolemia/dehydration if present**

See Dehydration and Intravenous Fluid Management, p. 228.

For *Shigella* and *Campylobacter,* give antibiotics but exclude *E. coli* $O_{157}H_7$ and *Salmonella*

Treat pseudomembranous colitis and *Entamoeba histolytica* with oral metronidazole

Call a gastroenterology specialist for suspected IBD

Admit the child if

He or she is dehydrated and not taking oral liquids, if there are signs of sepsis (tachycardia and hypotension not responsive to IV fluids), or if this is a chronic problem.

Consider admission to the PICU for suspected HUS.

INFANT WITH EPISODIC PAIN AND VOMITING—INTUSSUSCEPTION

S **What symptoms was the child having at home?**

Intussusception (a condition in which one portion of the bowel moves into one another, a.k.a. telescoping) initially presents as paroxysms of abdominal pain, with an infant screaming or crying. During these paroxysms, the infant will often appear to be straining, drawing the knees up to the abdomen.

Between paroxysms, the infant may appear to be well, playing and acting normally.

Later the pt is lethargic and occasionally even encephalopathic between paroxysms.

Emesis, especially bilious emesis, is very common.

The parent may also note bloody stools. These stools are often bright red blood mixed with mucus and are called currant-jelly stools because of their resemblance to dark reddish jelly.

How old is the pt?

It is more common in infants but can occur at any age and is extremely uncommon in neonates; 60% of all cases occur in the first year of life, usually between 4 and 10 months; 80% of all cases occur before the second birthday. 10% of cases occur in children over 5 years.

Has the child been recently ill with any other conditions?

It is often associated with a recent infection (especially adenovirus):

    – Otitis media   – Gastroenteritis   – Upper respiratory infection

Noninfectious predisposing events include:

    – Henoch-Schönlein purpura   – Bezoar   – Lymphoma

All of these conditions can cause enlargement of the terminal ileal lymph clusters known as Peyer patches, forming a lead point that is caught up in the peristaltic wave of the intestine and causes a proximal piece to be moved distally, often through the ileocecal valve.

O **Check the vital signs**

Tachycardia and tachypnea, secondary to pain. Fever can be very high, up to 106°F.

As noted above, these pts might have unstable vitals. If the tachycardia and tachypnea are associated with dropping blood pressures, call for help immediately.

Perform a PE, paying particular attention to the abdomen

A careful exam of the abdomen may reveal a tender sausage-shaped mass, usually in the RUQ. It may increase in size during a paroxysm of pain.

Intussusception usually begins at the ileocecal valve.

Dance sign is an empty RLQ on exam caused by intussusception of enough bowel to reach the transverse colon.

Perform a rectal exam

If the entire colon is intussuscepted, the advancing intestine may prolapse through the anus.

Look on the finger of your glove for bloody mucus (currant-jelly stool). This is highly suggestive, but its absence does not exclude intussusception.

Perform an abdominal x-ray series

There may be dilated loops of small bowel or a paucity of bowel gas. There may even be a soft tissue mass in the area of the intussusception.

Check a CBC

A WBC count between 10,000 and 18,000 is common.

If you are still not convinced, obtain an abdominal U/S

A tubular mass can be seen in longitudinal view and a doughnut-shaped mass in transverse view. Classical manifestation is a "target sign" (also known as "bull's eye" or "coiled spring") representing layers of intestine within intestine.

Intussusception

Intussusception is a common condition, but it can be lethal if misdiagnosed. When the bowel telescopes, it drags its mesentery with it, which becomes constricted in the tight loop of bowel. This leads to poor venous return, further swelling, and more constriction. The currant-jelly stool is caused by leaking of blood from this engorged bowel. If this process is allowed to continue, the bowel will eventually die and become necrotic from lack of blood supply and the oxygen it carries. Necrotic bowel must be removed or the pt will die.

Differential diagnosis

- Malrotation
- Enteritis
- Mesenteric adenitis
- Renal stones
- Acidosis (as in diabetic ketoacidosis)
- Gastroesophageal reflux disorder
- Pelvic inflammatory disease

- Volvulus
- Colitis
- Mesenteric ischemic
- Ileus

- Appendicitis
- Obstruction
- Biliary tract stenosis

- Bowel obstruction has a subdifferential including:
  - Stool
  - Stricture

  - Bezoar
  - Tumor/lymphatic tissue

  - Parasites

Intussusception can also be mistaken for meningitis because of the lethargy occurring between paroxysms and the associated high fever.

In pts who are out of the usual age range, or who are having a recurrent intussusception, evaluate for a possible pathologic lead point

Lead points include:
- Inverted appendiceal stump
- Duplication

- Meckel diverticulum
- Lymphoma

- Intestinal polyp
- Sarcoma

Rarely, intussusception will be the first sign of cystic fibrosis because it can happen to these pts when they become dehydrated.

Send the pt for an emergent barium or air-contrast enema

Before U/S, barium enema was the diagnostic procedure of choice. It shows barium leaking around the intussuscepted bowel in a coil-spring appearance; however, it was also noted that the hydrostatic pressure built up behind the telescoping bowel often reduced the intussusception.

If performed within the first 48 hours, reduction occurs in approximately 75%–80% of pts. After 48 hours, this number drops to 50%.

Air contrast has reduced the rates of perforation from 0.5% to 2.5% with barium to <0.2%.

If the enema does not work, call an emergent surgery consult

The pt will require an emergent laparotomy to attempt surgical reduction. If reduction seems impossible during surgery, or if the bowel already seems necrotic, the intussusception will be excised and an end-to-end anastomosis performed.

Ileo-ileal intussusception (rare) is unlikely to reduce with enema, and most require surgery.

CHEMICAL INGESTIONS

S **Ask the parents if they know what their child took**

All of the following differ in threat to life and type of supportive care required. Some of these toxins even have an antidote:
- Medications
- Cleaning agents
- Alcohol
- Plants
- Hydrocarbons (like gasoline)
- Illicit drugs
- Lead paint

If the parents identify the toxin as a medication, but do not know what type, or state that multiple open pill bottles were found, ask what kinds of meds are in the house or what kinds of medical conditions the people who live in the house have

This line of questioning will help narrow down the field of possible drugs. If possible, have someone bring in the pills and bottles that are left.

When did the ingestion occur?

Many actions you may take depend on how long it has been since the ingestion.

If the pt is an adolescent, it is important to ask if the ingestion was intentional

Perform a HEADSS exam with the parent(s) out of the room (see Well-Child Care: Adolescent, p. 142).

Has the child had any symptoms?
- Change in mental status
- Vomiting
- Fevers
- Seizures
- Headaches

O **Evaluate the pt's general appearance**

Often the pt will either appear well (most common) or altered/obtunded. Emergently evaluate the obtunded pt, and if the gag reflex is not present or the Glasgow Coma Score <8, intubate.

Perform a rapid, but general PE. Attempt to identify certain "toxidromes," recognizable clusters of symptoms and signs that occur with certain poisonings

Anticholinergics and sympathomimetics: Pupillary dilation (mydriasis), tachycardia, low-grade fever, urinary retention
- *Anticholinergics* (belladonna, atropine, Jimson weed): Flushing, dry mucous membranes, altered mental status, decreased bowel sounds
- *Sympathomimetics* (cocaine, methamphetamine): Diaphoresis, increased bowel sounds

Cholinergics (insecticides, succinylcholine, pilocarpine) opposite of anticholinergics: Diaphoresis, pupillary contraction (miosis), wheezing, bradycardia, diarrhea, hyperactive bowel sounds, urinary incontinence, excess pulmonary secretions.

Salicylates: Tinnitus, nausea, anion gap acidosis, vomiting, tachypnea (to the point of respiratory alkalosis), ketonuria.

Opiates (morphine, fentanyl): Nystagmus, miosis, decreased mental status, bradypnea.

Tricyclic antidepressants (amitriptyline, nortriptyline, imipramine): Seizures, acidosis, coma, hypotension, tachyarrhythmias, prolonged QRS complex.

Phenothiazines (haloperidol, chlorpromazine): Dystonia, fever, rigidity, tremor, oculogyric crisis, prolonged QT, coma.

Caustic ingestion (lye, acid, cleaners): Check mouth/lips for evidence of burns.

Check labs

Check serum and urine toxicology screens (include acetaminophen and aspirin levels if unknown ingestion) and also check liver and renal function.

Check chem 7 for acidosis. Calculate anion gap = $Na - (Cl + HCO_3)$. Normal is <15.

Check an ABG to assess acid-base balance. A low bicarb, with a high pCO_2, may suggest compensation. High pCO_2 or low pO_2 suggests respiratory failure, a need for intubation.

Check an abdominal x-ray
Rarely, pill fragments are visible. These include:
- Calcium
- Iron
- Iodine
- Heavy metals
- Enteric-coated tabs
- Other foreign bodies

Check an ECG
Evaluate for arrhythmias or conduction delays.

A Chemical ingestion
Approximately 50%–60% of all poisonings are in children younger than 6 years.
   Toddlers are most common.
Highest rate of suicide attempts is in adolescents. Many attempt poisoning.

Differential diagnosis
A conscious pt may report ingestion and look otherwise well, in which case you investigate the type of ingestion and attempt to limit possible toxicity.

> For a comatose pt in whom you have suspected or reported ingestion, be sure to consider other causes of acute coma, such as (mnemonic VEGO TIPS MD):
> - Hypo*V*olemia
> - *E*lectrolyte abnormalities
> - Hypo*G*lycemia
> - Hyp*O*xia
> - *T*amponade/Hypo*T*hermia
> - *I*nternal Bleed (head, abdomen, leg)
> - *P*neumothorax/*P*ulmonary embolism
> - *S*eizure
> - *M*I
> - *D*rugs

P Call your local poison control center

Give activated charcoal 1–2 g/kg to bind organic toxins
Ineffective against alcohols and things that do not contain carbon, such as caustics, arsenic, bromide, potassium, ethanol, methanol, ethylene glycol, heavy metals, iron, iodine, and lithium.
Syrup of Ipecac is no longer recommended. Have activated charcoal at home instead.
Gastric lavage ("pumping the stomach") is not commonly used anymore but may be used up to 1 hour after ingestion. Do not use with hydrocarbons or caustics.

Antidotes
- Acetaminophen: N-acetylcysteine
- Benzodiazepine: flumazenil
- Coumadin: fresh frozen plasma, vitamin K
- Digitalis: specific Fab antibody fragments
- Heparin: protamine sulfate
- Isoniazid: pyridoxine
- Methemoglobinemia: methylene blue
- Organophosphates: atropine/pralidoxime
- Arsenic, lead: penicillamine
- Carbon monoxide: oxygen (hyperbaric)
- Cyanide: sodium nitrite
- Ethylene glycol/methanol: ethanol
- Iron: deferoxamine
- Mercury: BAL
- Narcotics: naloxone
- Phenothiazines: diphenhydramine

All suicidal pts must be admitted for psychiatric hold
See Well-Care Child: Adolescent, p. 142.

FOREIGN BODY

S What was the foreign body and when and where was it placed?

Children place foreign bodies (FBs) in just about any orifice

Usually the nose in <3 years of age

Usually the ear in 3–8 years of age

Starting from the top: Ears, nose, mouth (trachea or esophagus), urethra, vagina, anus, other (trach, g-tube)

O Do the appropriate general and then focused physical exams and imaging

In younger children, especially in infants, sometimes there is a history of an FB, but often there will just be symptoms of respiratory distress, drooling, crying with pain, or vaginal discharge, etc. In these cases, it is wise to keep foreign body on your differential.

Esophageal (round on AP, flat on Lat): The FB on chest or lateral neck x-ray is seen in the coronal plane. Usually accompanied by dysphagia, drooling, or substernal chest pain.

Tracheal/bronchial (tracheal or laryngeal FBs are seen in the sagittal plane: flat on AP, round on Lat): Presents as cough, stridor, hemoptysis, aphonia, or respiratory distress. Decreased breath sounds or wheeze on one side suggests bronchial foreign body (usually the right mainstem bronchus because it branches at less of an angle than the left). Auscultate and percuss lung fields and then get a chest x-ray and AP and lateral neck x-rays looking for tracheal or bronchial foreign body.

Ear/nose: Unilateral nose or ear pain or foul-smelling discharge or bleeding. Check nose or ears with otoscope for foreign body.

Vaginal: Vaginal bleeding or foul-smelling discharge. Do vaginal exam and consider KUB or U/S to help confirm the diagnosis.

A Foreign body ingestion versus placement

Infants put everything in their mouths, so it is the adult caretaker's responsibility to keep things small enough to choke on away from the baby.

Older children usually will just say they were playing and it happened, but sometimes you will get a response that they were suicidal or another child did it to them.

Consider implications of where and what was found in the child

Infants:

- Oral foreign body: Consider issues of poor supervision, but recognize that it may happen with even the most careful parent.
- With foreign body anywhere else, such as the ear, nose, vagina, g-tube, or tracheostomy, consider abuse (anyone with access to the child such as a caretaker or an older child), especially in children less than 4 months old because they are not usually capable of placing the foreign body themselves.

Older children:

- For a foreign body placed in the rectum, urethra, or vagina (unless it is toilet paper, which is common), consider sexual abuse by anyone with access to the child.
- With repetitive foreign body placement anywhere, consider depression, abuse, or other psychological problem.

P Remove foreign body

Ear canal: Foreign bodies can be removed with a wire loop, alligator forceps, irrigation (except if suspect tympanic membrane perforation or vegetable matter), or suction. Be careful not to manipulate too much because inflammation can cause the ear canal to swell and make extraction very difficult. If extraction is not made with the first or second attempt, refer to ENT. If it is a live insect, drown it in mineral oil before extraction.

Nasal: Foreign bodies can be removed by first anesthetizing with lidocaine spray and then decreasing inflammation/swelling with phenylephrine drops. Then, when the swelling is decreased, pass a small Foley catheter beyond the foreign body, inflate the balloon, and pull gently back out of the nose. If this does not work, refer to ENT.

Esophageal: Foreign bodies need to be identified as sharp or dull by x-ray (or history if not radiopaque). If it is sharp, get another chest x-ray/KUB to verify passage to stomach and then repeat x-rays to verify passage. Have the pt return if any signs of abdominal pain, vomiting, or distention. If the FB is dull, make sure it is not a battery (these can be toxic). If not, instruct to return only if vomiting or abdominal pain occurs. If it is a battery or sharp object and it is stuck in the esophagus, arrange for endoscopic removal. If the battery or sharp is in the stomach, recheck in 24 hours to assure that it passes the pylorus, but return sooner if there is increasing abdominal pain or vomiting.

Trachea: Keep in position of comfort until ENT or Pulmonary can remove FB. Prepare to manage airway if the pt develops severe airway obstruction.

If you suspect abuse or neglect, refer the child to Protective Services

Do not feel guilty about referring a possible innocent parent to Social Services; even a suspicion may be enough to save a child's life.

If you suspect depression or a suicide, admit the pt for a psychiatric hold and call a child psychiatry consult

If depression is missed, there is a risk that a teen will succeed at suicide in the future.

If you suspect good parents with bad luck, provide preventive education

EDEMA—NEPHROTIC SYNDROME

S **Where is the edema?**

– Periorbital	– Abdominal	– Lower extremities
– Scrotal	– Vulvar	– Scalp

When did the edema begin?
Usually, the edema is worse in the mornings and has been slowly getting worse each day.

When the child urinates in the toilet, does he or she make bubbles or foam?
If there is protein in the urine (proteinuria), urine will be foamy.

Does anyone in the family have renal disease or kidney problems?
If the pt has a strong family history of renal problems such as renal failure or kidney transplant, it is important to take that into account when evaluating.

Does the pt have any other associated symptoms?
Signs such as fever, rash, arthritis, or arthralgias suggest systemic disease such as:

– Lupus	– Vasculitis
– Juvenile rheumatoid arthritis	– Crohn disease

O **Perform a good general exam**
Plot carefully on the growth curve and evaluate for possible failure to thrive.
Look carefully at the vital signs for hypertension or other clues of renal disease.
Look also at the temperature and exam for signs of infection.
Look specifically at the areas that become edematous in nephrotic syndrome (NS), such as periorbital, scrotal, sacral, ankles, and earlobes (soft, doughy earlobe suggests NS).

Order the appropriate tests for workup of the three main criteria of nephrotic syndrome
Proteinuria: Check a spot and/or 24-hr urine for protein to creatinine ratio.
Hypoalbuminemia: Check the blood albumin level.
Edema: On physical exam.

Perform a urine dipstick
The presence of large protein suggests the diagnosis of nephrotic syndrome.
Blood may or may not be positive, but remember that hematuria with mild to moderate proteinuria is more consistent with nephritis than nephrosis.

Draw blood for CBC with differential, BUN/Cr, and a lipid panel
The CBC will reveal both elevated hematocrit and signs of infection.
NS is associated with hyperlipidemia, often considered a fourth criterion.
BUN/Cr rule out renal insufficiency/failure.

Rule out TB
So that status can be ascertained before starting steroids

Check for possible alternative or secondary causes with
Antinuclear antibody (systemic lupus erythematosus)
Antineutrophil cytoplasmic antibody and complement (vasculitis)
HIV (AIDS)
Hepatitis B serology
ASO (poststrep glomerulonephritis)

Obtain a renal ultrasound to evaluate kidney size

Nephrotic syndrome

In NS, a glomerular lesion causes loss of protein in the urine.

This leads to proteinuria and hypoalbuminemia. The serum oncotic pressure drops and fluid leaks into the tissues, causing edema. The liver attempts to produce more protein to compensate for increasing production of lipoproteins and clotting factors, leading to hyperlipidemia and hypercoagulability. Urinary immunoglobulin G and M (IgG and IgM) loss cause immune deficiency.

Usually, children (especially males 2–7 years of age) present with generalized edema (without hypertension); otherwise asymptomatic with the following labs:
- Proteinuria: >40 mg/hr/m^2; >50 mg/kg/24 hr; Prot:Cr >2.0
- Hypoalbuminemia: Serum albumin <2.5 g/dL
- Hypercholesterolemia: Total chol >200

Minimal change disease (MCD) is the most likely cause. Other idiopathic causes are mesangioproliferative and focal segmental glomerular sclerosis.

Immune complex causes such as membranous nephropathy, membranoproliferative glomerulonephritis.

There are also secondary causes such as infections (malaria, syphilis), malignancy (lymphoma), autoimmune (lupus, Henoch-Schönlein purpura, serum sickness), and toxins (heavy metals).

Differential diagnosis

Heart failure: More likely to have rales on lung exam, and urine protein will be negative.

Renal failure: Edema is less likely, and an elevated BUN/Cr is essential.

Cirrhosis: Abdominal/lower extremity swelling, no proteinuria, and no facial/earlobe edema.

Benign proteinurias include transient proteinuria and orthostatic proteinuria.

 Refer to the nephrologist

Treat pts without a biopsy initially as if they had MCD (>75% of cases will be MCD and will respond to the therapy). Give prednisone 60 mg/m^2 per day or 2 mg/kg per day (max 60 mg/d) for 4–6 weeks with a slow taper over the next 2–5 months; 90% of pts will respond in <3 weeks. Parents and patients are taught to monitor urine protein levels by dipstick. Prednisone is continued at the same daily dose until 30 days after proteinuria has disappeared before taper starts.

Even if they respond initially, about 80% will require prednisone off and on over the next several years. A relapse is 3 consecutive days of a urine dip with protein of ≥2+.

If they continually relapse, other agents such as cyclophosphamide or cyclosporin can be used.

The nephrologist will consider biopsy if the pt fails to respond to immunosuppressants or if:
- There is a strong family history of nephritis or renal failure.
- There are signs of nephritis, such as hypertension, hematuria, and renal insufficiency.

Use furosemide to control edema; add albumin if hemoconcentration causes hematocrit >50%

Albumin helps prevent intravascular volume depletion during diuresis.

Prevent complications

Infection: Particularly susceptible to infections from encapsulated organisms such as pneumococcus. Give the vaccine and monitor carefully for infection. Treat presumptively if the pt arrives with signs of spontaneous bacterial peritonitis:
  – Ascites   – Abdominal pain   – Fever

Thrombosis: Children with NS are prone to venous thrombosis, so monitor for complications such as pulmonary embolus and renal vein thrombosis.

EASY BRUISING OR MUCOSAL BLEEDING—ITP

S **Where is the child bleeding from and for how long?**

Nosebleeds are common in children; however, bleeding from both nostrils, the gums, or vaginal and anal mucosae is not.

Cover menstrual histories with all adolescent girls.

Chronic bleeding implies a genetic cause, whereas acute bleeding is consistent with an acquired process.

Does the child also have a rash?

What the parents call a rash may actually be petechiae or purpura.

Does anyone in the family have a problem with bleeding or bruising?

Family history may imply a genetic link.

O **Evaluate the pt's vital signs**

Tachycardia suggests significant anemia or hypovolemia.

Fever may imply an infectious process, and sepsis should be considered emergently.

Evaluate the pt's color

Pts with hemoglobin level less than 9.0 are generally pale. Good places to check for this are:

– Conjunctiva   – Palate   – Palms of the hands

Look at the mucosae from which the pt has been bleeding

The nares should be examined for areas of crusted blood that would suggest recent bleeding.

Examine the gingiva for evidence of inflammation suggesting a common gingivitis. Mucosa that is bleeding because of a lack of clotting ability usually will not appear inflamed.

Examine for lymphadenopathy and splenomegaly

These may imply either a malignant process or an autoimmune phenomenon.

Examine all sites of bruising

Look for patterns. Bruises that look like household items (electrical cord, belts, etc.) or knuckles may imply child abuse. Bruises of coagulopathy should be patternless.

Look for areas of subcutaneous bleeding

Petechiae: Small, pinpoint, red, nonblanching macules, which represent subcutaneous capillary bleeding, most commonly appear on the legs, but may also appear on the palate, face, and torso.

Purpura (bruises): Larger nonblanching areas of subcutaneous blood.

Perform appropriate labs

CBC with a differential

PT

PTT

Peripheral smear for examination

A **Immune thrombocytopenia (ITP)**

ITP is characterized by isolated thrombocytopenia with platelet count <100,000/microL with normal white cell count and hemoglobin; prior terminology referred to this as idiopathic thrombocytopenia purpura. Nosebleeds, gum bleeding, petechiae, and purpura with a very low platelet count. A high mean platelet volume (MPV) implies autoimmune platelet destruction. Platelets are larger when they first emerge from the marrow and shrink as they age. In ITP platelets are rapidly destroyed after their release from the bone marrow; therefore the average platelets are larger than if they were to remain in circulation for their entire 5- to 7-day life span. All other cell lines on the CBC should be normal.

Differential diagnosis

Leukemia: Thrombocytopenia is accompanied by anemia and/or leukopenia or leukocytosis. Check for any circulating immature WBC forms (metamyelocytes, myelocytes, promyelocytes, or blasts). However, even in the absence of these, leukemia should still be considered, because it can occur with any CBC. It should be noted, however, that it would be extremely rare for the platelets on a leukemic blood smear to be large (increased MPV) like those in ITP. It is far more likely that they would be small or normal sized.

Disseminated intravascular coagulation (DIC): Both PT and PTT are elevated, often occurring in sepsis. Check the peripheral smear for fragmented RBCs. Without these, DIC is highly unlikely.

Vitamin K deficiency: An isolated elevated PT that is common in neonates and pts with chronic intestinal malabsorption.

Hemophilia: An isolated elevated PTT with a lifelong history of muscle and joint bleeds.

Von Willebrand disease: The most common genetic cause of bleeding; it can cause easy bleeding without the lab findings noted above in hemophilia.

Mucosal infection such as gingivitis, vaginitis, proctitis, etc.

Child abuse: Bruising in strange patterns, occult fractures, retinal hemorrhage frenulum tears.

P Admit the pt immediately for workup

Do not transfuse platelets unless the pt has signs or symptoms of an acute, life-threatening bleed (e.g., intracranial).

• Giving platelets to a pt who has an autoimmune destruction of platelets may drive this autoimmunity and cause increased destruction, like adding wood to a fire.

Start intravenous immunoglobulin (IVIG) 1 g/kg over 12 hours

IVIG will bind to the Fc receptors on macrophages in the spleen, thus preventing platelet destruction.

For immediate life-threatening bleeding, it is recommended that patients receive IVIG, methylprednisolone and platelet transfusion

Platelets should be transfused at a dose of 10–30 mL/kg and reassessed immediately following. Methylprednisolone should be given at a dose of 30 mg/kg per day (up to 1 g),

If suspect or cannot rule out leukemia, a bone marrow biopsy must be done to diagnose the type of leukemia, or differentiate it from ITP

With a diagnosis of leukemia, the bone marrow will be infiltrated with a clonal population of blast cells, whether they are lymphocytic or myelogenous. Production of all other cell lines will be decreased.

In ITP, the marrow should appear normal with increased numbers of megakaryocytes (the cellular precursor to platelets).

Place the pt on fall precautions and activity restrictions because minimal trauma may result in an intracranial hemorrhage

Note that hemorrhage, although a risk, is less likely if the pt has ITP because the young, large platelets are hyperfunctional and not many are required for clotting. In children with platelet count less than 30,000/microL avoid contact and collision sports and restrict activities that have substantial risk for traumatic injuries.

Patients should also avoid antiplatelet and anticoagulant medication.

If bone marrow biopsy is normal and IVIG ineffective, start prednisone 1–2 mg/kg qd

Immunosuppressive steroids should decrease immune activity against platelets.

FEVER WITHOUT ASSOCIATED SYMPTOMS

S ### How old is the child?

The risk of having a severe infection but still appearing well differs by age:
- <28 days of age: high risk
- 29 days to 3 months of age: moderate risk
- 3 months to 3 years of age: low risk
- >3 years of age: minimal risk

Workup is focused on not missing meningitis or other serious overwhelming infection (sepsis).

If the child is <3 months, it is important to ask about the method of delivery (vaginal or Cesarean section) and if mother was diagnosed with any perinatal infections

The older the pt, the less likely he or she will be infected by group B streptococcus or herpes simplex, but it is important to note. Neonates are at high risk.

Are there any sick contacts in the home or is the child at day care?

Upper respiratory tract infections (URIs) are highly contagious. Other sick children in the home or at day care may have exposed this child to a common pathogen.

Did the parent take the child's temperature, and if so, how was it taken?

Studies show that parental report of tactile fever usually correlates well with an actual fever.

Rectal temperature is more reliable than axillary. As a general rule, rectal temperature is 1 degree hotter and axillary temperature is 1 degree cooler than oral temperature.

O ### Check the vitals

Even if you have a history of fever, it is still important to document a fever.

Check the oxygen saturation

A pulse oximetry reading <95% is sensitive for pneumonia in the age group including neonates up through 3 months. All children with low O_2 sats should have a chest x-ray.

Evaluate the child's general appearance

If the child is well-appearing and comfortable, be reassured.
If the child is irritable and inconsolable by the parents, consider meningitis.

Perform a thorough PE. Look for obvious signs of infection

Rash: Might indicate viral exanthem, impetigo, or cellulitis.
Rales or rhonchi: On the lung exam, sounds like wet Rice Krispies or Velcro, respectively. Suggests atelectasis, fluid overload, or pneumonia.
Bulging fontanelle: Indicates increased intracranial pressure. With fever, consider meningitis.
Oral blisters: Common in a toddler or infant, these are likely to indicate herpangina (back of the oropharynx) or gingival stomatitis (front of the oropharynx).
Erythematous, purulent, enlarged tonsils: Common in children between 5 and 12 years of age; streptococcal pharyngitis may be asymptomatic. See Fever with Sore Throat, p. 202.
Erythematous, bulging, nonmobile, tympanic membrane suggests otitis media.

Assuming that all of the above indicatory PE findings are negative, what to do next depends, as noted above, on the age group. General labs that are usually ordered include CBC with differential, ESR, CRP, blood cultures, U/A and urine culture, CMP, HIV, TB testing, and CXR

Less than or equal to 28 days: CBC with differential, blood culture, urine by in and out catheter for U/A and urine culture, lumbar puncture (LP), sending the cerebrospinal fluid for cell counts, glucose, protein, and culture. No matter the results, the pt will be admitted.

29 days to 3 months: CBC with differential, blood culture, in and out catheter urine for U/A and culture.
- *No LP* (per the Rochester Criteria): If U/A is negative, and the WBC is between 5 and 15 without bands.
- *Perform LP:* If the white count is <5 or >15 or there is bandemia, all of which are shown to be indicators of sepsis in this age group.

3 months to 3 years: CBC with differential, blood culture, urine by in and out catheter (may cease to do this on males after 1 year of age) for U/A and culture. Perform LP in this age group only if you see signs suggesting meningitis on PE such as fever with meningismus and/or altered mental status.

Older than 3 years: Labs as indicated by PE or HPI.

A   **Fever of unknown origin. Specific diagnosis differs by age group**

Rule out sepsis: Less than or equal to 28 days.
Fever without source: 29 days to 3 months.
Rule out occult bacteremia: 3 months to 3 years of age. Usually caused by *Streptococcus pneumoniae* and usually resolves without treatment, but may develop focal infections such as meningitis.
More than 3 years old: Overwhelming infection is less likely because of mature immune system.

Differential diagnosis

Neuro: Meningitis, encephalitis, spinal abscess
Resp: Pneumonia, bronchitis, tracheitis
CV: Endocarditis
FEN/GI: Salmonellosis, appendicitis
Renal/GU: Cystitis, pyelonephritis
Heme/ID: Leukemia/lymphoma, HIV/TB/Syphilis, any infection

P   **<28 days: admit and observe**

If the LP results remain negative and the pt develops symptoms of a viral URI, or the fever resolves, no treatment is indicated. May discharge.

If there are indeterminate or (+) LP or CBC results, start vancomycin and cefotaxime IV until the cultures are negative.

If the patient is too unstable from respiratory or hemodynamic standpoint to undergo lumbar puncture, start empiric antibiotics. Can start ampicillin and (cefotaxime or gentamicin) and acyclovir. Add vancomycin in infants with concern for MRSA or septic shock.

29–60 days: if baby is well appearing, CBC is normal, and the parents are reliable, send pt home with a 24-hour recheck. Otherwise admit

If the LP was done and was negative, give a dose of ceftriaxone IV or IM and send the pt home with a 24-hour recheck.

If the LP was positive for meningitis, admit and start the same regimen as above.

If unable to get LP and patient is unstable, admit and start empiric antibiotics: ceftriaxone or cefotaxime and ampicillin and vancomycin and acyclovir (if concerning for HSV infection)

If well appearing but with significant historical risk factors, elevated WBC or abnormal CXR, start empiric antibiotics: Rocephin or cefotaxime.

61–90 days of age and baby is unstable, admit and start

Ceftriaxone or cefotaxime and vancomycin empirically

3 months to 3 years and the baby is well appearing

If WBC >15, give ceftriaxone and send home with a 24-hour recheck.
If WBC <15, may send home without antibiotics but with a 24-hour recheck.

>3 years of age: reassure the parents. Provide Tylenol (10–15 mg/kg) or ibuprofen (10 mg/kg), but instruct them that fever is a benign entity

The medication should only be used to alleviate the child's symptoms of fever.

Parents should return child to the hospital if irritable, lethargic, or feeding poorly

FEVER WITH IRRITABILITY AND VOMITING—MENINGITIS

S **How old is the child and what symptoms is he or she having?**
Nonspecific: Fever, irritability, decreased feeding, vomiting, lethargy.
Meningitic symptoms (less common): Bulging fontanelles, seizures.
In older children (after about 1 year), symptoms of meningitis include headache, neck
  stiffness, spontaneous vomiting, photophobia, seizures, altered mental status (AMS),
  focal neurologic deficits, and lethargy.

O **Carefully examine the child, looking for signs of meningitis and source of the fever**
Vitals: Fever and tachycardia are likely. Hypotension is an ominous sign.
AMS: Confusion, lethargy, somnolence, coma.
Stiff neck: Ask pt to touch chin to chest.
  • Brudzinski sign is positive if on passive neck flexion the knees bend or there is leg
    pain.
  • Kernig sign: Flex the hip 90 degrees and try to straighten leg at knee; test is positive
    if unable to straighten leg.
Skin lesions: Petechiae (small, nonblanching red spots) and purpura (coalesced spots
  into bruises) may indicate a fulminant infection, such as one with meningococcus.
Look for any site from which a bacterial infection could have invaded into the
  meninges:
  • *Sinusitis:* Facial tenderness and halitosis
  • *Otitis media:* Bulging, erythematous tympanic membrane
  • *Mastoiditis:* Postauricular swelling that pushes the pinna forward

Obtain appropriate labs and studies
CBC with differential and blood culture. Indications of a bacterial infection include
  elevated WBC, neutrophilia, and bandemia.
Obtain U/A and urine culture to rule out urinary tract infection, also a possible
  diagnosis.

Deciding to perform a lumbar puncture (LP)
If you suspect meningitis, it is imperative that you perform an LP. Contraindications
  include failure to obtain informed consent from the parents and signs of increased
  intracranial pressure (ICP), such as bulging fontanelle, papilledema, and focal neurologic deficits.
If you suspect increased ICP, obtain a head CT to assess ventricular patency.

Interpreting the LP results
Check opening pressure in older children. Normal is 15–22 cm H_2O.
Color: Yellow cerebrospinal fluid (CSF) is called xanthochromia (breaking down RBCs
  turns the CSF yellow, suggesting their long-term presence). Cloudy CSF suggests
  infection.
Tube 1: Send for a culture and Gram stain.
Tube 2: Send for protein and glucose levels. Protein is normally between 15 and 50. A
  protein >50 is the most consistent sign of an abnormal LP. Normal glucose is about
  two-thirds of the serum glucose (~60–80). In bacterial meningitis, it is likely to be low.
Tube 3: Send for cell count. This will give you:
  • RBCs: Vary (0–1000s) depending on how traumatic the LP was. However, the pres-
    ence of xanthochromia may indicate herpes or subarachnoid hemorrhage.
  • WBCs: Normal is <20 in newborns, <8 in older pts. Add ~1 WBC per 500 RBCs.
  • Differential: Predominant cell type is a clue as to the type of infection.
Tube 4: Save this tube for any *special tests* indicated by history, exam, or the results
  from the other three tubes. Special tests include tuberculosis (TB) culture, viral poly-
  merase chain reaction, and India ink for fungus.

Meningitis. Etiologies include

Neonates (<28 days old): Group B strep, *E. coli*, *Listeria monocytogenes*.

Older children: *S. pneumoniae* and *Neisseria meningitides*. *Haemophilus influenzae* type B used to be a common and life-threatening cause, but it is extremely rare since the advent of the vaccine.

Viral meningitis is a possibility in all age groups. Enterovirus is the most common pathogen, and it occurs most frequently in the summer. It is essentially benign.

A history of TB exposure should be present to make a diagnosis of TB meningitis. It can cause meningeal obstruction and often fatal hydrocephalus.

Before performing an LP, consider the differential diagnosis

Acute enteritis: Fever and vomiting followed by diarrhea within 8 hours.

Urinary tract infection: Can cause fever and vomiting but not irritability.

Pneumonia: Usually a cough will be present. Check a chest x-ray.

Subarachnoid hemorrhage: Blood in the CSF causes meningeal inflammation. Symptoms may mimic meningitis. Fever and head CT should help differentiate the two.

Now perform the LP and put all of the CSF clues together (Table 12-2)

TABLE 12-2   Typical Cerebrospinal Fluid Findings in Central Nervous System Infections

Infection	WBC	Diff	Glucose	Protein	Color
Preemie	<16	Normal	60–80	15–120	Clear
Normal	<8	Normal	60–80	15–50	Clear
Bacterial	>500	PMNs	0–20	>100	Cloudy
Partially Txd	>500	Variable	20–40	>100	Variable
Viral	>10	Lymphs	60–80	50–150	Usually clear
Herpes	>10	Lymphs	60–80	50–150	Bloody, xanthochromic
TB	20–200	Lymphs	0–10	200–2 g	Usually cloudy

 Admit this pt for treatment. For suspected bacterial meningitides, consider an ICU admission. Initiate treatment in the ER

For possible bacterial infections:
- In preemies, start ampicillin, cefotaxime, and vancomycin.
- In neonates, start ampicillin and cefotaxime and gentamicin. +/− dexamethasone.
- In children, start cefotaxime or ceftriaxone, vancomycin, and dexamethasone.

If you suspect herpes, start acyclovir IV, continue for 21 days if workup +.

For possible fungal, TB, or other chronic infections, start antibiotics and await confirmation of diagnosis before treatment unless high clinical suspicion and the pt is unstable.

As always with sick pts, IV fluids and respiratory support are mainstays of treatment

FEVER WITH PRODUCTIVE COUGH—PNEUMONIA

 Is there fever and productive cough?

A temperature over 101.3°F with a productive or productive-sounding cough of abrupt onset is most typical for pneumonia. Shortness of breath and tachypnea are also common.

How long has this been going on?

If the cough is chronic or without fever, consider alternative diagnoses such as asthma or pertussis.

Does the child have any underlying diseases, which may place him or her at higher risk for certain types of pneumonias?

Cystic fibrosis: Staphylococcal and *Pseudomonas* infections become more likely.
Asthma: CAP and atypical pneumonias.
Sickle cell disease: Consider acute chest syndrome.
AIDS: Consider *Pneumocystis carinii* pneumonia, cytomegalovirus, or fungus.
Neurologic impairment: Such as cerebral palsy, be suspicious for aspiration pneumonia.

Where is the child from and has the child traveled anywhere recently?

American Southwest: Consider coccidioidomycosis and, although unlikely, Hantavirus.
American Midwest: Consider histoplasmosis or blastomycosis.
Developing countries: Consider salmonella, measles, and tuberculosis.

 Examine the pt

Do standard exam with emphasis on the lung fields.

Look for signs of respiratory distress

Look for poor air movement, use of accessory muscles of respiration, or tachypnea.

Listen to lungs for any focal area of sound change

- Wheeze (high-pitched, almost whistle-like) – Decreased air movement
- Rhonchi (course, Velcro-like breath sounds) – Crackles (fine Rice Krispies–like sounds)

Percuss lung fields for any signs of consolidation

If there is dullness, consider effusion or infiltrate. Tympany, a loud, hollow sound, suggests pneumothorax or obstructive disease such as asthma. If you have difficulty interpreting percussion, consider performing:

• Whispered pectoriloquy (pt whisper syllables such as A while you listen and auscultate the lung fields)
• Tactile fremitus (pt says "ninety-nine" while you palpate the chest and back)

In both of the above exams, increased transmission of the sound occurs with pulmonary consolidation, as in pneumonia, and decreased transmission occurs with free air (pneumothorax) or obstructive disease (e.g., asthma).

Obtain a chest x-ray (CXR)

Look for signs of consolidation or effusion.

A **Pneumonia**

Inflammation of the lungs with infiltrate on CXR

Pneumonia can be broken down into three main types

Community-acquired pneumonia (CAP):

• *Lobar pneumonia:* As the name suggests, an entire lobe or part of a lobe is filled with pus and appears white on CXR. Most common etiology is *S. pneumoniae*, but *H. influenzae* and *Klebsiella pneumoniae* are also common.
• *Atypical pneumonia:* Characterized by hazy bilateral or patchy interstitial infiltrates on the CXR. Typical etiologies are *Mycoplasma pneumoniae*, *Chlamydia pneumoniae*, or *psittaci*. Common in adolescents and can be accompanied by rashes or joint pain.

* *Viral pneumonia:* Can look like either of the two above, but usually causes minimal infiltrates. Common etiologies are influenza, respiratory syncytial virus, and adenovirus.

Nosocomial (hospital-acquired) pneumonia: Consider *Pseudomonas aeruginosa*, *Staphylococcus aureus*, or whatever bacterial outbreak is occurring in your institution.

Aspiration pneumonia: If the pt is neurologically or developmentally impaired, *S. aureus* and anaerobic organisms are most common.

Differential diagnosis

Even if there is an infiltrate on the CXR, you should consider any one of the following not only as possible alternatives to your diagnosis but also as possible comorbid conditions.

* *Asthma:* Chronic cough, worse at night, wheezing, chest tightness, shortness of breath.
* *Acute bronchitis:* May have the white count and infection symptoms, but lack an infiltrate on CXR. *H. influenzae* is the most likely etiology.
* *Viral upper respiratory infection (URI):* Milder symptoms including nasal and pharyngeal complaints.
* *Pertussis:* Chronic cough, paroxysmal cough, posttussive emesis, whoop (if older than 6 months), and URI symptoms.
* Consider immunodeficiency or cystic fibrosis (regardless of race) if the pt has had multiple/frequent pneumonias.

P   **<30 days old, most usually have viral pneumonia (e.g., RSV). Does not usually need antibiotics unless secondary bacterial infection suspected. If so, admit and treat with ampicillin 100 mg/kg/d divided q6h and cefotaxime 100 mg/kg/d divided q6h**

Admit any baby less than 30 days old with a fever.

Likely bacteria are group B strep, *E. coli*, *Listeria*, *S. pneumoniae*, *H. influenzae*.

>30 days old, treat with ampicillin/sulbactam 200 mg/kg/d divided q6h IV, then when pt improves, amoxicillin/clavulanate 40 mg/kg/d divided q8h to finish a 10-day course. If bacteria not known, empiric therapy can be started with ceftriaxone 50–100 mg/kg/d in one or two divided doses

Likely bacteria are *S. pneumoniae*, *S. aureus*, *Moraxella*, *H. influenza*, and *Neisseria meningitidis*.

If you suspect an atypical pneumonia such as mycoplasma or *C. pneumoniae*, consider azithromycin 10 mg/kg (max. 500 mg) on first day and then half of that dose for the next 4 days

Admit for

Any signs of respiratory distress or unstable vital signs

Persistent oxygen requirement

FEVER WITH BARKING COUGH—CROUP

S **What is the time course of the symptoms? Are there any associated symptoms?**

Typically, croup starts with a low-grade fever and a mild runny nose for up to a week, followed by hoarseness, fever, and a barking cough or stridor. Pts usually present on the second or third day of the illness.

Is there any change in the stridor with position change?

If the stridor (hoarse cough) changes with position, consider foreign body.

Is the child toxic-appearing or drooling?

If the child is toxic-appearing (looks extremely sick and very tired), and especially if the child has been drooling in tripod position, consider epiglottitis.

Is the cough productive or dry?

Productive coughs tend to be intrapulmonary processes, whereas dry coughs tend to be intrapulmonary or upper airway.

Have the parents noticed any signs of respiratory distress?

- Unable to speak in full sentences
- Accessory respiratory muscle usage
- Subcostal retractions
- Tachypnea
- Suprasternal retractions
- Abdominal breathing
- Nasal flaring

How old is the child?

Croup can occur at any age but usually occurs between 3 months and 3 years.

O **Evaluate the vital signs and pulse-ox**

Expect a low-grade fever, although high fever does not rule out croup. Lack of fever may indicate a foreign body aspiration.

Be concerned about a child with tachypnea and tachycardia.

Be *very* concerned about a child with slow respirations or bradycardia.

Pulse-ox should be greater than or equal to 95% on room air.

Observe and listen to the child from the door (being careful not to agitate the child). What do you see and hear?

Note the mental status of the pt, which can range from agitation to obtundation.

Notice the child's color for any signs of cyanosis.

Auscultate, looking for decreased air movement.

Assess work of breathing by looking for signs of respiratory distress such as subcostal, intracostal, and supraclavicular retractions, and nasal flaring.

Listen for an intermittent barking cough that sounds similar to the sound produced by a seal.

Listen closely for stridor. Stridor at rest is a worrisome sign.

If the diagnosis is uncertain, obtain a posteroanterior (PA) chest and lateral neck x-rays

Croup will display a narrowing of the subglottic airway on PA chest x-ray with some local haziness. The lateral neck films will help rule out epiglottitis and retropharyngeal abscess.

A **Acute Laryngotracheobronchitis or croup**

An acute subglottic inflammatory process (the narrowing of the area below the glottis causes the stridor), which is almost always viral in nature. Parainfluenza (types 1–3) causes most of the cases. Influenza, adenovirus, respiratory syncytial virus, and measles are less common causes.

Assess the degree of stridor and of respiratory distress

If the pt has stridor at rest, poor air movement, cyanosis, severe retractions, and/or tachypnea to a significant degree, or worse, tiring out and obtundation, monitor carefully and watch for possible respiratory failure.

Differential diagnosis

Carefully consider and rule out:

- *Foreign body aspiration:* Afebrile
- *Epiglottitis:* Toxic-appearing, febrile, no cough, drooling
- *Retropharyngeal abscess:* Dysphagia, neck stiffness
- *Bacterial tracheitis:* Toxic, copious tracheal secretions
- *Acute asthma exacerbation:* Cough, wheezing, no stridor
- *Spasmodic croup:* Spontaneous resolution

P Initial treatment is always cool mist for 20–30 minutes

The aim of all therapy is to shrink the edema (increase the size of the airway). Cold, humidified air induces local vasoconstriction. Have the parent hold the mask slightly away from the child's face, again so as not to agitate the child.

Add oxygen to the mist, 4 L/min of flow. Follow the pulse-ox

If the pulse-ox is less than 95%

Start epinephrine 1:1,000

If the pt has stridor at rest, or stridor persists after cool mist:

Racemic Epi 0.5 cc in 3 cc normal saline can also be used, but there is no difference in effect and it is more expensive.

Administer dexamethasone (a corticosteroid) 0.6 mg/kg, maximum 16 mg

If the pt has moderate to severe croup, but responds to cool mist

Significantly decreases inflammation for several hours and prevents late phase of allergic reaction

Monitor patient

Patients who respond to treatment should be observed for 3–4 hours after medication. Children who remain comfortable and have no stridor at rest, good pulse-ox, good air exchange, normal color, normal level of consciousness, and can tolerate PO can be discharged.

Parental advice on discharge

Most children with croup do not need to be admitted, and it will usually resolve spontaneously within 3–5 days.

Follow-up with PCP should be arranged within the next 24 hours.

Admit for

Persistent signs of respiratory distress despite treatment or suspicion of tracheitis, epiglottitis, retropharyngeal abscess, or foreign body.

FEVER WITH WHEEZING COUGH—BRONCHIOLITIS

S **How old is the child?**

Bronchiolitis is an inflammatory obstruction of the small airways, usually caused by
respiratory syncytial virus (RSV). Other possible etiologies are:

- Parainfluenza virus
- Adenoviruses
- Mycoplasma
- Other viruses

Bronchiolitis tends to occur in children younger than 2 years, with most cases occurring between 3 and 6 months. If child is older than 2 years, consider an alternative
diagnosis.

What time of year is it?

Bronchiolitis usually occurs between December and June.

Is anyone else at home sick?

Often, someone else at home will have upper respiratory infection (URI) symptoms. The
disease is much milder in older hosts because they have larger-diameter airways and a
more mature immune system.

**Is the child male, bottle-fed, attending day care, around a smoker, or in a
crowded home?**

These are all risk factors for bronchiolitis.

What are the child's symptoms?

RSV usually begins with runny nose, sneezing, and low-grade fever, and progresses after
1–3 days to a paroxysmal wheezy cough and eventually shortness of breath and respiratory distress. If there are other systemic symptoms, such as vomiting or diarrhea,
consider alternative diagnoses.

 Perform a PE

Listen to the lungs carefully for rhonchi, crackles, and wheezing.

Look carefully for signs of respiratory distress:

- Accessory respiratory muscle usage
- Tachycardia
- Nasal flaring
- Subcostal retractions
- Tachypnea
- Cyanosis
- Suprasternal retractions
- Abdominal breathing

If disease progresses enough, may have poor air movement followed by lethargy and
apnea.

Liver may be palpable as a result of lung hyperinflation.

Pulse oximeter

Often the oxygen saturation will be less than 94%.

Arterial blood gas

It will commonly show hypoxia, hypercapnia, and acidosis.

Chest x-ray

Initially it will be normal. Some will have:

- Hyperexpansion
- Peribronchial cuffing
- Segmental consolidation

**Swab the nasopharynx and send for an RSV enzyme-linked immunoassay or
culture**

To confirm, not rule out, the diagnosis. A negative test only means RSV was missed or
another virus is responsible.

There are epidemiologic factors to consider here as well. It is important to know when
the first case of RSV arrives in your hospital every winter.

Bronchiolitis

A viral infection of the small airways leading to inflammation and obstructive asthma-like symptoms, including wheezing and hyperexpansion. Because resistance to flow in a tube is inversely proportional to the radius to the fourth power, and only young children have such small airways, this usually only occurs in children younger than 2 years. After this, airways are too large for simple inflammation to incur sufficient change to laminar airflow.

RSV is the most common etiology; others include influenza, parainfluenza, and adenovirus.

Differential diagnosis

Asthma: Especially if there is a family history of asthma, repeated episodes of bronchiolitis, sudden onset of URI symptoms without a prodrome, or good response to a single dose of albuterol. There is unlikely to be a fever.

Chronic aspiration caused by tracheoesophageal fistula or neurologic deficit: Consider if respiratory difficulty occurred with feeds preceding the recent episode.

Cystic fibrosis: Frequent/chronic pneumonias. Check sweat chloride.

Laryngotracheomalacia: History of prematurity with intubation or stridor since birth.

Bronchopulmonary dysplasia: History of prematurity with intubation and chronic wheeze.

Heart failure: See Heart Failure, p. 18.

Tracheal or bronchial foreign body: Sudden onset, no prodrome, a lack of fever, and unilateral breath sounds should make you consider this diagnosis.

Pertussis: Pt looks well between paroxysmal coughing jags; also, the prodrome is longer.

Bacterial bronchopneumonia: Poor response to just supportive measures, infiltrate on chest x-ray (CXR).

Chlamydia trachomatis pneumonia: Affects children 1–4 months old with more cough and less wheezing or fever. There are usually patchy infiltrates bilaterally on the CXR.

P **Give humidified oxygen**

Moist air lubricates mucus and the oxygen can penetrate to the alveoli.

Racemic epinephrine by handheld nebulizer is not shown to be effective but still is often used.

Positioning the infant with the head of the bed slightly elevated and with the neck slightly extended (sniffing position)

This will improve air entry.

Inhaled bronchodilators are not routinely suggested

But for severe symptoms, a one-time trial of inhaled bronchodilator can be warranted.

Give IV fluids at about 1.5 times maintenance rate

Hydration will increase clearance of respiratory secretions.

Oral feeding may risk respiratory distress. Consider nasogastric feedings also.

Anticipatory guidance

Symptoms begin over day 2 or 3, peak at day 3–5, and resolved over 2 or 3 weeks. Intake and output needs to be monitored. Review nasal suctioning with parents.

If interstitial pneumonia on CXR, consider starting a macrolide antibiotic

This will cover atypical organisms such as *Mycoplasma* and *Chlamydia*.

Admit

If supplemental oxygen is required to maintain oxygen saturation.

If the pt cannot tolerate feeds because of respiratory difficulty.

If there are signs of respiratory distress.

Consider bilevel positive airway pressure or intubation with mechanical ventilation if respiratory distress worsens despite aggressive treatment

This will merit transfer to the ICU.

FEVER WITH RUNNY NOSE, DRY COUGH—VIRAL URI

S **Has the child had any fever?**

(+) fever suggests infection: Pneumonia, sinusitis, otitis media.

(−) fever suggests noninfectious etiology: Asthma, foreign body.

Is the child behaving normally?

If the child is lethargic, toxic (extremely ill) appearing, or obtunded, these are all signs that the child may have more than just the common cold (URI).

If the child has a fever, cough, and runny nose, but is otherwise behaving normally and playing, this is probably only a viral URI and nothing needs to be done.

What are the associated symptoms?

Ask if there are any symptoms (run through your review of systems) to see if anything would lead you to believe:

• Common cold: Cough, rhinitis, sore throat
• More than just a cold: Ear pain, drooling, shortness of breath, bad breath, vomiting, voice change

O **Evaluate the vital signs**

Although children can commonly have fevers to any degree, a low-grade fever (less than 102.5°F) is more indicative of a rhinoviral infection.

Mild tachycardia may be present with fever, but tachypnea would be unusual.

Assess the general appearance of the child

The child should appear nontoxic because these URIs are rarely severe. Signs of respiratory distress, such as retractions and nasal flaring, should not be present.

Perform an exam of the eyes, nose, ears, throat, and lungs

Eyes: Red eyes with swollen conjunctiva likely indicate conjunctivitis, which is common in toddlers who rub nasal secretions into their eyes. It will usually be bilateral with scant discharge. A unilateral, markedly red eye with gross purulent discharge suggests bacterial conjunctivitis.

Nose: Nasal passages should be red, swollen, congested, and full of mucus ranging in color from clear to green. Pale, boggy-appearing mucosa suggests allergic rhinitis.

Ears: Tympanic membranes should be nonerythematous, with normal landmarks and light reflex (cone-shaped reflection of the light on the anterior inferior quadrant). A bulging, red eardrum, with distortion of the normal landmarks or light reflex with decreased movement to insufflation suggests an acute otitis media.

Mouth and throat: May appear mildly red, but the tonsils should not be red or have any pus on them if they are visible at all. There should be no lesions on the roof of the mouth.

Lungs: Despite the cough, the lungs should sound clear with good air movement. Extra sounds such as the following should prompt further workup of a pulmonary process such as pneumonia or asthma:

• Wheezing: Expiratory whistling high-pitched noises
• Rhonchi: A harsh sound like the one made by Velcro
• Rales: Crackles like the sounds made by wet Rice Krispies

Percuss the lung for dullness. If it is found, check to see if the area of dullness transmits sound through either egophony or tactile fremitus. If the dullness transmits sound, then it is a consolidation; if not, it is an effusion (collection of liquid).

A **Viral upper respiratory tract Infection (URI)**

This is the most minor of infection and one of the most common reasons for pediatric ER visits. It is characterized by involvement of the eyes, nose, and throat with minor symptoms in each area. The most common bacterial complications of these illnesses are:

• *Otitis media:* Characterized by a red, bulging tympanic membrane with decreased movement to insufflation. In children who are old enough to express it, there should be reported pain. Common pathogens are *S. pneumoniae*, *H. influenzae*, and *Moraxella catarrhalis*. Mastoiditis, characterized by mastoid pain and anterior displacement of the pinna, is a rare complication.

- *Sinusitis:* Occurs when the small meatus that drains the sinuses become obstructed for prolonged periods by inflamed nasal mucosa. Should be considered any time a viral URI continues to have fever for longer than 1 week. Characterized by tenderness to palpation of the forehead over the eyes or of the cheekbones, postnasal drip, and halitosis.

Differential diagnosis

The H&P should rapidly rule out the following more serious infections:

    – Pharyngitis   – Epiglottitis   – Meningitis   – Pneumonia   – Sepsis

P   If the pt lacks evidence of a bacterial process or complication, reassure the parents

Antibiotics are only for bacterial infections, so in the case of viral URIs or colds, they are completely useless. As a result, the benefits of taking the medicines do not outweigh the risks of adverse reactions and developing microbial resistance, so antibiotics should not be used.

Fever control: Many parents are only in the ER because of fever. Reassure the parents that fever is a benign condition that cannot harm their child. Fever is only the body's reaction to infection. The infection, not the fever, can be dangerous, but if you are comfortable that it is a viral URI, then the fever poses no risk. To make the pt more comfortable, acetaminophen or ibuprofen can be given.

Cough suppressant: Many parents want to stop their child from coughing, but coughing clears the airway. In the end, it is beneficial to the pt. If the parents insist, any guaifenesin-dextromethorphan combination at bedtime will suffice to suppress coughing.

If otitis media is present, start amoxicillin, 90 mg/kg/per day divided in two doses for 5–7 days for children ≥2 years of age, or 10 days for children <2 years of age

Most children get better without antibiotics, but if you diagnose acute otitis media, standard practice is to treat. If the fever persists after 7 days, switch to amoxicillin with clavulanate.

If sinusitis is suspected, give the same dose of amoxicillin, but duration is 10–14 days

Antibiotic penetration of obstructed sinuses is difficult, so longer therapy is necessary.

There are no admission criteria for these illnesses unless you suspect sepsis or meningitis

FEVER WITH SORE THROAT—PHARYNGITIS

S **How old is the child?**

Different age ranges represent increased risk of different pharyngitides:

- Infants and toddlers are at risk for herpangina. These pts have blisters on their tonsillar pillars and often high fever. The blisters are painful, so the pts will not want to eat.
- 5–15 years of age is the usual range for strep throat (streptococcal pharyngitis), but it can occur at any age. It is extremely uncommon before 2 years and less severe after 20 years of age.
- From 15 years through adolescence and young adulthood, mono (mononucleosis) is a common cause of pharyngitis.

What symptoms is the child having?

Common symptoms associated with pharyngitis (sore throat) are:

| – Headache | – Abdominal pain | – +/– Nausea/vomiting | – Rhinorrhea |
| – Fever | – +/– Dysphagia | – Cough | |

One way to differentiate strep throat from other upper respiratory infections (URIs) is that cough and rhinorrhea are usually not present in strep throat.

O **Examine the throat**

There are many different ways a sore throat can appear on PE:

- *Herpangina* (caused by coxsackievirus): Generalized redness with painful ulcers toward the back of the mouth (tonsillar pillars and soft palate)
- *Herpes simplex virus I* (HSV-1 usually occurs around the mouth and HSV-2 usually occurs around the genitalia, but both can do both): Causes ulcerations more anterior in the mouth (gingiva, lips, and tongue).
- Both strep throat and mono present as exudative pharyngitis: Beefy redness restricted to the pharynx, with enlarged tonsils, with or without the presence of pus.
- Peritonsillar abscess presents as unilateral tonsillar enlargement and uvular deviation, especially if associated with a muffled voice.

Finish a general PE, looking for these other common signs

Scarlatiniform rash (scarlet fever) is a velvety or sandpaper-like rash with Pastia lines and circumoral pallor; diagnostic of strep.

Tender anterior cervical lymphadenopathy is common in all of these illnesses.

Blisters on the hands and feet are common with coxsackie infections (hand, foot, and mouth disease).

Splenomegaly is associated with infectious mono.

Prominent cough, rhinorrhea, or otitis media make strep throat, mono, and herpangina less likely.

Perform necessary lab tests

Rapid strep test and throat culture.

Monospot and Epstein-Barr virus (EBV) titers. CBC with differential should show lymphocytosis with atypical lymphocytes in mono.

A **Pharyngitis**

Caused by infectious inflammation of the throat or pharynx.

Differential diagnosis

Strep throat caused by group A strep or *Streptococcus pyogenes*. Scarlet fever is associated with a toxin-producing strain.

Strep throat diagnosis mnemonic: A PUFL MN (a puffle man); the more of these criteria that are positive, the more likely it is to be strep throat:

- *A*ge (5–15 year)
- Ø *U*RI symptoms (no cough/rhinorrhea)
- *M*ay to *N*ovember (peak incidence)
- *P*haryngitis (w/ beefy red tonsils)
- *F*ever
- *L*ymphadenopathy (tender cervical)

CENTOR criteria also gives an idea of which patients would benefit from testing.

Dependent on four factors: Tonsillar exudates, tender anterior cervical lymphadenopathy, fever, absence of cough.

One point is given for each criterion. Patients with a score ≥3 may benefit from testing.

Herpangina and hand, foot and mouth disease are caused by coxsackieviruses and can be diagnosed by the ulcers located posteriorly in the mouth and pharynx.

Herpes stomatitis (usually HSV-1) causes ulcers in the more anterior portion of the mouth.

Mononucleosis is a syndrome usually caused by EBV. It is characterized by exudative pharyngitis, low-grade fevers, fatigue, lymphocytosis, and splenomegaly.

Interpret the rapid strep and throat culture

Diagnostic if the rapid strep or throat culture is positive.

If the rapid strep is negative, you may wait for the throat culture results to treat, or you may treat immediately if your clinical suspicion for strep throat is high (more of the above criteria = remember A PUFL MN).

If the throat culture is positive, either start or continue treatment.

If throat culture is negative, remember that some false negatives exist and continue to treat if your clinical suspicion remains high.

Rule out strep throat to avoid its complications and sequelae

Treating strep throat reduces incidence of complications such as peritonsillar abscess and cervical lymphadenitis and sequelae such as rheumatic fever (responsible for irreversible heart valve lesions) and glomerulonephritis. Initiate therapy within 9 days of the onset of symptoms to prevent rheumatic fever.

P Treatment with penicillin V-K (treatment of choice) for 10 days

If <27 kg: 250 mg two or three times daily; If >27 kg: 500 mg two or three times daily.

Although bacterial resistance has emerged as a problem with other bacteria worldwide, group A Strep remains remarkably sensitive to penicillin. It will continue to be the drug of choice until resistance is more commonly seen.

If the pt is allergic to penicillin, treat with azithromycin

Azithromycin can be given but is considerably more expensive. In addition, resistance develops rapidly, so it should be reserved only for those pts who are truly allergic to penicillin. Dose: 12 mg/kg (max 500 mg/dose) on day 1 followed by 6 mg/kg/dose (max 250 mg/dose) once daily on days 2 through 5.

Herpangina and mono are viral illnesses requiring only supportive care

Children with herpangina should be encouraged to take cool liquids to avoid dehydration.

Adolescents with mono should get plenty of rest and refrain from kissing and sharing glasses or cans of soda.

FEVER WITH DYSURIA—URINARY TRACT INFECTION

S **Obtain a general history of the complaint**

Urinary tract infections (UTIs) can present in almost any age group in many different ways.

- It can present as simple dysuria without fever; usually described as a burning with urination, frequent urinations with minimal urine produced, and a generalized discomfort.
- UTIs can also present with just fever, especially in the neonatal and infancy periods.

Culture urine when the pt has fever and no source (see Fever Without Associated Symptoms, p. 190).

Does it burn when the pt urinates?

(Dysuria) This is one of the most common symptoms of UTI.

Is the pt waking up at night to urinate or having small, frequent urinations?

Urinary frequency is another symptom of UTI, and nocturia is a good way of assessing it because children usually do not wake up more than once or twice, if at all, to go to the bathroom at night.

Does the pt have any associated symptoms?

Flank pain is associated with pyelonephritis (infection that has ascended to the kidneys).

Vomiting is common in UTIs in infants. In older children, it is likely to indicate pyelonephritis.

Pyelonephritis is also associated with higher fevers and chills.

Severe abdominal pain when the pt cannot hold still may indicate an associated renal stone. This is the opposite of what is seen in appendicitis, where pts try to hold very still.

Has the pt had UTIs before? If so, how many and how often?

Multiple UTIs suggests a urinary tract abnormality, poor hygiene, or possible sexual abuse.

If pt is a female child, how does she wipe herself?

Wiping back to front is a risk for UTIs.

Is pt sexually active?

Sexually active females have an increased risk for UTIs.

O **Evaluate the pt's general appearance and vital signs**

Pt may appear uncomfortable, but should not appear ill or toxic. Mental status and BP should be normal, and the pt should not be tachycardic unless febrile or in pain.

Pt's age and sex

Infants are at high risk for UTIs (males more than females).

Males: 6 months to 1 year of age, the risk of a UTI in anatomically normal males drops to almost zero. UTI symptoms in adolescent boys is more commonly sexually transmitted infections.

Females: The risk of UTI in females peaks from 6 months to 2 years of age and then again in adolescence.

Perform a focused and directed PE

Check for costovertebral angle (CVA) tenderness on the flank at about the 10th through 12th ribs (pyelonephritis).

Tenderness just above the pubic symphysis is suprapubic tenderness suggestive of cystitis.

Look for lesions and discharge on genital exam.

Obtain a urine sample

Perform in-and-out catheterization for young children. Bag specimen (sealing a bag over the genitalia) is not useful for culture to rule out UTI because of frequent contamination.

In children who are toilet trained, obtain a clean-catch specimen. Have the pt clean the genital area with several moist sterile towelettes; let the first portion of urine go into the toilet, and then catch the middle portion in the specimen cup.

Obtain a U/A (dipstick or lab) and send a specimen for culture

Positive nitrite and leukocyte esterase indicate UTI. Bacteria produce nitrites while sitting in the bladder, and white cells produce leukocyte esterase. Very young infants hold almost no urine in their bladders, so these tests are less sensitive. This is why a culture is also necessary.

Microscopic blood can be caused by UTI but not without a positive nitrite or leukocyte esterase.

Positive glucose suggests diabetes mellitus, a risk factor for pyelonephritis at any age.

 ### Urinary tract infection

Infections range from a simple cystitis (bacteria growing in the bladder) to a pyelo-nephritis (bacterial infection of the kidney). Pyelonephritis is more common with anatomic abnormalities of the urinary tract but can occur in completely normal hosts.

Differential diagnosis

The differential of the main features of cystitis are:
- *Dysuria:* Trauma, chemical irritant, stricture, foreign body
- *Frequency:* Diabetic ketoacidosis, polydipsia, microbladder
- *Suprapubic tenderness:* Trauma, tumor, appendicitis
- *Fever:* Sepsis, bacteremia, meningitis

The differential of the features of pyelonephritis are:
- *CVA tenderness:* Appendicitis, trauma, renal colic
- *Vomiting:* Central nervous system (CNS) abnormality, CNS bleed, enteritis

 ### Early and aggressive antibiotic therapy (within 72 hours of presentation) is necessary to prevent renal damage. Empiric treatment recommended, guided by local resistance patterns. Oral cephalosporin should be first line in treatment of UTI in children without genitourinary abnormalities

Amoxicillin and TMP-SMX should be used with caution because of high rate of resis-tance of *E. coli.* Fluoroquinolones are effective and resistance is rare in children but should be limited for multidrug-resistant, gram-negative bacteria. Treatment duration should be 3–5 days for immune-competent children without fever, and usually 10 days for children presenting with fever.

Admit all pts younger than 2 months for urosepsis. Admit all pts with pyelonephritis who are not tolerating oral intake for IV antibiotics

At less than 2 months of age, it is difficult to contain infection, so the pt is more likely to develop sepsis.

Females more than 5 years of age and all males, and any pts who are now having a repeat episode of pyelonephritis, require a workup for urinary tract abnormalities

Repeat urine culture: 3 days into their treatment.

VCUG: After a negative culture, the pt may have a vesiculocystourethrogram (VCUG), which will reveal most abnormalities, such as ureteral reflux and posterior urethral valve.

Renal U/S: To rule out hydronephrosis, scarring, or dysplasia.

Start prophylactic antibiotics (usually Macrobid or Bactrim) on any child with a uro-logic abnormality such as posterior urethral valves, history of recurrent UTI (three febrile UTI in 6 months or four total UTI in 1 year) and then refer to Urology.

FEVER WITH RASH—VIRAL EXANTHEM

S How long has the child had the rash?
Time course of the rash may help in the diagnosis of the illness.

How long has the child had fever, and what relation does it have to the rash?
Fever usually precedes a rash. Most rashes that coexist with fever are secondary to viral illnesses. Therefore, many of them have a prodrome of fever.
A high fever (greater than 104°F) for 5 days or more preceding the rash should make you suspicious of Kawasaki disease (see Kawasaki Disease, p. 208).

Does the pt have any associated symptoms?
Scarlet fever: Sore throat (streptococcal pharyngitis) with sandpaper rash and Pastia lines.

> *Rheumatic fever:* J♥NES is a good mnemonic:
> * *J*oints: migratory polyarthritis   * ♥ Carditis   * *N*odules (subcutaneous)
> * *E*rythema marginatum: Pink macules
>   coalesce into serpiginous pattern
> * *S*ydenham chorea

Meningococcemia: This is an emergency. Headache, purpuric rash on legs, photophobia, altered mental status (AMS), vomiting
Epstein-Barr virus (EBV, mononucleosis): Fatigue, lymphadenopathy, sore throat
Measles: Cough, conjunctivitis, coryza (runny nose)
Viral gastroenteritis: Can occasionally develop a rash
Erythema multiforme may be associated with cough because mycoplasma is a common etiology

Is the child taking any medications?
Many medications can cause a rash and fever as an allergic reaction. Mononucleosis causes a salmon-pink rash on the trunk in response to amoxicillin or ampicillin.

What is the distribution of the rash?
The pattern or distribution of the rash can help form your differential diagnosis.

Has the child had all of his or her vaccinations? Ask to see the card documenting this
An up-to-date vaccine card would not rule out measles, rubella, and varicella (all common viral causes of rashes), but they become far less likely.

O Evaluate pt's general appearance
It is important to note when the pt is "toxic" appearing:
    – Extremely ill   – Poor spontaneous activity   – Pallor
    – Irritability   – AMS
With fever and rash this would suggest sepsis, meningococcemia, or some other dangerous condition and learning to recognize the difference is extremely important.

Describe the rash. Be sure to use gloves while touching lesions
The rash should be characterized regarding its location on the body, as noted above, and if it forms any patterns, such as sun-exposed areas.
The rash should also be characterized by lesion type (Table 12-3).

TABLE 12-3   Lesion Types

Lesion	Flat	Round, Raised	Nonblanching	Fluid-Filled
<5 mm	Macules	Papules	Petechiae	Vesicle
>5 mm	Patches	Plaque	Purpura	Bullae

Nodules are dermal (deeper), whereas papules/plaques are epidermal (shallow).

Viral exanthem

Erythema infectiosum (fifth disease): Etiology is Parvovirus B_{19}.
  • Red rash on each cheek (a slapped-cheek appearance)
  • Followed by generalized red maculopapular rash, which becomes lacy in appearance

Varicella (chicken pox): Etiology is varicella-zoster virus.
  – Highly contagious   – Generalized distribution   – Pruritic
  – Three different lesions: pink papule,
    vesicle (dewdrop on a rose petal), and
    scabbing ulceration. All three lesions
    should be seen on a pt at once

Roseola infantum (exanthem subitum, sixth disease): Etiology is human herpes virus 6.
  – High fever, 2–3 d   – Well-appearing   – Febrile seizure
                                      child   common
  – Fever followed by erythematous rash
    with small macules and papules
    surrounded by a pale ring appears.
    Distribution is usually on the neck,
    trunk, and behind the ears

Measles (rubeola): Etiology is a paramyxovirus, rare since vaccine.
  • Prodrome is triad: Cough, coryza, conjunctivitis.
  • Rash is red, maculopapular, starts on the forehead and ears, then spreads over body.
  • Koplik spots present on the buccal mucosa immediately preceding rash.

Differential diagnosis

Scarlet fever: Etiology is complication of group A Strep (GAS) pharyngitis.
  • Red, sandpaper-like (small papules), generalized, with Pastia lines in the flexion
    creases.

Rheumatic fever: Sequelae of GAS infection; see J♥nes Criteria above.

Impetigo: A localized streptococcal or staphylococcal skin infection.
  – Localized to face or extremities   – Macules become vesicles   – Honey-crusting

Cellulitis: A spreading streptococcal or staphylococcal skin infection.
  – Violaceously red, swollen, hot to the touch   – Usually on the limbs

Meningococcemia: A systemic infection caused by *N. meningitides*
  • Purpura fulminans (most severe form): Complicated by disseminated intravascular
    coagulation, causing petechiae and ecchymoses. Rapidly fatal without treatment.

Erythema multiforme: An immunologically activated rash that appears as target lesions
  on the skin, sometimes accompanied by mucosal inflammation (Stevens-Johnson
  syndrome).

Kawasaki disease: See Kawasaki Disease, p. 208.

 Treatment for most viral exanthems is supportive, whereas treatment for bacterial infections almost always includes antibiotics

Aspirin is contraindicated to prevent Reye syndrome.

Admit pts with measles with pneumonia or encephalitis, or any suspected meningococcemia

Obtain an echocardiogram and consult Cardiology if you suspect rheumatic fever

Lifetime penicillin prophylaxis could be required to prevent further GAS infections. If
  no carditis develops, prophylaxis needed for 5 years or until 21 years of age, whichever is longer.

FEVER WITH RASH, CONJUNCTIVITIS, AND LAD—KAWASAKI DISEASE

S **What symptoms is the child having?**

Kawasaki disease (KD) has a constellation of symptoms that will help make the diagnosis. The pt must have fever (usually higher than 101.3°F) for 5 days and four of the following five criteria:
- Bilateral nonpurulent conjunctivitis
- Oral lesions (oropharyngeal erythema, dry erythematous cracked fissured lips)
- Cervical lymphadenopathy (least common)
- Erythematous truncal rash
- Hand and feet changes (swelling of the digits and later periungual desquamation)

How old is child?

KD usually occurs between 6 months and 6 years. Never seen in children older than 8 years.

O **Examine pt's general appearance and check vital signs**

If the pt is afebrile or not irritable, he or she is unlikely to have KD.

Perform a generalized PE, paying particular attention to the following areas

Eyes: The bulbar conjunctiva should be erythematous and swollen but without discharge.

Oral cavity: The lips are often red, swollen, and cracked. Oropharynx may be diffusely erythematous, and there is often a strawberry tongue (red with stippling like a strawberry).

Neck: Only 60% have the cervical lymphadenopathy, but when present it is usually striking. It can be unilateral or bilateral, and a single lymph node should measure >1.5 cm. It will likely be tender to palpation, but it should not be fluctuant because this is a nonsuppurative adenopathy.

Skin: There is no specific rash in KD, so it is often referred to as a polymorphous rash. It is usually erythematous and can resemble the rashes of measles (maculopapular), scarlet fever (sandpaper-like), erythema multiforme (target-shaped lesions), etc.

Hand and feet changes: The palms and soles may be erythematous or indurated (hard to the touch). They are often swollen, and desquamation (peeling) of the digits is often seen, but usually in later stages of disease.

Look for these other PE signs

Heart murmur: Associated with rare acute mitral insufficiency

Jaundice: Rare obstructive jaundice secondary to hydrops of the gallbladder or hepatitis

Check the labs. There are no diagnostic studies for KD, but the following are suggestive

Thrombocytosis: Usually in the range of 600,000 to more than 1 million.

Elevated WBC: May be elevated to between 20,000 and 30,000. Erythrocyte sedimentation rate and CRP may also be elevated.

Sterile pyuria: U/A shows WBCs without infection.

Aseptic meningitis (although not the kind commonly referred to when discussing a viral or fungal etiology): If a lumbar puncture was performed, WBCs are often present, again without infection. It is common although not frequently checked.

A **Kawasaki disease**

A medium-vessel vasculitis with characteristic symptoms as noted above. Etiology is unknown, but many suspect an undiscovered infectious cause.

Avoidable sequelae

Treatment is fairly benign, but the consequences of untreated disease can be life-threatening.

This disease is often described in three stages:
- *Acute stage:* Most of the above signs and symptoms associated with this stage.
- *Subacute stage:* The fever, rash, and lymphadenopathy resolve and the vasculitis begins, causing coronary artery aneurysms (ectasias). This typically occurs between days 11 and 24 of the illness. Myocardial and endocardial inflammation can occur in 20%–25% of pts. When these coronary artery aneurysms are associated with thrombocytosis, the pt is at risk for coronary artery obstruction and myocardial infarction.
- *Late stage:* Coronary artery obstruction (myocardial infarction) occurs in this stage if the aneurysms do not resolve.

Treatment does not completely prevent aneurysms, but the risk is dramatically reduced. Infants with KD (6 months to 1 year) might not display even four of five criteria (atypical KD) but should be treated anyway, because their risk of aneurysm is even higher.

Differential diagnosis of fever, rash, and conjunctivitis +/− lymphadenopathy

– Toxic shock syndrome	– Scarlet fever	– Rocky Mountain spotted fever
– Lyme disease	– Measles	– Erythema infectiosum
– Rubella	– Roseola	– Epstein-Barr virus
– Enterovirus	– Adenovirus	– Stevens-Johnson syndrome
– Serum sickness	– Systemic lupus erythematosus	– Drug reaction

P Admit and immediately begin treatment with intravenous immunoglobulin (IVIG), 2 g/kg over 8–12 hours qd and high-dose aspirin, 30–50 mg/kg/daily divided into four doses

IVIG-only therapy has been shown to decrease the risk of coronary artery aneurysm. Aspirin will provide both anti-inflammatory and antithrombotic effects.

Patients are monitored for at least 24 hours following completion of IVIG to confirm resolution of fever.

Perform an echocardiogram

If it is normal, the pt may have an appointment to repeat an echocardiogram in 2–6 weeks to evaluate for coronary artery involvement.

After the child is afebrile 4–5 days, the aspirin dose can be decreased

3–5 mg/kg once a day and can be discharged on this dose. This will continue the anti-thrombotic effects.

If the follow-up echocardiogram is negative for coronary lesions, the aspirin can be stopped. If coronary abnormalities are detected, the aspirin will be continued indefinitely. A pediatric cardiology specialist should determine the pt's treatment.

Remember that children on aspirin are at risk for Reye syndrome

An autoimmune hepatitis with associated nonketotic hypoglycemia if they contract influenza or varicella. Instruct parents to call their pediatrician at the first sign of illness.

RASH WITH PRURITIS

S **Which is first: the itch or the rash?**
Atopic dermatitis, a form of eczema, is sometimes called the itch that rashes, but this phenomenon could also occur in systemic disease such as liver, kidney, or endocrine disorders.

Does the itching prevent sleep?
Scabies, eczema, and urticaria can all be severe enough to awaken the pt from sleep.

Where is the rash?
Scabies spares the head and neck and occurs especially at the interdigital webs and other areas known as intertriginous zones:
- Penile shaft
- Wrists
- Elbows
- Groin
- Natal cleft
- Axillae

Atopic dermatitis occurs in the popliteal and antecubital fossae, around the eyes and ears, and in the various skin folds and creases.

When did the rash start?
Scabies is often chronic, with pruritus sometimes continuing for weeks after treatment.
Urticaria is often acute but can recur.
Atopic dermatitis tends to be chronic with a difficult-to-remember start date.

Does anyone else have the rash?
Scabies can occur in multiple family members, but often the first case in a family will precede the others by about a month, about the time it takes for someone to become sensitized to the infestation.

Does anyone in the family have allergic disease?
A strong family history of asthma, allergies, eczema, or other allergic problems is suspicious or at least supportive of the diagnosis of atopic dermatitis.

Are there any associated symptoms?
If pts are having any malaise, fatigue, weight loss, or other systemic symptoms, then consider illnesses such as cancer, autoimmune, liver, renal, and endocrine diseases.
If pts are having urticaria, angioedema, and symptoms of shortness of breath or impending doom, consider anaphylaxis and treat with urgency (see Anaphylaxis, p. 160).

What medicines is the child taking?
Medication reaction is another thing to consider when pruritic rash exists.
Antibiotics such as penicillins, cephalosporins, and sulfa drugs are all common culprits.

O **Carefully examine the rash and note its distribution**
Scabies: Look for burrows on the wrists, penis shaft, elbows, axillae, between fingers, feet, groin, perineum, and natal cleft.
Atopic dermatitis: Look for a dry, scaly rash in the folds and creases of the body, areas such as the antecubital fossae, popliteal fossae, and around the ears and eyes.
Urticaria and the other pruritic rashes do not seem to follow a particular distribution.

Test for dermatographism by running the back of your pen on the pt's arm with some pressure. If a wheal forms at the site within minutes, the test is positive
Suggestive for urticaria/allergic rash

Consider the following lab tests
BUN/Cr: Elevated BUN suggests uremia, which can cause itching.
Liver tests and hepatitis panel: An elevated bilirubin can cause itching.

All of these rashes can be diagnosed by exam

Scabies: Burrows in interdigital webs, at the wrists, penis shaft, elbows, feet, groin, perineum, natal cleft, and axillae.

Atopic dermatitis: A dry, scaly rash in the fossae and folds of the body. One of the most common rashes in childhood, it occurs in up to 10% of children. It is often associated with asthma and allergic rhinitis.

Urticaria: Pruritic wheals that tend to rise up and resolve within hours, only to rise up at a different site. They usually resolve with antihistamines.

Molluscum contagiosum: Papules with umbilicated centers, which spread from place to place on the skin with scratching. They are viral in origin.

Miliaria rubra: Patches of erythema with small papulovesicles; a common heat rash.

Lichen planus: Flat-topped papules and hypertrophic plaques on wrists, low back, eyelids, shins, scalp, and the head of the penis.

Differential diagnosis

Secondary to systemic diseases such as cancer (especially cutaneous T-cell lymphomas), liver disease (cholestasis), chronic renal failure, drug reactions, polycythemia, insect bites, parathyroid dysfunction, psychogenic pruritus, and opiate withdrawal.

P **Scabies: apply permethrin cream to all of skin for 12 hours; wash sheets and clothes in hot water**

This should ensure death for all of the infecting organisms. It is highly contagious, so consider treating all family members.

Atopic dermatitis: apply moisturizing creams several times a day and pat (do not rub) dry after bathing

If this is ineffective, short courses of mild topical steroids should alleviate symptoms.

Urticaria: give antihistamines and try to find the cause

Viral is the most common cause, but it is more likely that the cause will never be found.

Molluscum contagiosum: advise pt (parent) to avoid scratching because it will spread the lesions

The lesions may be removed but often resolve spontaneously in a matter of months.

Miliaria rubra: expose affected area and allow it to dry and cool

Lichen planus: treat with topical corticosteroids

Drug allergy: if it is suspected, stop the medication and wait to see if the rash improves

HENOCH-SCHÖNLEIN PURPURA

S **Is there a rash, joint pain, abdominal pain, and blood in the urine?**
If so, it is very likely you have diagnosed Henoch-Schönlein purpura (HSP). At the very least, you should have rash and joint pain or abdominal pain.

What does the rash look like?
The rash should look like purple, well-circumscribed bruises that do not blanch.

Which joints hurt?
Usually it is the knees or ankles and it is symmetric.

Ask the pt to describe the abdominal pain
Usually described as crampy or colicky.

Any vomiting or blood in the stool?
Vomiting with abdominal pain occurs occasionally. It can be confused with appendicitis.
Blood and mucus in the stool are both common.

Is there any blood in the urine or any foaming of the urine in the toilet bowel?
Asymptomatic hematuria and/or proteinuria are common.

Has the child had any colds recently?
Many children report a recent upper respiratory infection, suggesting that a viral infection may lead to an immune disruption that causes HSP.

O **Perform a careful PE**
Perform a good general exam, looking specifically to eliminate things such as sepsis, idiopathic thrombocytopenic purpura (ITP), and lupus.

Does the rash look typical for HSP?
Purpuric (nonblanching, bruise-like lesions +/− palpable) on the lower extremities.
Petechiae (nonblanching pinpoint red lesions) could suggest ITP or other platelet disorder.
Macular rashes or any blanching rashes should suggest alternative diagnoses.
Malar rash on the face suggests systemic lupus erythematosus (SLE).

Is there any focal abdominal tenderness?
Abdominal pain that localizes to a particular area (e.g., RLQ) suggests alternative diagnoses such as appendicitis, especially if there is guarding or peritoneal signs (see Abdominal Pain, p. 172).

Are there any signs of arthritis?
Although mild joint swelling may occur, warmth and redness suggest alternative diagnoses.

Check pertinent labs
U/A: In HSP may see hematuria (either gross or microscopic) and/or proteinuria. If there is a suspicion of sepsis, send the urine for culture.
BUN and Cr to evaluate renal function.
CBC, and if the suspicion is high enough for sepsis, also send a blood culture.
IgA is elevated in 50% of pts with HSP. May help confirm the diagnosis.
Anti ENA-4 panel (anti-dsDNA, anti-Smith, anti-Ro, and anti-La) and antinuclear antibody (ANA) if suspect SLE.
Skin biopsy showing leukocytoclastic vasculitis can confirm the diagnosis.
PT, PTT, antiphospholipid antibody to rule out other causes of easy bruising.

Henoch-Schönlein Purpura (HSP)

An IgA-mediated small-vessel vasculitis characterized by four classic findings:
- Purpuric rash on the lower extremities
- Symmetric arthralgia of the large joints of the lower extremities
- Crampy abdominal pain with vomiting
- Asymptomatic hematuria

Symptoms can vary, but at minimum, the rash is required for diagnosis.

A biopsy of the skin should show a leukocytoclastic vasculitis.

Differential diagnosis

Several alternative diagnoses have already been mentioned. Of these, the most important to rule out either by H&P or with labs and further studies is sepsis, especially
meningococcal.

Other diagnoses to consider are:
- ITP: Petechiae, mucosal bleeding, thrombocytopenia

- SLE: A good mnemonic is MD NO PARISH ANA ("Dr., don't let ANA die"):

• *M*alar rash	• *P*hotophobia	• *ANA +*
• *D*iscoid rash	• *A*rthritis	
• *N*euro (like seizures, psychosis)	• *R*enal (like proteinuria)	
• *O*ral ulcers	• *I*mmune (like false + VDRL, anti-dsDNA)	
	• *S*erositis (pleuritis, pericarditis)	
	• *H*eme (like thrombocytopenia, leukopenia)	

- Other vasculitic processes, such as Goodpasture disease or Wegener granulomatosis,
  may lead to hematuria, abdominal pain, or other nonspecific complaints.
- *Juvenile rheumatoid arthritis:* See Limping in Child without History of Trauma,
  p. 216.
- *Appendicitis:* RLQ abdominal pain with peritoneal signs, vomiting, and fever
- *Tuberculosis:* Fever, night sweats (enough to need to change the bedsheets), chronic
  nonproductive cough, hemoptysis, and weight loss
- *Mesenteric:* Can cause crampy abdominal pain.
- *TTP/HUS:* Microangiopathic hemolytic anemia, renal failure, +/− mental status
  changes
- *Leukemia:* Can present with many of the same symptoms as HSP, so checking a CBC
  is a good idea for many reasons. CBC may show blasts.

Child abuse: Can also cause many of the same symptoms of abdominal pain, lower
extremity bruising, hematuria, and joint pain (see Physical Abuse, p. 222).

 Observe without treatment

After the diagnosis is made, the child is followed for possible loss of renal function and
to rule out more dangerous things on the differential diagnosis, but usually the symptoms resolve without incident.

May start prednisone 1 mg/kg/d if the pt needs symptomatic relief and if in severe pain

The worst outcome is usually related to worsening of renal function, even to the point
of renal failure. In these cases, there is no proven treatment but prednisone, cyclosporine, and even renal transplant. All have been tried, but there is no consensus
regarding proper treatment.

BITES AND STINGS

S **What bit/stung the child?**

Insects that sting: Bees, wasps, hornets, yellow jackets, ants
Insects that bite: Mosquitoes, fleas, lice
Arachnids that sting: Scorpions, ticks
Arachnids that bite (spiders): Black widow, brown recluse
Venomous snakes: Rattlesnakes, cottonmouth, copperhead, diamondback
Nonvenomous snakes: Garter snake, gopher snake, king snake
Mammals: Human, bat, rat, cat, dog

Where was the child when bite or sting occurred?

- Grassy area with shrubs: ticks
- In dark areas or in or near firewood piles: spiders or scorpions
- Ocean or beach: jellyfish or stingray

How old is the child?

The same amount of venom that may only cause minor symptoms in an adult could kill a small child.

Does the pt have any other problems or complaints?

Fever is a concerning symptom suggesting superinfection of the bite.
Anaphylaxis (see p.160): Should be addressed emergently if suspected.
Spider bites: Pain, swelling, paresthesias, headache, nausea, abdominal rigidity.
Snake bites: Severe swelling can cause compartment syndrome. See Limb Trauma, p. 220.
Stingray/jellyfish stings: Nausea/vomiting, syncope, paralysis, muscle cramps, seizure.
Scorpion stings: Nystagmus, mydriasis (blurred vision), hypersalivation, dysphagia, diaphragmatic paralysis (trouble breathing), restlessness, seizure.

O **Perform a general PE**

Inspect all areas carefully, especially areas with hair, for foreign bodies such as ticks or stingers.
Inspect skin for rashes, bites, or breaks.

- *Tick bites:* Look carefully for the tick, because it may still be there.
- *Cat or snake bites:* Are puncture wounds (high risk for infection).
- *Spider bites:* Often cause visible small breaks in the skin with central pallor.
- *Stingray stings:* May be pale, red, or blue, and swollen with local lymphadenopathy.
- *Jellyfish stings:* cause a red, raised, pruritic, painful rash.
- *Insect stings:* Look for a stinger and local angioedema.
- *Scorpion stings:* Cause a purpuric plaque, which progresses to ulceration and necrosis (the amount of venom is represented by the diameter of the lesion) with lymphatic streaking.
- If the child has been in a fight, look at the fingers and hands and ears for closed-fist, finger tendon, and ear cartilage injuries.

With breaks in the skin, look specifically for signs of infection such as redness, streaking, warmth, or swelling around the wound. Look for pus or discharge from the wound.
X-ray the area of injury, looking for embedded foreign bodies or broken bones.
Check labs: With envenomations for signs of infection or hemolysis (CBC), electrolyte abnormalities (lytes), hypoglycemia (glucose), rhabdomyolysis (CK), renal failure (Cr), and bleeding diathesis and/or hepatic injury (liver enzymes, PT, PTT).
ECG (if arrhythmia) and echocardiogram (if heart failure) with severe envenomations.

Animal-induced injury with or without envenomation. Avoidable sequelae include

Ticks: Tularemia, babesiosis, ehrlichiosis, Lyme disease, tick paralysis, Colorado tick fever, Q fever, relapsing fever, Rocky Mountain spotted fever.

Mosquitoes: Equine encephalitis, dengue fever, yellow fever, malaria.

Stings or venoms: Anaphylaxis or systemic toxicity of the venom.

Human bites: Closed-fist injuries can lead to septic joints, disabling damage to tendons.

Animal bites: Dog bites are high risk because they cause crushing injury. Consider treatment for rabies, especially with bats, skunks, raccoons, foxes, or any wild carnivore. Domesticated animals are less likely to cause rabies. With any dirty, open wound, consider tetanus (See Limb Trauma, p. 220).

P **Remove all ticks and stingers**

Grab as close to the skin as possible. Pull out slowly with forceps, and then clean the site thoroughly.

Soak stingray injuries in tolerably hot water to reduce pain. Wash jellyfish stings in normal saline or acetic acid to inactivate stingers

Plain water will release more toxin.

For human or animal bites, use lidocaine to numb the wound and clean thoroughly

Irrigate with copious amounts of clean water and debride the wound.

Leave the wound open (unsutured), unless it is on the face.

Consult a hand surgeon if the injury occurred to the hand.

If suspicion is high enough, such as unprovoked wild animal attack, vaccinate

Rabies is required for bats, rodents, and animals foaming at the mouth (dogs in the United States are unlikely to carry rabies).

Evaluate need for tetanus vaccination or immune globulin. See Limb Trauma, p. 220.

Give Augmentin for 3–7 days with high-risk bites. Reevaluate in 24–48 hours

High risk: Punctures, wounds with redness/warmth, wounds in immunosuppressed pts.

Give instructions to return sooner if signs of infection are noticed. If swelling is occurring around the wound, elevate and decrease use of the affected limb and remove constricting clothing or jewelry. If extensive necrosis or compartment syndrome occurs, consult a surgeon

This will be most common with venomous stings and bites.

Rule out or treat anaphylaxis

Hymenoptera venom is a common cause. See Anaphylaxis, p. 160.

Give antivenin if snake, spider, or scorpion type can be identified and is available. Contraindicated treatments include cutting and attempting to suction venom, and using ice, alcohol, or tourniquets

If rhabdomyolysis (spider bites) occurs, hydrate heavily with normal saline IV. If that fails then consult renal for dialysis.

Treat pruritus with antihistamines

LIMPING IN CHILD WITHOUT HISTORY OF TRAUMA

S **How old is the child?**

This changes your differential somewhat. Toddlers and children will usually have an infection, whereas adolescents will usually have slipped capital femoral epiphysis (SCFE), Osgood-Schlatter, or a rheumatologic disorder such as juvenile rheumatoid arthritis (JRA).

Where is the pain?

The location of the pain can give you an idea about where the pathology is, and this can help with the differential diagnosis. Keep in mind that knee pain can be referred hip pain and vice versa. If the child has either hip or knee pain, perform a good PE to discern the actual source of the pain. If the pain is not over a joint but instead over a long bone, consider osteomyelitis, fracture, or even cancer.

Is there any fever?

The presence of fever in a child with a limp helps promote diagnoses such as septic joint, osteomyelitis, and JRA.

The absence of fever suggests diagnoses such as SCFE, Osgood-Schlatter, and Legg-Calve-Perthes disease.

Has the child received steroids recently?

This increases the risk of avascular necrosis of the hip.

O **Perform a good PE**

After reviewing the vital signs and performing a good general PE, look specifically and carefully at the musculoskeletal exam for any signs of:

- *Septic joint:* Pain, swelling, warmth, redness, and decreased range of motion (ROM) over a single joint
- *Osteomyelitis:* Pain, swelling, warmth, and redness over an area of skin overlying a bone
- *JRA:* Swelling, warmth in any or several joints, lymphadenopathy, hepatosplenomegaly
- *SCFE:* Pain on internal rotation
- *Legg-Calve-Perthes:* Pain (in hip or knee) with weakness and decreased ROM in the hip
- *Osgood-Schlatter:* Pain and localized swelling at the tibial tuberosity

Order the appropriate labs and studies

Get an x-ray series (x-ray of *two or more* views, usually anteroposterior [AP] and lateral) of the joint.

SCFE: Get an AP and frog-leg view of the pelvis, looking for an "ice cream sliding off the cone" appearance to the epiphysis of the greater trochanter.

Legg-Calve-Perthes disease: Take an x-ray or MRI of the affected hip, looking for disruption, or worse, destruction of the femoral head.

To help differentiate septic joint, JRA, and osteomyelitis, obtain a CBC with diff, CRP, blood culture, ESR, ANA, and rheumatoid factor (RF).

If the joint has palpable fluid, aspirate it and send for cell count and culture.

Osgood-Schlatter: No imaging is necessary if classic findings present on exam.

A **Evaluate the cause of limping**

Septic joint: Fever with a single joint swollen, hot, and red. Elevated WBC, CRP, and ESR with a predominance of neutrophils and possibly bands on the peripheral smear. Blood culture and aspirate culture may or may not be positive. Joint aspirate should have >50,000 polymorphonuclear neutrophil leukocytes.

Osteomyelitis: Disruption of the cortex of the bone on x-ray with overlying erythema and fever. Blood cultures will likely be positive. Gram-positive organisms are most likely.

JRA: Note there are three types:
- Pauciarticular: <4 joints. If ANA is positive, there is increased risk of uveitis.
- Polyarticular: >4 joints. Similar to early rheumatoid arthritis, especially if RF is positive.
- Systemic (Still disease): More systemic with less joint complaints.

- Mnemonic: WAFFL ME CHARMS.

• *W*eight loss	• *A*nemia	• *F*atigue
• *F*ever	• *L*ymphadenopathy/leukocytosis	• *A*nemia
• *M*yalgias	• ↑ *E*SR	• *S*erositis
• ↑ *C*RP	• *H*epatosplenomegaly	
• *R*ash	• *M*orning stiffness	

SCFE: Hip or knee pain with decreased ROM and pain on internal rotation at the hip with classic x-ray findings. Very often associated with obesity.

Legg-Calve-Perthes: Pain in the hip or knee with disruption or destruction of the ball of the ball-and-socket joint of the hip. Most common in the 3- to 4-yr-old age group.

Osgood-Schlatter: Tender nodule at the tibial tuberosity and knee pain, worse with running.

Differential diagnosis

Fracture: Although there is no history of it, trauma still may have occurred and either the child is not telling the parent, the parent is not telling the clinician, or it seemed insignificant.

Cancer: Consider bone tumor if there is a localized swelling or mass in the leg, and the x-rays show a cyst, mass invading the bone, or other suspicious lesion. Consider lymphoma or leukemia if the pt has other masses, hepatosplenomegaly, lymphadenopathy, or blasts on the peripheral smear. In the latter cases, pain comes from rapid bone marrow expansion.

P ### Consult Orthopedics emergently for suspected septic joint

Surgical treatment is required to save the joint. Do not wait to start antibiotics.
- Septic joints can easily progress to sepsis, especially in younger children.

Start cefazolin if osteomyelitis is suspected

Chronic therapy and removal of infected orthopedic hardware will be required.

If JRA is suspected, call pediatric rheumatology for further workup and treatment

Rule out cancer and infection before starting steroids.

For SCFE and Legg-Calve-Perthes, refer to Orthopedics for surgical intervention

No weight bearing until after surgery.

Treat Osgood-Schlatter with NSAID therapy

This should effectively decrease the inflammation of the tibial tuberosity.

Reduce and cast all fractures and refer to Orthopedics for those fractures that may require surgery

Refer to Child Protective Services if abuse is suspected (see suspected physical abuse, p. 222)

Refer all suspected malignancies to Oncology

HEAD TRAUMA

S **How did the head trauma occur?**

Mechanism of injury is important in judging expected severity (fall from couch versus third floor).

Consider child abuse if a story sounds strange, changes, or is inconsistent with the injury.

Did the pt lose consciousness?

Loss of consciousness (LOC) suggests significant injury. Talk to someone who witnessed the event. Ask if the child cried immediately or if he or she seemed awake the entire time.

If there were no witnesses and the pt is old enough to answer questions, ask what he or she remembers about the incident. Amnesia to any part of the event suggests LOC.

Did the pt have any posttraumatic events, such as a seizure or vomiting?

Contact seizures: Seizures that occur within seconds of the injury. They are benign.

Early posttraumatic seizures: Seizures that begin >1 minute after the trauma are clinically significant. Observe pt for risk of further seizures.

Vomiting: Short-term vomiting is also benign. Vomiting that persists for more than 4 hours after the event is concerning.

Other posttraumatic events include:

- Headache (probably most common)   – Dizziness
- Cerebrospinal fluid leakage from the ears or nose (likely indicates a basilar skull fracture)
- Waning LOC

O **Evaluate pt's level of consciousness**

This is probably the most important part of the PE in this pt. If pt is a well-appearing conscious child or adolescent brought in by a concerned parent, there is probably not much to worry about. However, if pt displays altered LOC even if Glasgow Coma Scale (GCS) is 15 (normal), careful observation and often interventions must be taken.

The GCS will help you assess pt (Table 12-4).

The maximum score is 15, the minimum is 3.

If pt has a GCS of 8 or less, the pt is unlikely to be able to protect own airway and should be intubated.

TABLE 12-4   Glasgow Coma Scale

Eyes Open	Motor	Verbal
4 = Spontaneously	6 = Obeys commands	5 = Oriented
3 = To Speech	5 = Localizes to pain	4 = Confused
2 = To Pain	4 = Withdraws from pain	3 = Words
1 = Closed	3 = (Decorticate) Flexor posturing	2 = Sounds
	2 = (Decerebrate) Extensor posturing	1 = Nonverbal
	1 = No movement	

Look at vital signs

Cushing triad: A late sign of increased intracranial pressure (ICP) with bradycardia, hypertension, and abnormal respirations.

Examine head for signs of trauma

Hematoma: Feels like a hard, ovoid mass. It should be tender to palpation.

Step-off: Might indicate a depressed skull fracture.

Laceration: May need to be sutured or skin-clipped.

Fundoscopic exam: Look for sharp optic disc margins. Blurred margins suggest increased ICP. Retinal hemorrhages suggest shaken baby syndrome.

Ears: Hemotympanum (blood behind the tympanic membrane [TM]) or a ruptured TM with clear liquid discharge is both consistent with a basilar skull fracture.

Battle sign: An ecchymotic line (bruise) behind the ear that usually appears several hours after the trauma. It also suggests basilar skull fracture.

Raccoon eyes: Periorbital ecchymoses that also suggest basilar skull fracture.

Septal hematoma: A surgical emergency. Look in the nose for a bulging dark red or black septum.

Perform a complete neurologic exam, provided the pt is conscious

Note any focal neurologic findings. Mnemonic is C MR CGR ("See Mr. Cougar"):
- *C*ranial nerves
- *M*otor
- *R*eflexes
- *C*erebellar
- *G*ait
- *R*homberg
- *S*ensory

Although it is still controversial, depending on how high risk the patient is, determines if a patient needs neuroimaging. Bear in mind that clinical decision rules are not intended to replace clinical appearance or judgment

In children younger than 2 years, perform head CT if suspected skull fracture, suspicion of child abuse, focal neurologic findings, altered mental status, bulging fontanelle, persistent vomiting seizure following injury, definite LOC for longer than a few seconds, or if associated with clinically important traumatic brain injury (ciTBI). Patients at intermediate risk can be managed with close observation for 4–6 hours after the injury, but head CT needed if any worsening of condition. Intermediate risk includes vomiting that is self-limited, LOC that is less than a few seconds, history of lethargy or irritability but resolved, behavioral change reported by caregiver, injury caused by fall of more than 3 feet, patient ejection or high-risk mechanism of injury, nonfrontal scalp hematoma, nonacute skull fracture, unwitnessed trauma, or age younger than 3 months with non-trivial trauma.

Imaging should be avoided in children <2 years if at low risk for brain injury. They must meet all following criteria: normal mental status, no parietal/occipital/temporal scalp hematoma, no LOC >5 seconds, no skull fracture, normal behavior, no high-risk mechanism of injury.

In children greater than 2 years of age: CT needed for high-risk ciTBI (focal neurologic findings, skull fracture findings, seizure, persistent AMS, prolonged LOC).

Observation recommended (with possible CT if worsening symptoms) in children >2 with: vomiting, headache, questionable LOC, or injury caused by high-risk mechanism of injury.

Imaging should be avoided in children >2 years if at low risk for brain injury. They must meet all following criteria: normal mental status, no LOC, no basilar skull fracture findings, no vomiting, no severe headache, no high risk mechanism of injury.

 Blunt head trauma

Concussion: A normal head CT with mild persistent symptoms, headache, dizziness, etc.

Contusion: Found on head CT as a point of edema with or without bleed.

Epidural hematoma: Caused by a ruptured intracranial artery, usually the middle meningeal artery. Clinically characterized by an initial LOC, followed by a lucid interval, followed by waning consciousness. It shows up as a lentiform-shaped bleed on the head CT, compressing the brain. There may be midline shift of the brain.

Subdural hematoma: Caused by torn bridging veins between the brain and the dura. Characterized by a unilateral crescent-shaped bleed on CT scan, exerting minimal pressure on the brain.

Skull fracture, basilar, depressed, or nondepressed: Basilar skull fractures have a 10% risk of meningitis. Depressed skull fractures have an increased risk of seizures.

P **All of the above diagnoses, with the exception of concussion, require a neurosurgical evaluation. Pts with concussions may be sent home**

Parents should be given instructions to return if their child's consciousness wanes or changes, if the vomiting returns, or if the child has diplopia or ataxia.

Athletes who participate in contact sports should have a mandatory week off from activity. Two concussions within 1 week put them at risk for sudden death.

Admit to a monitored bed all pts with

GCS <15, early posttraumatic seizure, skull fractures, all bleeds, persistent vomiting, dizziness, or abnormal neurologic exam.

LIMB TRAUMA

 What was the mechanism of the injury?
This will tell you how the accident happened, what limb was involved, etc.
The story will also be important in ruling out child abuse.

Can the child move the limb? If the leg is involved, can the child bear weight?
The ability to move or bear weight may give some indication about the severity of the injury.

O **Begin with a rapid but thorough general PE**
It is important not to miss other possible sites of trauma. These could indicate that the injuries are more extensive than previously thought or that there is a pattern of the injuries that could be consistent with abuse.

Examine the affected limb
The limb may be swollen, red, and warm at the site of trauma. It will almost certainly be tender. Point tenderness may indicate a fracture.
Skin breakage or obvious deformity might indicate a compound fracture.
Check to see if the limb has passive mobility and if the child will let you move it.
Nursemaid elbow: Subluxed radial head caused by a traction injury on the arm of a toddler. The child will be holding the arm extended and internally rotated and will refuse to move it. X-rays are unnecessary unless you suspect a fracture. To reduce, hold the radial head, rapidly supinate, and then flex the forearm; if that does not work, try pronation and then flexion. A click or pop is usually heard with successful reduction. It may take a few minutes for the child to start using the arm.
Perform a neurovascular examination distal to the site of injury. Check that pulses are equal to the contralateral side. Digits should be warm with brisk capillary refill after pressure, actively mobile by the pt, with no pain on passive movement, and have sensation.

Look carefully for broken skin
If the skin is broken, look carefully for both fracture and foreign body.
Skin breakage puts the pt at risk for infection, including cellulitis and osteomyelitis.

Obtain x-rays of the affected limb in multiple views
Order at least two views (AP and lateral usually called a "series," e.g., "right-hand series") of the affected area. Fractures and dislocations are not always seen on a single view.
In a toddler or infant with lower extremity trauma in which the site of injury is not obvious on PE, the entire lower extremity must be imaged.
If child indicates knee or hip pain, x-ray both joints. Pain can refer from one joint to the other.

A **Limb trauma. Assess for fracture**
Traumas with no point tenderness and negative x-rays and intact neurovascular exams are likely to be sprains or ligamentous injuries.

Fracture type
Fractures can be:

- Transverse (perpendicular to the bone's length)
- Longitudinal (parallel to the bone's length)
- Compound (fracture associated with a break in the skin)
- Torus (buckling of the bone)
- Spiral (twisting injury)
- Oblique (diagonal)

The next three fractures only occur in pediatrics.
- *Greenstick:* Bone bends, leaving cortical disruption on only one side.
- *Bending:* Bone looks slightly more curved than it should.
- *Salter Harris (SH):* Fractures of the growth plate

There are five types of SH fractures. A good mnemonic is **SALTER**. For the mnemonic to work, think of the femur at the knee where "above" means toward the side of the growth plate with the metaphysis (the long part) and "below" means toward the short end of the bone.
- Type I: (Same) no change in appearance of growth plate.
- Type II: (Above) fracture occurs Above the growth plate (most common, ~70%).
- Type III: (Low) fracture occurs beLow the growth plate.
- Type IV: (Through) fracture goes Through the growth plate (both above and below).
- Type V: (Emergency Room or Rammed) fracture obliterates space of growth plate.

Evaluate for possible compartment syndrome or significant neurovascular injury

Compartment syndrome: The swelling in one or more of the soft tissue compartments in the limb (spaces between facial planes) causes compression of the nerves and blood vessels in the compartment, leading to neurovascular damage. Pain on passive movement of the digits (most sensitive and specific), pallor, paresthesia, and absent or weak pulses all suggest the diagnosis.
- 4P's is a good mnemonic: Pain (with passive movement of digits), paresthesia, pallor, pulselessness

Consult Orthopedics emergently for a fasciotomy if you suspect compartment syndrome.

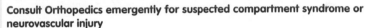

Consult Orthopedics emergently for suspected compartment syndrome or neurovascular injury
Waiting may cost the pt a limb.

Cast simple fractures and provide Orthopedic follow-up

For complex fractures (such as open fractures), involve Orthopedics on a nonemergent basis
Without orthopedic intervention, SH fractures have increased risk of poor growth because of the damage to the growth plate.

Recommend home treatment with rest, ice, compression, and elevation (RICE) and an NSAID like ibuprofen for all sprains or ligamentous injuries

Suspected child abuse should be reported to the appropriate authorities

See suspected physical abuse, p. 222

Check the vaccination card and give tetanus prophylaxis if necessary (Table 12-5)
If the pt received all childhood vaccinations and has had the last one within the last 5 years, then he or she needs nothing. If the pt has a small, contaminated wound and parents do not know the vaccination history, then the American Academy of Pediatrics recommends both Td and TIG be given.

TABLE 12-5   Vaccinations

DtaP	Small Clean Wounds		Contaminated or Large Wounds	
Series	Td	TIG	Td	TIG
<3 doses or unknown	Yes	No	Yes	Yes
≥3	No if in last 10 yr	No	No if in last 5 yr	No

SUSPECTED PHYSICAL ABUSE

 Did the parents seek medical care in a timely fashion?
One of your first clues to abuse is a delay in seeking care for a serious injury.

Does the story match the injury?
Think about whether the injury sustained is possible by the mechanism proposed.

Is the story inconsistent or vague in some way?
Another red flag for child abuse is different versions of the story from different people, or worse, different versions of the story from the same person. If the parents have no idea how this happened, that is also cause for suspicion or at least further investigation. Make sure to ask open-ended questions.

Is the child developmentally capable of the injury?
The child cannot have climbed up the stairs if he or she is not even rolling over yet.

Interview the child alone
If children are old enough to tell the story themselves, they should be allowed to do so.

Who has access to the child?
It does not necessarily have to be the person who brought the child to the hospital who is at fault. There could be an aunt, uncle, cousin, friend, stepparent, or parent's significant other who was the abuser.

 Carefully observe general evaluation of the child
Are clothes appropriate for season? Are clothes clean and in good repair? Full examination should be done with clothing removed.

Carefully observe the interactions of the child and parent
If the parent does not show appropriate concern for the degree of the injury or exhibits inappropriate, angry, or abusive behavior with the child or siblings, that should be noted.

Examine the child carefully for signs of abuse
Reluctance to use or move an extremity should be sought.
Look for retinal hemorrhages, trauma to genitals, mouth (frenulum tears in a premobile infant), signs of neglect (malnourishment).
Look for bruises in patterns caused by hands, hangers, extension cords, belt buckles, cigarette, iron, spatula, and so on.
Look for areas of local tenderness and or swelling over bones suggesting fractures, especially ribs, head, and extremities.
Bruises at different stages of healing or in atypical locations such as face, ears, upper arms, hands, thighs, feet, chest, abdomen, back.

Look for other skin lesions
Burns from immersion in hot water or brandings from hot objects such as the following are all injuries to be further investigated: irons, lighters, cigarette butts.
Also look for abrasions or bruising from gags, tourniquets, and other restraints.
Look carefully at the inside of the mouth/palate, anus, and genitalia for other signs of abuse (see Considering Sexual Abuse, p. 224).

Obtain a skeletal series looking for fractures
If you suspect abuse, it is often prudent, in younger children, to obtain a skeletal survey on which you may find multiple ages of fractures.

Consider head and abdominal CT
If the pt has altered mental status, has any focal neurologic deficit, or is an infant, obtain a head CT emergently to rule out an intracranial hemorrhage.
If there is any abdominal bruising or tenderness, consider an abdominal CT to rule out splenic, hepatic, duodenal, or other intra-abdominal injury.

Check pertinent labs

With significant soft tissue injury, check a CK and Chem 7 to rule out rhabdomyolysis.
With abdominal trauma, check an amylase and a lipase to rule out traumatic
pancreatitis.

If pt is an infant, obtain an emergent ophthalmologic exam

Infants are at risk for retinal hemorrhages if they are shaken. This is diagnostic of abuse.

Consider parental and child risk factors for abuse

Parental risk factors: Drug use, alcoholism, history of being abused, poverty, psychosis,
prior abuse.
Risk factors for children: <3 years, chronic illness, not the abuser's birth child, congenital anomaly.

Assess for signs of abuse on x-ray

Many fractures can be consistent with abuse, but what you have to decide is whether the
history matches the degree of injury.
Two patterns of fracture that are nearly always indicative of abuse:

- Multiple, unexplained fractures in a symmetric pattern in various stages of healing
  in the ribs and long bones.
- Bucket handle fractures: Metaphyseal chips are seen on the lateral and medial aspect
  of the long bone. This fracture is usually caused by violent shaking of the extremity.

Fractures that are highly suspicious include:

- Transverse or oblique fractures of the humerus or femur without a good story
- Rib fractures in children less than 5 years of age. These are highly suspicious
  because they are rarely present even after falls or car accidents.

Differential diagnosis

Accidental trauma: Sometimes the child actually did trip and fall.
Mongolian spots: Nontender flat blue nevi that the pt has had since birth.
Ricketts and osteogenesis imperfecta: Lead to fragile bones/multiple fractures of different ages.
Bleeding diatheses (e.g., hemophilia): May have very significant bruises from minor
trauma.
Cultural practices: Cupping and coining are examples of practices from other countries
in which objects are heated and rubbed on the skin. The marks they leave may appear
severe, but because they are performed with the intention to heal, they are not considered abuse.

Decide if you suspect child abuse

You are obligated to report the suspected abuser to the appropriate state government
agencies as well as to law enforcement. The pt should be admitted to the hospital for
protection. Suspicion of abuse is enough to warrant a report. Abuse usually recurs
and escalates with each episode, so next time the pt may not survive to make it to the
hospital.

Carefully document the H&P and PE

Write down direct quotes without grammatical corrections. Have the pt point to any
body part named and describe where pt points. If pictures would be useful, take them.
Be sure to include a picture of the face and to time and date the photograph.

SUSPECTED SEXUAL ABUSE

S **Who is the reporting party and how was the abuse discovered?**

It is important to note whether the pt has told a parent about sexual abuse, versus the parent having suspicions aroused by physical evidence, or by the presence of another child being abused in the home. A child who is directly admitting abuse is likely to be telling the truth. If a child is going to lie, she or he will more often deny abuse.

Have you noted any behavioral changes in the child?

Young children may:
- Have a recurrence of   – Lose bowel/bladder control   – Become irritable
  bed-wetting   – Develop new feeding difficulties
- Become clingy

With older children, one might see:
- Drop in grades   – Loss of concentration   – Worsening peer relationships
- Depression   – Suicidal ideation   – Inappropriate sexual behavior
- Substance abuse

Has the parent found any suspicious physical evidence?

Often the parent will note discharge or blood in the daughter's underwear as a major physical sign. Other signs include:
- New recurrent abdominal pain   – Dysuria   – Genital bruising
- Lesions (verrucous, ulcerative, etc.) – Swelling   – Discharge

Find out the details of the alleged abuse, including who is accused, when and where did it happen, have there been multiple episodes, and, if so, for how long it has been going on

It is worth noting that as much as 80% of all child abuse is perpetrated by someone the child knows, and often someone they are close to, especially a family member.

Interview the pt

A child who has been abused may feel extremely vulnerable. Some tips on interviewing include the following:
- Begin by establishing rapport. This may be done by discussing nonthreatening topics, playing with toys, or drawing pictures.
- Use the child's language when naming body parts.
- Proceed from general to specific questions. Make sure not to lead the child with your questions. Ask "and then what happened?" rather than "Did he touch your privates?"
- Do not interrupt if a child reports abuse, just let her or him talk. When the child is finished, ask about details of sexual contact including penetration and pain.
- Be supportive and reassuring.
- If the child has not disclosed, be supportive. Relate that you understand that some of the complaints may be secondary to sexual abuse. Discuss secrets, fears, and touching.

O **Perform a general PE before examining the genitalia**

Look for signs of physical abuse, including unusual bruises or bite marks.

It is important to note that for a full and appropriate genital exam, your hospital's specialist team should be called. If one is not available, look for the following

Examine entire perineal region for lacerations, abrasions, bruising, or scarring. Pay particular attention to posterior vulvar fourchette, hymen, and anus.

Old injuries may have skin tags or scars.

Children heal extremely well, so absence of scars does not rule out a history of abuse. A normal exam does not rule out abuse.

It is important again to note that this exam should, whenever possible, be done by a specialist, with a handheld magnifier, a light, a camera, and a colposcope.

Before and throughout the exam, tell the child exactly what you are going to do. Make sure she or he is okay with everything you are doing before you do it.

Send urine for U/A with microscopy, chlamydial/gonorrheal ligase chain reactions, bacterial culture, and, in females older than 8 years, check a pregnancy test

Microscopy may reveal sperm if there was recent vaginal penetration with ejaculation.

If any of the tests for sexually transmitted infections or pregnancy are positive, this is very helpful in court to prove the abuse occurred.

Check blood for rapid plasma reagin (serum test for syphilis) and HIV if the parent consents

Although syphilis and HIV can be acquired congenitally, in this situation a positive test would be supportive of sexual abuse.

 Suspected sexual abuse

Sexual abuse is more common than usually thought. In their lifetimes, 1 in 3 women will suffer sexual abuse or rape. In males, the number is closer to 1 in 12. Perpetrators are usually males.

Differential diagnosis

Abuse must be ruled out before anything else. If you suspect abuse, it should be reported. Protecting the child from further abuse is the goal. To achieve this, it must be identified and proven. Although conditions such as Munchausen syndrome and Munchausen by proxy are possible, they are much less common and much less likely than abuse.

One scenario that can occur is the divorced parent accusing the other of sexually abusing the child. If the child denies the abuse and there are more physical findings, it is still nearly impossible to know whether the abuse is occurring or not, but in either case it should be reported and thoroughly documented.

 After the exam, it is the medical professional's job to act as a counselor

It is critical that the child's interaction with the medical professional be as positive an experience as possible.

It is important to address abused children's guilt, fear, and shame. Explain that it is not their fault and that they are in a safe environment now. Refer the family to family therapy

It can only be hoped that through therapy, the family will be able to heal these scars.

As far as reporting is concerned, state laws differ, but it can be assumed that your state makes the medical professional a mandatory reporter

Your state will most likely require both telephone and written reporting to Child Protective Services and the police.

Document everything thoroughly (when possible, use direct quotes without grammatical corrections), and photographs are also extremely helpful to prove a case in court.

PEDIATRIC WARD

INPATIENT CARE

S **Were there any problems yesterday or any overnight events?**

This is a good question for anyone who saw the pt the night before (e.g., parent, nurse, doctor).

Does the pt have any pain? Has the pain been well-controlled?

Assess whether the pt has pain, where it is, if it is well-controlled, and if it has changed.

When was the last urine output?

Ensuring number of outputs gives an idea of hydration status.

When was the last bowel movement?

Constipation is a common avoidable problem in the hospital.

How is the pt eating? Is he or she hungry?

This is a soft indicator that there might be more problems. Sick people lose their appetites.

Does the pt have any concerns or questions?

Gives an idea of how much the pt knows and an opportunity to inform or reassure.

Ask pt and parent about the child's condition and why he or she is in the hospital

Assesses the pt/parent's understanding so that you can explain more clearly if necessary. Maintaining good communication avoids problems and ultimately leads to more effective therapy.

O **Review the chart quickly**

Look at the notes (by consulting services, cross-covering doctors, the attending, etc.) that have been written since your last note so you will know about important changes or updates.

Look at the orders for any new orders since the last time you saw the chart. Find out why the changes were made. Be sure to know meds, what they are, and why your pt is on them.

Look at the nursing notes for any information that may not be in the doctor's notes.

Review the vital signs and ins and outs from the night before

Note any abnormalities in the vital signs, investigate possible causes, and notify the resident.

Examine the pt carefully

Keep in mind your initial exam of the pt and note any changes.

See Table 13-1 for abbreviations for the PE (see Abbreviations [p. xvi] for more—check with your local hospital service for approved/accepted abbreviations).

In general: 1+ is < average, 2+ is about average, and 3+ is > average.

TABLE 13-1 Abbreviations for the Physical Exam[a]

VS = Vital signs	**P** or **HR** = Pulse/heart rate	**T** = Temperature
BP = Blood pressure	**R** or **RR** = Respiratory rate	**PS** = Pain score
Gen = General appearance	**HEENT** = Head, eyes, ears, nose, throat	
TM = Tympanic membrane	**NCAT** = Normocephalic atraumatic	
OP = Oropharynx	**AFSFO** = Anterior fontanelle soft flat and open	
EOMi = Extraocular muscles intact	**PERRLA** = Pupils equal, round, reactive to light and accommodation	
CV = Cardiovascular	**RRR** = Regular rate and rhythm	

SM = Systolic murmur	φ **M/R/G/C** = No murmurs/rubs/gallops/clicks
B = Bilateral	**Lungs CTA** = Lungs clear to auscultation
L = Left **R** = Right	+ **BS NT ND** = Positive bowel sounds nontender nondistended
<u>**Abd**</u> = Abdomen	**NFEG/NMEG** = Normal female/male external genitalia
NRT = Normal rectal tone	**CVA** = Costovertebral angle
<u>**Ext**</u> = Extremities	φ **C/C/E** = No cyanosis/clubbing/edema
TTP = Tender to palpation	**ROM** = Range of movement **MAE** = Move all extremities
CN = Cranial nerves	**DTR** = Deep tendon reflexes

Note: Exam headings are underlined.

Review the pt's laboratories and microbiology results
Again, note any abnormalities and investigate possible causes.

Look at all of the x-rays and other studies done on the pt
By seeing them yourself, you can better understand and relay the official report.

 Diagnosis: __, hospital day: __

Assess for improvement
If pt is not getting better, then the treatment plan may need to be reassessed.

Assess reason for continued hospitalization
If you do not have a good reason why pts are still in the hospital, then they should go home.

Know what needs to be done to get the pt home or out of the hospital
An efficient workup or treatment can only occur if you have a clear plan.

Be sure to address all of the pt's or parents' concerns
If the pt/parent is dissatisfied, usually you have missed something or they think you have. It is important to clear up the misunderstanding in either case.
Parents are often better able to observe changes in their children, so listen to them.

 Address any problems, pain, abnormal vitals, PE findings, labs, micro results, or studies found while gathering data to write your note
Note problems or abnormalities, and investigate possible causes.

Gather all of your data and write your note
Subjective: Things told to you by the pt, parents, nurses, or other doctors
Objective: Data such as vitals, ins and outs, PE, labs, micro, and studies
Assessment: Summarize diagnoses and whether they are improving, worsening, or static
Plan: Summarize what will be done for each of the problems the pt has
Record information such as medicines, IV fluids, diet, and hardware.
Organize the assessment and plan by problem list or by systems:
- Neuro = Neurologic
- Resp = Respiratory
- CV = Cardiovascular
- FEN/GI = Fluids electrolytes nutrition/gastrointestinal
- Renal/GU = Renal/genitourinary
- Heme/ID = Hematologic/infectious disease

Be sure to time, date, and sign your note.
The note should be a summary showing both what has and will happen.

DEHYDRATION AND INTRAVENOUS FLUID MANAGEMENT

S **When was the last time the child urinated? How many times in the last 24 hours?**

If it has been more than 6–8 hours since the child's last void, this is concerning and consistent with significant dehydration. Try to quantify how much less urine output (UOP) the pt has compared with normal.

Is the child making tears when he or she cries?

If the child is screaming and crying during the exam but not making a single tear, that will be another clue to the child's level of dehydration. Children less than 3 months of age may or may not produce tears, making this an unreliable marker in this age group.

Is the child having vomiting, diarrhea? How many times per day? Is the child febrile?

If the child is having continued losses, then it is important to keep track of them and replace them so that you do not fall even further behind than you already are.

Fever represents an increase in the metabolic rate and diaphoresis, thus increasing the insensible losses.

Is the child eating and/or drinking?

If the child is eating and drinking, you may be able to orally replace the fluids being lost, but otherwise you may have to rehydrate intravenously.

Has the child lost weight, and do the parents remember a recent weight to compare with today's?

If you are fortunate enough to have a weight from 2 days ago that is 10% higher than today's weight, then it is easy to assess the degree of dehydration. It is 10%. For example, if a child weighed 12 kg 2 days ago and now weighs 10.5 kg, then the degree of dehydration is 12.5%.

O **Do a focused PE to assess dehydration**

Signs to look for on PE to assess dehydration include:

- Hypotension (often a late and ominous sign)
- Altered mental status
- No tears when crying
- Sunken anterior fontanelle (children <18 mo)
- Tachycardia
- Dry mucus membranes
- Poor skin turgor
- Poor capillary refill

Check U/A, looking specifically for urine specific gravity (SG)

The more concentrated the urine (SG >1.020), the more dehydrated the child is likely to be.

Check serum electrolytes, BUN, and creatinine

Examine the lytes and replace any potassium or other electrolyte deficits. If there is hypernatremia, you can also calculate a **free water deficit = pt's wt × % dehydration**. The BUN/Cr ratio can also be a clue suggesting dehydration if the ratio of those two is greater than 10.

Examine for the cause of dehydration. It is often obvious (diarrhea, vomiting, or refusal to take any oral intake)

A **Assess degree of dehydration (Table 13-2)**

TABLE 13-2   Degrees of Dehydration

Dehydration	%	Signs/Symptoms	Urine Specific Gravity
Mild	5%	Dry mucus membranes, ↓UOP	1.020–1.030
Moderate	5%–10%	Tachycardia, sunken fontanelle and eyes	>1.030
Severe	>10%	AMS, orthostatic, poor capillary refill	>1.035

P Maintain your pt's daily fluid balance and rehydrate if necessary

In reality, many dehydrated children can be orally rehydrated. But if the child is unable to tolerate oral fluids or if he or she is NPO for a procedure, then IV fluids are required.

Bolus if orthostatic or hypotensive

If severe dehydration exists, then bolus 20 cc/kg normal saline until orthostasis is corrected or the pt begins to urinate. After doing this three times for a total of 60 cc/kg, consider changing to colloid or blood for continued volume replacement. These boluses should not be added to the calculated fluid deficit.

Calculate fluid deficit using the three components of fluid replacement

Initial deficit: Multiply the pt's weight by the assessed degree of hydration. So a 10-kg child who has severe dehydration has approximately a 1 kg = 1 L (remember that 1 L of water weighs 1 kg) deficit. This deficit should be replaced over 24 hours, with the first half going in over the first 8 hours and the second half going in over the next 16 hours.

Maintenance fluids: "4-2-1" rule:

100 cc/kg/d or 4 cc/kg/hr for the first 10 kg, 50 cc/kg/d or 2 cc/kg/hr for the second 10 kg, and finally, 20 cc/kg/d or 1 cc/kg/hr for each remaining kg.

- Therefore, a 43-kg person should receive 1,000 + 500 + 460 = 1,960 cc per day.
- The same 43-kg person should receive an hourly maintenance of
  40 + 20 + 23 = 83 cc/hr.
- 83 × 24 = 1,992, so the numbers are fairly close.

Ongoing losses: Usually, if a pt is vomiting or stooling large amounts, keep track of the amount of the losses and replace them cc/cc with normal saline.

In summary, if a 21-kg child is 10% dehydrated, calculate the fluid replacement as:

- Deficit: 21 kg × 10% = 2.1 L, first half in first 8 hours and second half in next 16 hours
- Maintenance would be 40 + 20 + 1 = 61 cc/hr

So for the first 8 hours, the rate would be 2,100 cc/2 = 1,050 cc/8 hr = 131 + 61 = 192 cc/hr. Over the next 16 hours, the rate should be 2,100/2 = 1,050/16 = 65.6 + 61 = 127 cc/hr with D5½ NS (with 20 mEq KCl/L added after the first void to ensure that the kidneys are working normally).

Total ongoing losses every 8 hours and give them back, cc for cc with normal saline over the next 2–4 hours.

If the child is less than 4 months old, consider using D5¼ NS as the fluid because the kidneys are not yet fully developed and less able to concentrate the urine

An exception to this is any child of any age with hydrocephalus, ventriculoperitoneal shunt, or other neurosurgical pathology. In these children, given the increased risk of cerebral edema with hypotonic fluids, use only NS or D5NS for fluids regardless of the age.

PAIN CONTROL

 Does the pt have any pain? Rate the pain on a scale of 1–10
Assesses the severity of the pain so you can address and assess pain relief.

Ask the pt to point with one finger to where the pain hurts most
Pain location will help immensely with the differential diagnosis.

Try to describe the pain: is it sharp, dull, crampy, or burning?
The description of the pain is useful when generating a diagnosis because certain etiologies of pain have very different character. Dull chest pain has different implications than sharp chest pain.

Does the pain travel anywhere?
Pain radiation can suggest neuropathic pain, such as pain radiating down the leg from a pinched nerve in the spine, or it can suggest pancreatitis or dissecting aortic aneurysm such as epigastric pain radiating to the back.

When did the pain start?
Abdominal pain for 5 years is less worrisome than abdominal pain for 1–2 days.

How long does each episode of pain last?
If pain lasts seconds, it is much less worrisome than hours.

How often do the pain episodes occur?
Pain occurring once a month versus once an hour is less worrisome.

Is the pain getting worse, better, or staying the same?
If the pain is getting worse, then you have less time to evaluate and treat it.

What is the pt usually doing when the pain starts?
The context or circumstances when the pain starts can be an important clue.

Does anything make the pain worse or better? With activity, lying still, or certain position?
Exacerbating factors are helpful information for generating the differential diagnosis.

Has the same pain ever happened before? If the pain occurred before, what was done about it and what was it caused by? How is the pain different this time?
If this pain is similar to a previously diagnosed episode, that diagnosis may be the same this time also, so it is worth knowing and considering.

 Perform a good general PE, but carefully examine the location of the pain
Neck pain: Look for signs of meningitis or trauma and rule out both. Consider checking a cervical spine film.
Extremity pain: Look carefully for masses, signs of infection (cellulitis), or signs of trauma.
Joint pain: Examine for loss of function, range of motion, or weakness, as well as for signs of arthritis.
Knee or hip pain: Examine both to assure that the knee pain is not actually referred hip pain.
Abdominal pain: Examine for peritoneal signs (see Abdominal Pain, p. 172).
Back pain: See if movement of the leg at the hip causes radiating pain to the toes, suggesting neuropathic pain from a pinched nerve (unlikely in children without a history of trauma).

 Carefully investigate the possible causes of the pain and address them
Exclude the most dangerous possibilities such as peritonitis or appendicitis.

Differential diagnosis
Organic pain: Secondary to an organic cause, usually related to tissue damage.

Neuropathic pain: Results from neuronal injury; usually causes burning and/or hypersensitivity.

Malingering: The pt is simply making it up. Often associated with avoidance of an adverse stimulus (e.g., school, juvenile hall, home if being abused) or for narcotic addiction.

P Treat the pain

Even if the pain is dangerous (e.g., appendicitis) be sure to treat the pain during the workup.

Abbreviations:

– po = by mouth	– pr = per rectum	– IV = intravenous
– IM = intramuscular	– SQ = subcutaneous	– prn = as needed
– q = each	– qhs = at bedtime	– qd = once a day
– bid = 2× a day	– tid = 3× a day	– qid = 4× a day

Mild Pain:

• Acetaminophen: 10–15 mg/kg/dose (adult 650 mg) po/pr q4h prn
• Ibuprofen: 10 mg/kg/dose (adult 200–800 mg) po q6h prn mild pain

Moderate Pain:

• Ketorolac (Toradol): 0.4–1 mg/kg/dose (adult 15–30 mg) IV/IM q6h prn mod pain (max. dose 40 mg/d, max. duration 5 days, use only > age 2 year)
• Naproxen: 2.5–10 mg/kg/dose (adult 500 mg po) q8–12h (max. 1,250 mg/d) prn mod pain (use only over the age of 2 year)
• Acetaminophen with codeine: 0.5–1 mg/kg/dose q4–6h (adult 2 tabs of the Tylenol #3 formulation) prn mod pain

Severe Pain:

• Hydrocodone/acetaminophen (Vicodin): 0.4–0.6 mg/kg/d divided tid or qid (adult, 2 tabs q4h) prn severe pain
• Morphine: 0.05–0.1 mg/kg po/IM/SQ/IV q4h prn severe pain

If the pt weighs >40 kg, check that you are not giving more than the adult dose.

Patient-controlled analgesia should be used with severe pain whenever possible. It is a safe and effective way of controlling severe in-hospital pain.

Consider long-acting oral morphine or fentanyl (Duragesic) patches, before discharging a pt, if need to control chronic severe pain, as in cancer.

If you have chosen to give narcotic analgesics, always consider the side effects

If coma or a serious decrease in respiratory drive occurs, administer naloxone (Narcan) 0.1 mg/kg/dose IV or IM. The half-life of Narcan is short, so you may need to repeat the dose.

Assume constipation will occur if the pt is using narcotics, and preventively start on a high-fiber diet and/or docusate or other anticonstipation regimen. If it still occurs, treat with milk of magnesia or magnesium citrate.

POSTOPERATIVE CARE OF THE APPENDICITIS PATIENT

S **What type of appendicitis did pt have?**

The type of appendicitis determines the postoperative course and management:

- *Acute appendicitis:* An infected appendix that has not yet perforated
- *Perforated appendicitis:* Appendix ruptures, releasing pus into the abdomen
- *Gangrenous appendicitis:* A necrotic appendix, treated as a perforated appendicitis postop

Ask the pt to rate his or her level of pain

Narcotics are usually required. Assess pain control frequently postop.

Acute appys tend to have less pain (due to less preop inflammation) than perf'd appys.

Has the pt passed gas or had a bowel movement yet?

Passing gas (flatus) or stool indicates gut motility, a sign of recovery. Acute appys tend to experience increasing motility within 48 hours postop. Perf'd appys may take longer.

Is the pt hungry? Does the pt think he or she can eat, or does he or she still feel nauseated?

Postop ileus: When the bowel is manipulated during surgery, it causes a period of immotility during which the pt will not be hungry and may have nausea and vomiting.

Small bowel obstruction: Presents postop as frequent bilious (green) emesis and a distended abdomen. Obtain a KUB, place a nasogastric tube to suction, and get an emergent surgical consult. This is more common in pts with perf'd appys.

Recovery: When the pt begins to have flatus and regains appetite, he or she can be advanced meal by meal from ice chips to clear liquid to a regular diet.

Is the pt ambulating?

Walking should be encouraged. If the pt is not walking around by postop day 2, there is a risk for complications such as atelectasis and deep vein thrombosis (DVT).

O **Check for fever**

In a postop acute appy, fever most likely indicates ongoing infection.

- Pts with perf'd appys can be expected to spike fevers for several days as their bodies deal with the contaminated peritoneal space caused by the rupture of the appendix.

Also consider the postsurgical causes of fever mnemonic, five Ws:

- *W*ind (atelectasis)
- *W*ater (UTI)
- *W*ound (wound infection)
- *W*onder drugs (drug fever)
- *W*alking (DVT)

With that in mind, get the appropriate workup: chest x-ray, urine, blood, and wound cultures.

If fever is not present, assure that the pt is not tachycardic

If pain control is good, then tachycardia is concerning for intravascular volume depletion, which is common in perf'd appys because of third spacing. If it occurs, be sure to replace the volume.

Perform a PE, with a focus on the pt's lungs, abdomen, and extremities

Lung exam: Should have equal breath sounds bilaterally, with good air entry without rales, rhonchi, or decreased breath sounds. If the lung exam is abnormal, check O_2 sat and chest x-ray.

Abdominal exam: Perform gently; check carefully for distention (may be associated with scrotal or labial edema). Examine wound site for dehiscence, erythema, or drainage.

Extremities exam: Examine for edema or abnormal capillary refill time (>2 seconds).

Check the labs

Acute appys might only require 1 day of labs postop to make sure the WBC count decreased appropriately, representing resolution of the infection.

Perforated appys require the following labs daily:

- Chem 7: Will give you information about this pt's fluid status. Hyponatremia with an elevated BUN is consistent with a pt who has third-spacing fluid.
- CBC: Persistently elevated WBC count represents ongoing infection and often correlates with continued fevers.

 A   Acute or Perforated appendicitis, postop day __

Ensure that you assess the four following areas:
- *Pain:* Well-controlled?
- *Fever:* Ongoing infection versus one of the five W's
- *Gut motility:* Signs such as flatus and hunger represent recovery, and signs such as emesis and distention suggest ileus and possibly even obstruction.
- *Prevention:* Ensure that your pt is walking and using the incentive spirometer to improve gut motility and avoid fever from atelectasis and DVTs.

P   Management includes antibiotics, pain control, IV fluids, and supportive care

Antibiotics

Acute appy: Start a second-generation cephalosporin for 24 hours postop.
Perforated appy: Cover for all potential organisms in the colonic flora:
- Gram-positive (*Enterococcus*)
- Aerobic gram-negative coliforms
- Anaerobic organisms

Traditionally, ampicillin, gentamicin, and metronidazole are used. Broad-spectrum single agents such as piperacillin-tazobactam, ticarcillin-clavulanate, or carbapenems may also be used.
Perforated appys should be on antibiotics for at least 5 days postop and longer if the pt is still febrile.

Narcotics can help with pain control. Analgesia can be supplemented with ketorolac or acetaminophen. Start with parenteral analgesics and switch to oral when the child is drinking well

Acute appys: Most need <1 day of morphine and then a few days of acetaminophen with codeine by mouth.
Perforated appys: Usually need morphine by patient-controlled analgesia for several days.

IV fluids

All appys should have increased rate of fluid intravenously, usually starting at twice the maintenance rate, and decreasing to 1.5 times the maintenance. When the pt tolerates diet, without vomiting, the IV may be hep locked.

Other supportive care

Pts should be given incentive spirometry and encouraged to use it 10 times per hour while awake to prevent atelectasis.

POSTOPERATIVE CARE OF THE PYLORIC STENOSIS PATIENT

S **How is the baby doing since his or her surgery?**
Allow the parent to tell you all of their concerns regarding the postoperative period.

Ask the parents if they think the baby is in any pain
Pyloromyotomies are small surgeries with small incisions and are often performed in <20 minutes; however, even with a small upper abdominal incision, parents will often perceive pain in their child.

Is the baby vomiting at all?
It is good to reassess the chief complaint and address any concerns the parents may have.

How is the baby tolerating the new feeding schedule?
The new feeding schedule (see below) can be initiated on the first postoperative day. It is an important assessment of the success of the surgery. Asking this question is an important follow-up to the last question. Even if the pt is not vomiting, he or she may not be ready to eat yet.

O **Check the baby's vital signs**
Tachycardia (HR >160 in this age group) may indicate pain.
The baby should be afebrile, with normal respirations and blood pressure.

Check the baby's intake and output to make sure he or she is tolerating feeds, receiving enough IV fluids, and producing urine
The baby's ins and outs should be balanced, with the intake being slightly greater than the output. If the total fluid output is small (<1 cc/kg/hr), consider giving an IV fluid bolus of 10–20 cc/kg of normal saline over 1 hour.
Check to see if the pt is tolerating the new feeding schedule. Emesis should be recorded.

Perform a general PE
Do a focused exam unless the pt is symptomatic. A comprehensive exam was done on admission, and things such as red reflex, testicular exam are unlikely to change.
Lungs: Rales or rhonchi may represent aspiration during surgery or postoperatively.
Heart: Heart murmur should be absent. Murmur may represent significant blood loss, which is highly unlikely with this kind of surgery.
Capillary refill: Should be less than 2 seconds because this pt should be well hydrated.

Now gently examine the abdomen. Check the wound
The wound should be approximately 1.5–2 cm long in the epigastrium and clean. There should be no surrounding erythema or discharge from the wound. These signs may represent the beginning of an infection.
Gently palpate the abdomen in an area away from the wound. It should not be distended or exquisitely tender. The baby may not even cry. Distention and exquisite tenderness should make you think of peritoneal inflammation.

Blood should be checked at least once postoperatively with a CBC and BMP
Again, the CBC should confirm minimal blood loss. There should be virtually no change in hemoglobin or hematocrit levels since admission.
The BMP should have normalized. On admission, the baby can have some severe metabolic derangements, including alkalosis, hypokalemia, and hypochloremia. The BUN-to-creatinine ratio may have been greater than 20:1. With hydration, these numbers should return to normal.

If aspiration is suspected, a chest x-ray should be obtained

Status postpyloromyotomy, postop day __

Your assessment should also mention the resolution of metabolic derangements and how the pt is doing with feeds.

Also watch for complications of the surgery, such as wound infection, peritonitis, postop fever, and recurrence of the original problem (rare).

P **Begin refeeding the pt on the first postoperative day, usually within 6 hours of surgery. He or she should be hungry**

Moderate regurgitation is common due to pyloric and antral spasm, and gastric irritation. Feeding should begin with an electrolyte solution such as Pedialyte. Start with only 5 cc.

If the pt tolerates this without emesis, 10 cc of Pedialyte may be given 2 hours later.

If there is still no emesis, you may switch to 10 cc of half-strength formula 2 hours later. This may be increased to 15 cc 2 hours later.

If the pt tolerates 15 cc of half-strength formula, you may now switch to full-strength formula. Repeat 15 cc.

Now, every 2 hours the amount may be increased: 20 cc, then 30 cc, then 45 cc, and finally 60 cc. Once the pt tolerates 60 cc, feed regularly every 3 hours.

If the pt has emesis with any of the doses of feed, feeds should be held for 4 hours and then restarted at the last tolerated dose.

Stop IV fluids when feeds are tolerated (at least 2 feeds of ≥60 cc).

Control pain with acetaminophen. 15 mg/kg rectal q4h PRN. Can use minimal amounts of IV narcotics if needed

Once the pt is tolerating regular feeds of formula or breast milk, and pain is not an issue, pt may be discharged

There should be follow-up in a surgery clinic to check the wound and remove sutures as needed, and follow-up with a general pediatrician at the regular 2-month visit.

INPATIENT CARE OF THE ORTHOPEDIC PATIENT

S **Does the pt have any pain? If so, where and how much does it hurt on a scale of 1–10?**
Make sure that if your pt has pain, the etiology is discovered and the pain is controlled.

Can the pt wiggle or move his or her toes/fingers?
If the child is unable to move the toes/fingers of the cast limb and this is a new problem, this may signify neurologic damage or compartment syndrome (see below).

Can the pt feel his or her toes/fingers?
If the pt cannot feel the toes/fingers or has abnormal sensation, check for other signs of compartment syndrome.

Have the pt's toes/fingers changed color or do they feel numb or cold?
If the fingers or toes are turning blue or black, or they feel unusually numb or cold, check for pulses proximally. If they are diminished or nonpalpable, emergently notify the orthopedist and possibly vascular surgeon.

Has the pt been using the incentive spirometer?
Use of the incentive spirometer will decrease the incidence of atelectasis and possibly of postoperative pneumonia, so encourage its use.

O **Examine the pt**
Perform a good general PE.

Look at the vitals for any worrisome signs
Infection: Fever could be a sign of infection.

> If the fever spike is near surgery, consider the postsurgical causes of fever mnemonic: five W's:
> - *W*ind (atelectasis)
> - *W*ater (UTI)
> - *W*ound (wound infection)
> - *W*onder drugs (drug fever)
> - *W*alking (DVT)

With that in mind, get the appropriate workup. Check a chest x-ray; get urine and blood cultures, and wound cultures if appropriate.
Internal bleeding: Tachycardia can be a sign of nervousness, pain, or worse, hypovolemia. If tachycardia occurs, monitor it closely. If it persists and pain is not the cause, consider giving an IV fluid bolus. If the bolus improves the tachycardia, consider the possibility that the pt is still bleeding. Pts can bleed into places such as the abdomen, thigh, chest, or subgaleal space with little outward sign of the problem except persistent tachycardia. If you suspect this, notify the resident immediately.
Pulmonary embolus: Tachycardia, with or without hypoxia and nervousness, could suggest a pulmonary embolus from fat or clot. If the suspicion is high enough, get a CT scan of the chest with contrast. Call the orthopedic surgeon before starting heparin or other anticoagulants.

> **Look at the digits distal to the fracture, cast, or splint for signs of compartment syndrome**
> These are icy cold, *p*allor, *p*aresthesias (tingling or abnormal sensation), *p*ulselessness, or especially severe *p*ain with passive movement of the toes or fingers of the affected limb.
> - Mnemonic = four P's. See Limb Trauma, p. 220.

Look for signs of infection
Look for cellulitis (warm, red, swollen, tender skin) or purulent discharge near any hardware. Monitor carefully for possible development of osteomyelitis. Check an x-ray (or MRI if clinical suspicion is high enough) of the affected limb for disruption of the cortex or soft-tissue swelling.

A **Status post __, postop day __**

Assess for pain control

See Pain Control, p. 230.

Assess for compartment syndrome

Increased pressure is usually caused by inflammation and swelling in a space enclosed by fascial planes. When the pressure exceeds that of local arterial blood flow, ischemia results. Evaluate carefully and remember the four P's (see above).

Assess for internal bleeding

Look carefully for:
- – Persistent tachycardia
- – Hypotension
- – Drop in hematocrit
- – Local swelling
- – Pallor

Assess for infection

It is important to rule in or out osteomyelitis because the treatment for this is chronic antibiotics, and the longer it goes unrecognized, the harder it is to eradicate.

Consider offering physical therapy (PT) and/or occupational therapy (OT)

Usually the answer to this offer is yes. Call PT and OT to see if they can offer any help with the pt's rehabilitation.

P **Control the pt's pain**

See Pain Control, p. 230.

Treat compartment syndrome if it is present

The treatment is to surgically release the pressure by opening the space enclosed by fascia = fasciotomy. If this needs to be done emergently, notify the orthopedic surgeon.

Resuscitate the pt and control/stop internal bleeding if it is present

If you suspect internal bleeding, stabilize/resuscitate the pt with normal saline boluses 20 mL/kg up to three times and then start transfusing blood. In the meantime, emergently contact the surgeon for possible surgery to achieve hemostasis.

If you suspect infection, obtain blood cultures, x-rays, MRI, and other studies as appropriate

Based on the results of the workup for fever, x-ray, U/A, blood, urine, or wound culture, treat the infection appropriately. If osteomyelitis is diagnosed (often on MRI), the pt will need long-term treatment (at least 6 weeks) with antibiotics and possibly even surgical insertion of antibiotic pellets into the bone for better local delivery of the antibiotic.

Prepare pt for discharge

Keep the pain well-controlled. Get the pt as active as possible within the constraints of the injury. Consult PT and OT for tips and advice on how to do this, as well as exercises and strategies the pt can use to make the transition from hospital to home.

III
OBSTETRICS AND GYNECOLOGY

OBSTETRICS CLINIC

INITIAL VISIT

S | **Is the pt sure about the date of her last menstrual period (LMP)?**

LMP is customarily used to establish the estimated gestational age (EGA) and estimated date of confinement (EDC) (or "due date").

An accurate EGA/EDC is the single most important piece of information to be known about a pregnancy.

An *unsure* LMP warrants an ultrasound examination to establish EGA/EDC.
- A history of irregular periods or hormonal contraception use before conception may also warrant an U/S, especially if your physical examination of the uterus is inconsistent with proposed dates (see below).
- Methods to "date" a pregnancy of unknown age (e.g., ultrasound, physical exam) become progressively more inaccurate as the pregnancy advances.

- Therefore, it is crucial to establish the EGA/EDC early in pregnancy.

Review obstetric history
Identify any obstetric problems that may recur with current pregnancy.
Pts with previous pregnancies affected by NTDs should be on folate 4 mg/d.

Perform ROS and obtain PMH
Elicit a history of any potential medical problems complicating pregnancy or complications of past pregnancies.

Obtain PSH
Pts with previous C/S should be counseled regarding delivery options for current pregnancy:
      – Trial of labor   – Repeat C/S

Obtain social history
Alcohol, tobacco, and substance use should be identified and counseled appropriately.

Obtain family history
Pts with a family history of congenital anomalies, mental retardation, or metabolic diseases should be identified and referred for prenatal diagnosis (see Second Trimester Visit, p. 242).

Does the pt have any high-risk factors for gestational diabetes mellitus (GDM)?
GDM is a major contributor to morbidity in pregnancy (see Gestational Diabetes Mellitus, p. 254).
Identifying potentially affected individuals early can minimize complications.
The presence of any of the following high-risk factors warrants first trimester screening for GDM:
      – History of glucose intolerance   – First-degree relative with DM
      – Adverse obstetric outcomes usually associated with GDM

Does the pt have any risk factors for antiphospholipid syndrome (APS)?
The presence of any of the following warrants a workup for APS (see Antiphospholipid Syndrome, p. 250):
- History of recurrent abortion (three or more first trimester losses) or a single second or third trimester fetal loss
- Severe preeclampsia <34 weeks
- Severe fetal growth restriction
- History of thrombosis

O **Confirm a positive pregnancy test (β-hCG)**

Pregnancy can be confirmed with either a qualitative β-hCG (test is performed with a urine specimen and reported as positive or negative) or a quantitative β-hCG (test is performed with a blood sample and reported as a numeric value).

Is the EGA 10 weeks or older?

If so, attempt to elicit fetal heart tones by Doppler monitor.
Establishing heart tones helps confirm the EGA.

Perform PE

Careful attention should be paid to thyroid, cardiac, and pulmonary systems, which are most commonly associated with serious medical complications in pregnancy.
Uterine size should be confirmed to be consistent with EGA.
If your physical examination of the uterus is inconsistent with EGA, obtain U/S.

Is the pt obese? (BMI >30)

Obese pts have a higher risk of glucose intolerance and should also be tested for GDM in the first trimester.
Caloric requirements during pregnancy should be limited (total weight gain = 30 lbs).

Is glycosuria present on the office urine dip?

Some glycosuria is expected (caused by decreased tubular reabsorption), but a positive result on a second voided fasting urine warrants first trimester testing for GDM. If a patient has a history of GDM, also do first trimester testing.

A **Intrauterine pregnancy (IUP) at 8 weeks**

Differential diagnosis of an early IUP includes any form of abnormal pregnancy:
    – Ectopic pregnancy   – Missed abortion   – Molar pregnancy

P **Perform or schedule U/S if EGA is unclear**

Indications include unsure LMP or discrepancy on PE.

Draw the "prenatal" labs

Blood group, Rh status, and antibody screen; CBC, Rubella, RPR, HBsAg, and HIV
Perform Pap smear and gonococcus/*Chlamydia* cultures.
MSAFP and NIPT if between 15 and 20 weeks at initial visit (see Second Trimester Visit, p. 242).

Prescribe prenatal vitamins and iron supplementation

Folate is the most important element for its association with prevention of NTDs (recommended intake 0.4 mg/d).
Ideally, pts should be taking some source of folate supplementation for 3 months before conception.
Iron supplementation helps the mother maintain iron stores in the face of increased requirement during pregnancy.

Instruct and educate pt about common questions and complaints

Diet, sleep, bowel habits, exercise, bathing, clothing, recreation, and travel

Up to 30% of all pts will experience vaginal spotting during first trimester.

Schedule next appointment

For an uncomplicated pregnancy, see the pt every 4 weeks in the first trimester.

Consider referral to high-risk clinic

A pt with any medical problems should always be considered to receive care or consultation from a high-risk clinic.

SECOND TRIMESTER VISIT

S **If the pt was previously suffering from symptoms associated with the first trimester, are these resolving?**

Nausea and vomiting of pregnancy, fatigue, and associated symptoms should usually be declining by the second trimester. Offer antiemetics for vomiting.

Any persistent symptoms mandate workup for etiology.

Does the pt have any new complaints?

As the uterus enlarges, some women start to experience discomfort from the stretching of pelvic ligaments.

"Round ligament pain" is a common diagnosis during the second trimester. Preterm UCs should be worked up.

Does the pt belong to an ethnic group that has a high risk for specific genetic disorders?

Consider screening tests in the following populations:
- Eastern European (Ashkenazi) Jewish: Tay-Sachs and Canavan disease
- Cajun and French-Canadian: Tay-Sachs
- Caucasian: Cystic fibrosis, SMA

O **Check blood pressure**

Maternal blood pressure falls for the first 24 weeks of pregnancy and then returns to normal values by term, secondary to relaxation effect of progesterone on smooth muscle.

Diastolic pressure falls greater than systolic, widening pulse pressure.

Check urine dip for glucose and protein

Glucose >1+ (>100 mg/dL) may require earlier screening for GDM.

Proteinuria ≥2+ (≥100 mg/dL) requires urine analysis for infection and close observation of BP for preeclampsia.

Confirm appropriate maternal weight gain

Total weight gain for pregnancy should be about 30 lbs in women with a normal BMI.
In women with a BMI >30, the ideal weight gain is 12–15 lbs.
- 5 lbs should be gained in the first trimester.
- 1/2–1 lb/wk should be gained for the remainder of pregnancy.

- <10 lb weight gain by 20 weeks should prompt a nutritional review.

Elicit fetal heart tones with Doppler

This confirms ongoing viability of pregnancy.

Measure fundal height (FH)

This helps confirm ongoing fetal growth.
- If EGA <20 weeks, a rough estimate can be made by palpation.
- If EGA >20 weeks, assess by measuring fundal height in centimeters.

Measurement of FH in centimeters should equal EGA in weeks.

A **IUP at 17 weeks**

P **Offer prenatal screening**

Prenatal screening varies depending on what your facility offers. Examples include first trimester testing, second trimester testing, or combination of first and second trimester testing. Examples include the triple screen with nuchal translucency, the second trimester quad screen, the sequential screen, and the integrated test. The newest test is the NIPT (noninvasive prenatal test), that assesses the fetal karyotype from a maternal blood sample.

The expanded MSAFP test (a.k.a. "triple screen")

The expanded MSAFP test is a screening test used to detect NTDs and trisomies 18 and 21 in the general population.

- This test is available to *all* pregnant pts and is performed between 15 and 20 weeks.
- Detects 90% of NTDs and 60% of trisomies 18 and 21.
- The following markers are measured in maternal serum:
  - Alpha-fetoprotein (MSAFP)
  - hCG
  - Estriol

NTD screening uses the MSAFP value (alone).
- Algorithms are used that adjust for maternal weight and EGA.
- Results are reported as MOM.
  - MSAFP values >2.5 MOM are considered a positive screen and require further workup in the form of an amniocentesis and U/S (see more below).

MSAFP, hCG, and estriol are analyzed for risk of trisomies 18 and 21 (Down syndrome).
- Results vary by maternal age, with older women having a higher screen positive rate.
  - *Low* MSAFP (<0.7 MOM) and *low* estriol coupled with *elevated* hCG is considered a positive screen for trisomy 21 and warrants an amniocentesis and U/S for further evaluation.
  - A low value for all three analytes is considered a positive screen for trisomy 18.

Offer prenatal diagnosis to all pts with an indication

Prenatal diagnosis is a process by which pts at high risk for genetic abnormalities are worked up.

Process consists of genetic counseling followed by one or more of the following tests:
- CVS
- Ultrasound
- Amniocentesis
  - Amniotic fluid is obtained by transabdominal needle aspiration under U/S guidance.
  - Collected fluid (with its amniotic cells) may be analyzed for:
    - Chromosomes (for detection of trisomies) or microdeletion testing
    - Acetylcholinesterase and alpha-fetoprotein (both of which are elevated with NTDs)
    - Specific genetic defects

Pts with the following history should be offered prenatal diagnosis:
- Pts with a positive *screen* for either an NTD or trisomy
- Birth defects in previous pregnancies
- Genetic disorders
- Exposure to teratogens
- Suspected fetal anomalies
- Pregestational diabetes mellitus
- Patients who are ≥35 y/o by their EDC

- Women of advanced reproductive age have a higher risk for Down syndrome and therefore require a test that is more sensitive than the triple screen.

Schedule next appointment

For an uncomplicated pregnancy, see the patient every 2–4 weeks between 13 and 36 weeks.

THIRD TRIMESTER VISIT

S **Is the fetus moving?**
Any report of decreased fetal movement can signal fetal intolerance to the intrauterine environment and mandates some sort of antepartum testing (see below).

Is the pt experiencing any uterine contractions?
Any contractions <35 weeks should have workup for PTL (see Preterm Labor, p. 280).
Pts with contractions >35 weeks should have cervical exam to assess dilatation.

Does the pt have any symptoms of preeclampsia?
New-onset visual complaints, headaches, or abdominal pain should raise suspicion for preeclampsia, and blood pressure should be examined closely.

O **Check blood pressure**
BP should be carefully monitored in the third trimester for preeclampsia.

Because BP is usually decreased in pregnancy, even a high normal value should be rechecked.

Check urine dip for protein
Proteinuria ≥2+ (≥100 mg/dL) requires urine analysis for infection and close observation of BP for preeclampsia.

Confirm appropriate maternal weight gain
1/2–1 lb/wk should be gained throughout the third trimester.

Excessive weight gain may signal excessive fluid retention, which can be associated with PIH.

Elicit fetal heart tones with Doppler
Doppler heart tones confirm ongoing viability of pregnancy.

Measure fundal height (FH)
This helps confirm ongoing fetal growth.
After 20 weeks, the FH in centimeters should equal the estimated gestational age in weeks.

Order 1-hour post glucose blood sugar (PGBS)
At 24–28 weeks, pt should have a diabetes screen performed with a 1-hour PGBS.
 • Pts ingest a 50-g load of glucose (in the form of a flavored drink).
 • Serum glucose levels are measured 1 hour later.
Values above 140 mg/dL are abnormal and require further evaluation (see Gestational Diabetes Mellitus, p. 254).

Repeat CBC and RPR at 24–28 weeks

Administer anti-D immune globulin to eligible pts at 28 weeks
Anti-D immune globulin is administered at around 28 weeks to pts who are Rh negative with no antibodies currently in serum (see Isoimmunization, p. 260).

A **IUP at 28 weeks**
P **Instruct pt on potential experiences or problems**
All pts should be instructed to go to L&D immediately for evaluation of any symptoms of labor or rupture of membranes.
Decreased fetal movement (FM) can be a sign of fetal morbidity and requires evaluation (see AP testing below).

Schedule follow-up visit
Visits every 2–3 weeks until 36 weeks
Visits every week from 37 weeks until delivery

Check a GBS culture at 35–37 weeks

Group B streptococcus (GBS) can be found as part of the normal flora around the vaginal introitus and rectal area of some women.

Carriers may vertically transmit GBS to the neonate during labor and delivery, where it can cause septicemia, pneumonia, or meningitis during the first week of life.

- Such disease is known as early-onset GBS infection (to distinguish it from late-onset GBS infection, which is nosocomial or community-acquired).

Administration of antibiotics to GBS carriers during labor helps prevent early-onset disease.

- Penicillin 5 million units IV load, then 2.5 million units IV q 4 hours until delivery (Rec)
- Clindamycin 900 mg IV q 8 hours until delivery (Alt)

Consider antepartum (AP) testing

High-risk pregnancies have an increased amount of fetal morbidity and mortality.

AP testing provides an objective way to assess fetal well-being during the third trimester of pregnancy.

Currently accepted *indications for AP testing* include the following:

- Fetal: Decreased FM, postdates (EGA >40 weeks), PIH, IUGR, oligohydramnios, polyhydramnios, multiple gestations, previous fetal demise
- Maternal: CHTN, DM, SLE, CRF, APS, uncontrolled hyperthyroidism, hemoglobinopathies, cyanotic heart disease

The most popular method of AP testing is the combination of NST and AFI.

- The NST consists of monitoring the fetal heart rate for a 20-minute period.
  - A reactive NST, defined as two episodes of an increase in the fetal heart rate of at least 15 bpm for at least 15 seconds, is a reassuring sign of fetal well-being.
  - Absent accelerations (nonreactive NST) requires further evaluation (see below).
- The AFI is an ultrasonographic measurement of the amount of amniotic fluid.
  - Normal AFI is 5–25 cm

Other methods of AP testing are the contraction stress test (CST) and the biophysical profile (BPP).

- The CST consists of monitoring the fetal heart rate in the presence of induced contractions.
  - This assesses how the fetus responds to an environment of stress (contractions).
- The BPP is an assessment of fetal well-being based on five objective criteria:
  - NST, AFI, FM, tone, and breathing (assessed by U/S).
  - Each parameter is scored with a 0 or 2 (maximum score 10).
  - Subsequent management is based on score.

POSTPARTUM VISIT

S **How is the pt doing since delivery?**

This open-ended question gives the pt an opportunity to raise any concerns she may be having.
- Review delivery before beginning the conversation, noting any complications.
- This is an appropriate time to screen for *postpartum depression* or *psychosis*.

Is the pt breastfeeding?

Inquire about any problems.

Is the pt having any abnormal bleeding? Fevers?

Lochia usually stops by the third postpartum week but can be present in a minority of women at the time of the postpartum check (see below).

If the pt had a C/S, how is the wound healing?

Occasionally, pts complain about a tingling or burning sensation around the wound, which is the result of cut nerves.

Is the pt experiencing normal voiding and bowel movements?

Postpartum urge and stress incontinence usually improve with time.
Postpartum constipation can be a source of discomfort.

Has pt resumed sexual intercourse?

Atrophic vaginitis, changes in libido, fatigue, and general perineal discomfort can affect the resumption of relations in the postpartum period.

How is the pt's diet?

Encourage plenty of fluids for sufficient milk production and as prophylaxis or treatment for constipation.

What are the pt's plans for future pregnancies?

Knowing the future childbearing plans provides the basis for selecting an appropriate contraceptive.

O **Perform physical examination**

Breasts: Check for masses, engorgement, or signs of infection.
C/S wound should be dry, closed, and usually pink in color.
Pelvic
- External genitalia
  - Verify healing of any episiotomy or laceration from delivery.
  - Verify external genitalia are anatomically correct.
- Cervix
  - Observe for any lesions.
  - Review last Pap and repeat if warranted.
    - Previously abnormal Paps should have a workup completed postpartum.
- Uterus
  - Verify that uterus is involuted and nontender.
  - Verify that postpartum discharge from uterus (lochia) is absent or sparse.
  - There are three stages to lochia:
    - Lochia rubra: 3–4 days, mostly bloody and thick
    - Lochia serosa: 1–2 weeks, darker and thinner
    - Lochia alba: Several weeks, yellowish-white color
- Adnexa
  - Bimanual palpation for any masses

A **4- to 6-week postpartum check**

P **Prescribe contraception**

General rule for resumption of ovulation depends on lactation status:
- Nonlactating mothers → 4 weeks
- Lactating mothers (regular, with short intervals) → 6 months

See individual Family Planning SOAP notes for more detail.

- Barrier method
  - Popular postpartum contraception
- Hormonal methods
  - Can be started within the first few weeks postpartum
    - Oral contraceptives
    - Contraceptive patch
    - Intravaginal ring
- Injectable contraceptives
  - Abnormal bleeding patterns may be confused with lochia if given too early
- Intrauterine devices
  - Can be placed immediately postpartum
  - Acceptable for nulliparous and teenagers
- Diaphragm
  - Requires involution of uterus before fitting

Provide breastfeeding counseling

Several common complaints in the postpartum period can be alleviated with some simple interventions.

- Pain
  - Sore, cracked nipples
    - Counseling regarding infant latching/positioning
    - Air-dry nipples
    - Avoidance of creams and irritative soaps
  - Engorgement/plugged ducts
    - Frequent feedings
    - Warm compresses before and during feeding, cold compresses after feeding
- Infection
  - Counsel the pt on returning to office for assessment
  - Termination of breastfeeding not necessary

Order diabetes mellitus testing if pt had GDM

Pts who have GDM are at higher risk for overt diabetes and should be tested for glucose intolerance at their postpartum visit (see Gestational Diabetes Mellitus, p. 254).

Schedule follow-up

3 months

- For women starting a new contraceptive method, schedule a 3-month follow-up to address any difficulties with usage.

Annual

- All others can follow up for their annual well-woman exam.

ANEMIA

S **Does the pt have any symptoms of anemia?**
Symptoms of anemia include:
- Fatigue   – Lethargy
- Headache   – Paresthesias
- Pica (appetite for substances of no nutritional value, e.g., dirt, ice)

Is the pt at high risk for a nutritional deficiency?
Pregnancy may cause severe nausea/vomiting or anorexia, leading to folate deficiency.
Pts who eat diets lacking in green-leafy vegetables or animal protein may suffer from folate deficiency.
Strict vegetarians may lack Vitamin B_{12}.

What is the pt's ethnic background?
Certain ethnicities are at high risk for inherited hemoglobinopathies:
- African-American: Sickle cell
- Asian/Mediterranean: Thalassemia

Is the pt taking prenatal vitamins and iron supplementation?
All pregnant pts should be encouraged to take supplemental iron and vitamins (source of folate) during pregnancy.
- Supplemental folate is most critical during early pregnancy.
  - RDA: 400 µg folate
- Supplemental iron is most critical after 20 weeks.
  - RDA in uncomplicated pregnancy: 30 mg of elemental iron
  - RDA in multiple gestations or large habitus patients: 60 mg of elemental iron
Persistent anemia despite supplementation should alert clinician to the possibility of a hereditary anemia.

O **Perform physical exam**
Physical signs of iron deficiency include:
- Glossitis   – Pallor
- Cheilitis   – Koilonychia

What are the results of the pt's Hb/Hct and mean corpuscular volume (MCV)?
Normal Hb/Hct falls during pregnancy because of a greater increase of plasma volume (50%) relative to red blood cell mass (30%).
Iron-deficiency anemia and thalassemias usually have a lowered MCV.

What are the results of the serum ferritin?
Serum ferritin reflects the amount of iron stored in the body's tissues and is the best indicator of the degree of anemia in pregnancy.
- Normal ferritin levels in pregnancy are 55–70 µg/L.
  - Low ferritin is consistent with iron deficiency.
  - Normal ferritin is seen with *early* iron deficiency, thalassemias, or chronic disease.

Peripheral smear
Morphologic features of iron-deficiency anemia (microcytosis and hypochromia) are not as commonly seen as in the nonpregnant state.

For African-American pts, what is the result of the Hb electrophoresis?
Hb S should be obtained at their first visit (if missed, obtain now).

A **Anemia**
Anemia during pregnancy is usually defined according to the fifth percentile hemoglobin values for pregnancy (pts with values below the fifth percentile are considered anemic).
- Fifth percentile values of Hb during pregnancy are:
  - First trimester   11.0 g/dL
  - Second trimester   10.5 g/dL
  - Third trimester   11.0 g/dL

Iron-deficiency anemia is the etiology in 75% of cases in pregnancy. Inadequate folate is the second most common nutritional deficiency. Other causes include:
- Anemia of chronic disease
- Hereditary anemias
  - Hemoglobinopathies
  - Thalassemias

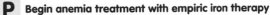

P Begin anemia treatment with empiric iron therapy

Because iron deficiency is the most likely etiology of anemia in pregnancy, start with empiric iron therapy.
- Iron-deficiency anemia requires 200 mg of elemental iron/day and can be given as any of the following:
  - Ferrous gluconate 325 mg (37–39 mg elemental iron)
  - Ferrous sulfate 325 mg (60–65 mg elemental iron)
  - Ferrous fumarate 325 mg (107 mg elemental iron)

Monitor response with reticulocyte count

Normally, a response to iron therapy in the form of an increased reticulocyte count can be observed 1 week after starting therapy.
- Response to treatment may take longer than in nonpregnant states.
  - An Hb response may be masked by physiologic progressive increases in plasma volume, which accompany normal pregnancy.
    - If present, an increase in Hb (1–2 g/dL) will be evident by 4 weeks.
  - With severe megaloblastic anemia, plasma volume is relatively decreased compared with a normal pregnancy, and treatment of the anemia can be associated with increases in volume that mask rising hemoglobin.

Work up nonresponders for other types of anemia

Serum electrophoresis may reveal thalassemia.

ANTIPHOSPHOLIPID SYNDROME

S **Does the pt have an *obstetric* history suspicious for antiphospholipid syndrome (APS)?**

The following obstetrical outcomes can be associated with APS:
- Recurrent pregnancy loss (three or more first trimester spontaneous abortions (SABs) with no more than one live birth or unexplained second or third trimester loss)
- Severe preeclampsia at <34 weeks' gestation
- Intrauterine growth restriction (IUGR) or uteroplacental insufficiency in the second or early third trimester

Does the pt have a past *medical* history suspicious for APS?

The following medical problems can be associated with APS:
- Nontraumatic arterial or venous thromboembolism
- Stroke, transient ischemic attack, or amaurosis fugax in a reproductive-age woman
- Systemic lupus erythematosus
- Hemolytic anemia or autoimmune thrombocytopenia

O **Does the patient's skin show evidence of livedo reticularis?**

This is a skin condition associated with APS characterized by reddish-blue skin changes visible on the extremities and intensified by exposure to cold.

Do the laboratory tests show thrombocytopenia or anemia?

Although both of these disease states have multiple etiologies, consideration should always be given to the association between APS and autoimmune thrombocytopenia or hemolytic anemia.

Does the patient have a false-positive serologic test for syphilis?

Patients with a false-positive rapid plasma reagin (RPR) should have testing for antiphospholipid antibodies (see Vulvar Ulcers, p. 336)

What are the interpretations of the APS serologic tests?

Two main tests are used to detect the presence of antiphospholipids:
- *Lupus anticoagulant* (LAC) is a functional assay "phenomenon" whereby coagulation is prolonged in vitro (even though thrombosis is promoted in vivo).
  - Multiple LAC assays are currently available:
    - Activated partial thromboplastin time
    - Dilute Russell viper venom time
    - Kaolin clot time
  - Results are reported as positive or negative.
- *Anticardiolipin antibody* test is an enzyme-linked immunosorbent assay test that detects antiphospholipids directed against cardiolipin.
  - Results are measured for IgM and IgG and are reported as low-positive, medium-positive, or high-positive. Low-positive results or isolated IgM are of questionable relevance and are not considered diagnostic.

A **Antiphospholipid syndrome**

Diagnosis is made by the presence of *both* of the following:
- Any of the above clinical features
- Positive testing for antiphospholipid antibodies (any of the following):
  - Lupus anticoagulant present on two samples, taken at least 12 weeks apart.
  - Anticardiolipin antibody (IgG or IgM) in medium or high titer (>GPL or MPL or >99th percentile) on two occasions, at least 12 weeks apart.
  - Anti-β2-glycoprotein-1 antibody (IgG and/or IgM) in titers >99% on two occasions, at least 12 weeks apart.

P **Educate patient regarding obstetric complications (and their symptoms) associated with APS**

Pregnancies affected by APS are at high risk for:
- Placental abruption
- Preterm delivery
- Preeclampsia

Pts should be given strict precautions about the *symptoms* of these potential complications:
- Painful bleeding (abruption)
- Preterm UCs (preterm delivery)
- H/As, visual or epigastric complaints (preeclampsia)

Start anticoagulation

Treatment is based on clinical history.
- For patients with a history of fetal death or recurrent abortion:
  - Daily low-dose aspirin
  - Daily unfractionated heparin in prophylactic doses (5,000–10,000 U bid)
  - PTT monitoring is not necessary
- For patients with a history of thrombosis or stroke:
  - Daily low-dose aspirin
  - Heparin to achieve full anticoagulation (10,000 U bid to tid)
  - PTT prolongation of 1.5–2.5 baseline
  - Heparin-induced thrombocytopenia may occur with full-dose heparin
  - Check platelet counts on day 5 and periodically for first 2 weeks
  - Heparin-induced osteoporosis can occur after 7 weeks of use

Serial fetal ultrasounds for growth every 4–6 weeks starting at 18–20 weeks' gestation

Pregnancies affected by APS are at high risk for IUGR.

AP testing beginning at 30–32 weeks' gestation

Pregnancies affected by APS are at high risk for abnormal fetal heart rate patterns.

CHRONIC HYPERTENSION

S **Has the pt been previously diagnosed with chronic hypertension (CHTN)?**

Review history, prior workup, and any complications (e.g., myocardial infarction, end-organ involvement).

With many pts, pregnancy is the first entry into the health care system and an opportunity to discover such chronic problems as hypertension.

Previously undiagnosed CHTN mandates a full workup (see below).

Is the pt currently taking any antihypertensive medications?

Review current and past medications, doses, and length of use.

Angiotensin-converting enzyme inhibitors are contraindicated during pregnancy because they can have teratogenic renal effects.

What is the pt's current activity level?

Activity restriction should be applied during pregnancy to avoid decreased placental perfusion.

O **Check BP**

BP measurements should be performed serially over periods of time to establish diagnosis and confirm degree of disease.

Severe CHTN (SBP ≥180 mm Hg or DBP ≥110 mm Hg) should alert clinician to possible reversible causes (see below).

Perform PE

Check for differences between radial and femoral pulses.

- Coarctation of the aorta is a rare, but easily detectable cause of hypertension. Check for signs of Cushing syndrome
- Thinning of skin, bruising, and muscle weakness/atrophy

What are the latest U/S results?

An early U/S (<20 weeks) establishes accurate dating of the pregnancy.

- This information is useful in managing complications associated with CHTN (pregnancy-induced hypertension [PIH], preterm labor [PTL]), which arise later in pregnancy.
- Comparison of subsequent U/S to this baseline is useful in evaluating suspected intrauterine growth restriction (IUGR).

Consider evaluation of renal function

Urine analysis to detect proteinuria

Serum creatinine to evaluate renal insufficiency

Renal insufficiency places the pt at greater risk for fetal loss and developing superimposed preeclampsia.

Doppler flow studies to detect renal artery stenosis

Consider lab studies to detect *primary* causes of CHTN

Potassium: Low in hyperaldosteronism

24-hour urinary catecholamines: Elevated with pheochromocytoma

Dexamethasone suppression test: Elevated plasma cortisol suggests Cushing syndrome

A **Chronic hypertension**

Mild CHTN: SBP ≥140 mm Hg or DBP ≥90 mm Hg before 20 weeks' gestation

Severe CHTN: SBP ≥180 mm Hg or DBP ≥110 mm Hg before 20 weeks' gestation

Reversible causes of hypertension should always be considered as etiologies and include:

- Renal disease
- Pheochromocytoma
- Coarctation of the aorta
- Cushing syndrome
- Primary aldosteronism

P   **Monitor BP serially and determine need for therapy**

BP is physiologically lowered during normal pregnancy, so patients with mild CHTN (most affected pregnancies) can sometimes discontinue medications and be followed closely.

- The primary purpose of BP surveillance and control is for maternal benefit (avoiding end-organ damage).

- Even though CHTN is associated with increased risk of preterm birth, placental abruption, superimposed preeclampsia, IUGR, and fetal death, treatment does NOT appear to reduce perinatal morbidity.

Treatment is customarily initiated for SBPs >180 mm Hg or DBPs >110 mm Hg.

- Methyldopa has been the most widely studied antihypertensive used during pregnancy and is recognized as safe.
  - Methyldopa 250 mg bid (max 2 g/d)
- Labetalol is also popular and safe.
  - Labetalol 100 mg bid (max 2,400 mg/d)

Obtain 24-hour urine

A 24-hour urinary protein collection will reveal any underlying proteinuria.

A baseline value (early in pregnancy) often helps evaluate for superimposed preeclampsia if signs develop later in pregnancy.

Refer to appropriate specialists

End-organ damage should be evaluated, especially with long-standing disease.

Refer the pt to the cardiologist, nephrologist, and ophthalmologist to assess the respective organ systems.

Monitor for signs of superimposed preeclampsia

Superimposed preeclampsia affects 25% of pregnancies with CHTN.

Monitor BP weekly beginning at 30 weeks.

Consider AP testing

Indications for AP testing should be individualized.

Initiate for signs of IUGR or preeclampsia.

Consider early delivery

Early delivery should be initiated for severe, uncontrolled CHTN or pts with prior bad obstetrical outcome.

GESTATIONAL DIABETES MELLITUS

S **Is the pt at high risk for gestational diabetes mellitus (GDM) *by history*?**
A history of any of the following places the pt at high risk for GDM and warrants first-trimester screening:
- A history of glucose intolerance
- A history of an adverse obstetric outcome usually associated with GDM, such as:
  o Macrosomia
  o Congenital anomalies (especially neurologic and cardiac defects)
  o Unexplained fetal demise
- A first-degree relative with diabetes

O **Does the pt have any *objective evidence* to place her at high risk for GDM?**
Any of the following objective findings place the pt at higher risk for GDM and warrant first-trimester screening:
- Hypertension
- Obesity (BMI >30)
- Advanced maternal age (≥35 y/o)
- Glycosuria on the office urine dip
- Previous pregnancy complicated by GDM

What is the result of the 1-hour glucose challenge test (GCT)?
Screening for GDM is done with a 1-hour GCT.
- Perform at 24–28 weeks for pts without risk factors (see above).
- The test consists of the pt ingesting a 50-g glucose load, usually in the form of a liquid suspension.
- One hour later, the pt's venous glucose level is measured.
- The pt does NOT need to be in the fasting state to perform the test.
  o An abnormal 1-hour GCT is 140 mg/dL or higher.
  o Some clinics use a cutoff value of 130 mg/dL, which improves sensitivity of the test.
  o In women who had a gastric bypass, the GCT is contraindicated because of the risk of dumping syndrome. For these patients, screen with a fasting glucose level.
All pts with an abnormal 1-hour GCT require a 3-hour glucose tolerance test (GTT).

What is the result of the pt's 3-hour GTT?
Diagnosis of GDM is done with the 3-hour oral GTT.
- This test consists of the pt ingesting 100 g of glucose.
- Venous glucose is measured during the fasting state and at 1, 2, and 3 hours after intake.
- Pts must be fasting and have eaten an unrestricted diet for 3 days before the test.
- Pts must be sitting during the test.
Values that *exceed* the following are considered abnormal:

– Fasting	95 mg/dL
– 1 hr	180 mg/dL
– 2 hr	155 mg/dL
– 3 hr	140 mg/dL

A pt with two or more abnormal values meets the diagnosis of GDM.

Review pt's blood sugar log book
Once diagnosis is made, sugar values are usually monitored and recorded in a log book. On every visit, the log book should be reviewed and the data recorded.
- Management decisions are based on trends (see below).

A **Gestational diabetes mellitus (GDM)**
GDM is a form of glucose intolerance that results from the anti-insulin action of human placental lactogen, a pregnancy hormone.

GDM is divided into two subgroups, A1 and A2, which are differentiated on the pt's fasting and postprandial blood sugars and the need for insulin.
- A1 GDM: *Therapeutic diet* controls fasting blood sugars to <95 and the 2-hour postprandial blood sugars to <120.
- A2 GDM: The pt cannot maintain these target values of fasting blood sugars <95 and 2-hour postprandial blood sugars <120 with dietary therapy and *insulin is initiated.*

P **Start the pt on dietary therapy, with total daily calories equaling 30 kcal/kg**

A nutritional counselor can be involved to individualize therapy.

Protocols for assessing blood sugar control vary from obtaining weekly fasting blood sugar values to qid home monitoring.

Monitor blood sugars

Blood sugars are either self-monitored (by the pt at home) or monitored by weekly fasting blood draw (in office).
- Self-monitored sugars are checked and recorded qid (fasting and 2 hours after each meal).
- Results are logged on a piece of paper to observe trends.

Start insulin for pts who have failed dietary therapy

Dietary therapy is usually considered failed when pt cannot keep fasting sugars <95 or 2-hour postprandial sugars <120 for 2 weeks.

To start insulin, first *calculate the total daily insulin* requirement, which is based on the pt weight in kg and gestational age as follows:

– First trimester	0.7 Units/kg
– Second trimester	0.8 Units/kg
– Third trimester	0.9 Units/kg

Next, *divide the total daily insulin* requirement into two doses as follows:

– Morning shot (2/3 of total daily)	2/3 NPH and 1/3 regular insulin
– Evening shot (1/3 of total daily)	1/2 NPH and 1/2 regular insulin

Ultrasound

Anatomic survey at 18–20 weeks

Consider serial ultrasounds to determine growth.

Start AP testing on A2 at 32 weeks

Twice-weekly AP testing should be started on all A2 GDM pts (see Third Trimester Visit, p. 244).

Scan A2 for estimated fetal weight (EFW) at 38–39 weeks

A2 GDM pts have an increased risk of macrosomia and require an U/S for EFW at term.

Deliver A2 at 38–39 weeks

Generally deliver A2 DM at 38–39 weeks.

Deliver A1 at 41 weeks

HYPERTHYROIDISM

S **Does the patient complain of any symptoms commonly associated with hyperthyroidism?**

– Fatigue	– Sweating
– Palpitations	– Weight loss or no weight gain
– Tremor	– Visual complaints
– Diarrhea	– Anxiety

Did the patient have similar complaints *before* becoming pregnant?

Many complaints associated with hyperthyroidism can also be common to a normal pregnancy.

Ascertaining whether the pt experienced these complaints before pregnancy may help distinguish etiology.

Additionally, in the first trimester, some normal pregnancies suffer from *transient hyperthyroidism*.

This phenomenon is secondary to the presence of human chorionic gonadotropin (hCG), a pregnancy hormone, which cross-reacts with the thyroid-stimulating hormone (TSH) receptor, to cause increased production of thyroid hormone.

This reaction peaks at around 10 weeks with the natural plateau in hCG levels and declines thereafter.

If pt has a *history* of hyperthyroidism, what is the etiology?

95% of pregnant women with hyperthyroidism have *Graves disease*.

This disease is characterized by TSH receptor antibodies (TSHR-Abs), autoantibodies that react with the TSH receptor to stimulate thyroid hormone production.

TSHR-Abs need to be monitored in most Graves disease pts during pregnancy (see below).

O **Review vital signs**

Tachycardia and weight loss (or no weight gain) are two of the most supportive signs of hyperthyroidism in pregnancy.

Presence of fever or a widened pulse pressure should alert the physician to the possibility of thyroid storm.

Does the pt exhibit any signs of hyperthyroidism on physical exam?

– Goiter	– Systolic flow murmur
– Hand tremor	– Exophthalmos
– Lid lag	– Onycholysis
– Proximal muscle weakness	

What are the results of the thyroid function tests?

Physiologic changes normal to pregnancy can alter certain thyroid function tests (Table 14-1).

- High levels of estrogen stimulate production of thyroid-binding globulin, which normally binds thyroid hormone.
- This, in turn, raises total T3 and T4, making interpretation of these values unreliable during pregnancy.
- TSH, free T3, and free T4 (the active hormones) are unaltered.

TABLE 14-1   Thyroid Function Test Results

	TSH	Free T3&T4	Total T4 & T3	T3 Resin Uptake
Pregnancy	↔	↔	↑	↓
Hyperthyroidism	↓	↑	↑	↓
Hypothyroidism	↑	↓	↓	↑

For pts with new-onset hyperthyroidism, are TSHR-Abs present?

Presence of TSHR-Abs confirms Graves disease.

For pts with Graves disease being currently medically treated or those previously treated with radioiodine or surgery, what are the titers of TSHR-Abs?

Even in the face of controlled or previously treated Graves disease, there may be high titers of TSHR-Abs in maternal serum.

High titers of TSHR-Abs can cross the placenta and react with the fetal thyroid gland to cause neonatal hyperthyroidism (rare).

Screen for such affected pregnancies by monitoring fetal heart rate for tachycardia and documenting fetal growth (see more below).

 Hyperthyroidism

The diagnosis of hyperthyroidism is made by detecting *low* TSH along with *elevated* free T3 and free T4.

Diagnosis of Graves disease is supported by findings of a goiter and ophthalmopathy and is confirmed by detection of TSHR-Abs.

Differential diagnosis includes:

- Toxic multinodular Goiter
- Thyroiditis
- Exogenous thyroid hormone
- Toxic adenoma
- Hyperemesis gravidarum (see p. 265)
- Gestational trophoblastic disease (see p. 344)

 Start antithyroid medication for newly diagnosed pts

The thioamides, methimazole and propylthiouracil (PTU), are the two currently accepted treatments for hyperthyroidism in pregnancy.

PTU is the preferred medication because of less transplacental passage.

• PTU 100 mg PO tid (titrate up to 800 mg/d)

• Rare side effect: Agranulocytosis, watch for fever and sore throat.

Monitor free T4 levels

Free T4 is used to monitor response to medications during pregnancy.

• Initial free T4 normalization takes 3–6 weeks.
• Once euthyroidism has been confirmed, check free T4 values every 2–3 weeks.
• Dosing can often be reduced as pregnancy progresses.
• One-third of patients can discontinue medication in the third trimester.

Consider AP testing

Initiate AP testing for pts with uncontrolled hyperthyroidism or high TSHR-Ab titers.

• AP testing traditionally consists of a nonstress test/amniotic fluid index (see Third Trimester Visit, p. 244).
• In pts with high titers of TSHR-Abs, consider U/S to assess fetal growth and to detect fetal goiter.

INTRAUTERINE GROWTH RESTRICTION

S **Does the pt have any risk factors for intrauterine growth restriction (IUGR)?**
Most cases of growth-restricted pregnancies have known risk factors, such as the
following:

– Previous IUGR	– Diabetes
– CHTN	– Anemia
– APS	– Other chronic illnesses (renal, pulmonary, heart)
– Multiple gestations	– Elevated MSAFP/hCG
– Low weight gain	– Smoking or substance abuse
– Malnutrition	– Exposure to teratogens
– Primary placental disease (previa, chorioangioma)	

Does the pt have a history of exposure to infectious agents?
Although accounting for <10% of all cases, the following infections have been associated
with IUGR:

– CMV	– Rubella
– Varicella	– Toxoplasmosis

Does the pt have a history of vaginal bleeding or preterm labor?
Both of these have been associated with increased risk of IUGR.

Has the pt had a previous ultrasound?
A baseline ultrasound, preferably before 20 weeks' gestation, can aid in the diagnosis of
IUGR by verifying that growth was appropriate in early gestation.

> Good dating of the fetus is the single most important piece of information in the management
> of IUGR.

O **What are the results of the fundal height measurement?**
Fundal height (FH) measurements are performed during *all* pregnancies as a *screening
tool*.
- After 20 weeks, the FH in centimeters should equal the estimated gestational age
  (EGA) in weeks.
  o Consider U/S if FH < EGA.

What are the findings on the current U/S?
When IUGR is suspected, serial U/S evaluations are performed.
- Several U/S parameters can be used to identify and manage the IUGR fetus:
  o Abdominal circumference (AC) or the head circumference/AC ratio

> The AC is the most sensitive single marker for IUGR.

  o Fetal weight
    • Fetal weights, plotted on a standardized growth curve, can be followed over time
      to assess growth.
    • A single U/S evaluation of the fetus has limited use, but IUGR is more suspected
      if the estimated fetal weight is < the fifth percentile.
  o Doppler velocimetry
    • Doppler velocimetry is an U/S technique that assesses blood flow through vari-
      ous organs.
    • In IUGR, placental blood flow *slows* and flow to the fetal brain (secondary to
      physiologic redistribution) *increases*.
  o Amniotic fluid index
    • IUGR pregnancies show oligohydramnios secondary to reduced perfusion of the
      fetal kidneys.

A Intrauterine growth restriction

IUGR is defined as estimated fetal weight (EFW) <10th percentile.
- Because some pregnancies with EFW <10th percentile will represent the lower end of the spectrum of a normal population, IUGR encompasses pathologic as well as "normal" small fetuses.
  o Pathologic IUGR is suspected when an EFW <10th percentile continues to fall off the growth curve over time.
    • Growth curves have several inherent inaccuracies (heterogeneous population of the United States, no adjustment for parity or maternal/paternal height).
  o EFW <5th percentile is associated with greater perinatal morbidity.

IUGR is classically divided into two categories:
- Symmetric, where all fetal U/S measurements are small: Usually occurs early in pregnancy and is associated with chromosomal or genetic problems.
- Asymmetric, where fetal head is "spared" and the rest of body measures are small: Occurs later in pregnancy and is the result of uteroplacental insufficiency (not enough blood and nutrients getting to fetus).

P Perform serial ultrasounds every 2–3 weeks

An interval of 2–3 weeks allows for accurate assessment of fetal growth.
Intervals shorter than 2–3 weeks are prone to misinterpretation secondary to the inconsistency of fetal growth and measurement errors intrinsic to the U/S.

Initiate AP testing

Pregnancies suspected of IUGR should undergo some sort of AP testing.
Nonstress test, contraction stress test, and biophysical profile are all acceptable (see Third Trimester Visit, p. 244).

Consider Doppler velocimetry

Umbilical artery Doppler velocimetry can be used to monitor the fetus.
- Absent or reversed end-diastolic flow of the umbilical artery is associated with adverse perinatal outcome.
- Normal end-diastolic flow in a suspected IUGR fetus is reassuring.

Plan timing of delivery

Timing of delivery weighs the risk of prematurity versus the risks of prolonging a gestation in a hostile intrauterine environment.
Decision is individualized and based on:
- Gestational age
- Findings on AP testing, U/S, and Doppler velocimetry
  o Generally, delivery for EGA >34 weeks or signs of advanced fetal compromise.

Consider administering steroids to benefit fetal lung maturity

If the pregnancy is likely to be delivered at <34 weeks as a result of IUGR, consider steroids.
Betamethasone 12 mg IM q 24 hours × 2 doses

ISOIMMUNIZATION

S **What is the father's Rh status?**

Paternal Rh status can be very important in managing pregnancies affected by Rh isoimmunization.

- If father is Rh negative and he is definitely the father, there is no risk of having an Rh-positive fetus.
- If the father is Rh positive or unknown status, an attempt to determine his genotype (heterozygous versus homozygous for the "D" antigen) can help counsel the pt on chances of having Rh-positive fetus.

What is the pt's past obstetric history?

Past pregnancies affected by Rh hemolytic disease provide prognosis for the current pregnancy.

- Good prognosis for current pregnancy with history of previously mildly affected fetus.
- Poor prognosis and high potential for recurrent severe disease with a history of hydrops fetalis.

O **What is the level of anti-D antibody?**

Anti-D antibody levels (maternal serum) reflect the degree of sensitization and the likelihood that the fetus will be affected.

Following levels serially will determine the need for amniocentesis.

Initial titer should be taken at first prenatal visit and then every 4 weeks starting at 20 weeks.

- Titers that are ≤1:8 may be followed conservatively with repeat titers every 2–4 weeks and serial ultrasound examinations to look for evidence of fetal anemia (see below).
- Titers that are >1:8 require serial amniocentesis.

What are the results of the U/S?

Beginning in the second trimester, serial U/S evaluations are done on the fetus to detect any signs of hydrops fetalis.

Ultrasonographic markers of hydrops include:

- Polyhydramnios
- Hepatosplenomegaly
- Pericardial and pleural effusions
- Bowel edema

What are the results of the amniocentesis?

Serial amniocentesis can begin at about 24 weeks in pregnancies *with titers >1:8*.

Analysis of amniocentesis to assess the degree of fetal anemia is performed by spectrophotometric density.

- Normal amniotic fluid has a density ranging from wavelengths of 525–375 nm.
- When bilirubin is present in the amniotic fluid (released from affected fetal RBCs), there is an increase in the wavelength to 450 nm.
- The difference between the density at 450 nm and that of normal amniotic fluid is called the ΔOD 450.
- This value is plotted on a graph called the Liley graph (see below).

A **Isoimmunization**

Isoimmunization refers to the process whereby maternal antibodies are directed toward antigen on fetal RBCs, resulting in hemolysis of fetal RBCs and fetal anemia.

- **Erythroblastosis fetalis** and **hemolytic disease of the newborn** are terms to describe this phenomenon.
- **Hydrops fetalis** is a term used to describe the end product of severe disease, which is characterized by severe anemia and secondary high-output heart failure and generalized edema.

The most common type of isoimmunization is with anti-D antibody and is known as **Rh isoimmunization**.

- "D" refers to an antigen that is part of a blood system called the Rhesus or Rh blood group.

o Other antigens in the Rh group are "C," "c," "E," and "e." Maternal antibodies result from exposure to foreign blood antigens from:
  • A previous pregnancy with a fetus that expressed blood antigens that differ from the mother's.
  • A previous blood transfusion that directly exposed the mother to foreign antigens.

P **Analysis of the Liley graph**

A Liley graph plots serial ΔOD 450 measurements against gestational age.

Plotting serial measurements follows the trend over time and is predictive of fetal anemia.

A Liley graph is divided into thirds or zones I, II, and III.
  • Zone I values represent mild disease and are usually followed up with a repeat value in 3–4 weeks.
  • Zone II values represent moderate disease and may be followed up with repeat testing every 1–4 weeks depending on the trend.
  • Zone III values signal impending fetal death and require intervention in the form of blood transfusion or delivery.

Plan delivery

Mild disease
  • Deliver at term.
Moderate disease
  • Follow trends on the Liley graph.
    o If rising, consider early delivery.
    o If falling, consider temporizing delivery (transfusing) until fetus is mature. Severe disease.
  • Consider **percutaneous umbilical blood sampling** (PUBS).
    o PUBS measures fetal hemoglobin and hematocrit directly.
      • Guides management of unclear pictures (Zone II) on the Liley graph.
      • Also helpful for gestations that are too early to be interpreted through the Liley curve.
  • Consider intrauterine transfusion.
    o Intrauterine transfusion is used to treat the severely anemic fetus.
      • Customarily begun when fetal hematocrit (determined by PUBS) is <25%.

MILD PREECLAMPSIA

S **Does the pt have any symptoms of preeclampsia (pregnancy-induced hypertension [PIH])?**

Most cases of mild preeclampsia do not have any symptoms.

Presence of symptoms raises suspicion for severe disease (see Severe Preeclampsia, p. 266).

Does the pt have any risk factors for PIH?

– Previous PIH	– CHTN	– Chronic renal disease
– DM	– African race	– Reproductive age extremes
– Nulliparity	– Multiple gestations	(<17 or >40 y/o)

O **What is the BP?**

BP in NORMAL pregnancy follows a predictable pattern of physiologic changes:

- First trimester — Decreases (systolic less than diastolic, increasing pulse pressure)
- Second trimester — Nadir at 24 wk
- Third trimester — Increases to term (any rise above nonpregnant values is abnormal)

Blood pressure should be measured with a correct and reproducible technique.

• Always measure with arm at the same height as heart.
• Use appropriate cuff size.
  ○ Larger cuffs for obese pts (cuffs fitting too tightly can cause abnormally elevated readings)

> SBP ≥140 mm Hg or DBP ≥90 mm Hg taken on two occasions at least 6 hours apart after 20 weeks' gestation meets the diagnosis of mild PIH.

Does the pt have any protein in the office urine dip or U/A?

Normally, there should only be trace protein in the urine of a pregnant pt.

Greater amounts may signify proteinuria levels that are diagnostic of preeclampsia.

The following terminology is frequently used when quantifying proteinuria in the office:

– 1+	30 mg/dL
– 2+	100 mg/dL
– 3+	300 mg/dL
– 4+	2,000 mg/dL

What is the pt's CBC and expanded chemistry panel?

The following laboratory findings support a diagnosis of PIH:

• Hemoconcentration (high or high-normal hemoglobin/hematocrit)
• Elevated uric acid

The following laboratory findings are signs of severe disease (see Severe Preeclampsia, p. 266):

• Low platelets
• Elevated liver enzymes

What is the result of the 24-hour urine protein and creatinine clearance?

A 24-hour urinary protein collection will quantify any proteinuria.

• A nonpregnant pt has a 24-hour excretion of 100–125 mg of protein.
• A pregnant pt excretes up to 150 mg of protein in 24 hours.

> Mild preeclampsia is diagnosed when proteinuria exceeds 300 mg in 24 hours.

Mild preeclampsia

Mild preeclampsia is diagnosed by the presence of the following:
- SBP ≥140 mm Hg or DBP ≥90 mm Hg
  o After 20 weeks of pregnancy on two occasions more than 6 hours apart
- Proteinuria of ≥300 mg in 24 hours

 Admit

All pts suspected of having mild preeclampsia should be admitted and observed.

Ultrasound

Perform U/S at time of admission to confirm estimated gestational age (EGA)
- Management of IUGR is based on EGA.
- U/S can be *used* as a baseline to compare with subsequent scans for fetal growth.

Monitor BPs

Pts should have BP monitored while on bed rest.
- Monitor BP hourly early in admission and then routinely if stable.
- Serial measurements help identify any progression toward severe PIH.

Monitor for symptoms of severe PIH (see Severe Preeclampsia, p. 266)

Inquire daily about any PIH symptoms that could signal worsening disease.

Follow labs and 24-hour urine collections serially

Monitor lab values at least once weekly.
- Identify any trends by charting values on a flow sheet.
- Draw labs immediately for any symptoms or signs of worsening disease. Periodic collection of 24-hour urine monitors for worsening proteinuria.

Monitor fetal well-being

Continuous fetal monitoring initially, and then daily to twice weekly surveillance (NST) for pts who remain stable while under observation.

Consider steroids

Administer antenatal steroids for gestations <34 weeks in anticipation of an early delivery.
- Steroids aid in pulmonary lung maturity.
  o Betamethasone 12 mg IM q 24 hours × 2 doses

Plan delivery

Delivery is the only definitive treatment for PIH.

Labor induction for all term gestations.
For preterm gestations, continue bed rest until one of the two outcomes is reached:
- Disease worsens: Progression to severe preeclampsia mandates delivery.
- Pregnancy reaches 35 weeks.

All pts should receive magnesium sulfate (MgSO₄) while *in labor* to prevent seizures.
- 4 g IV load and then continuous push at 2 g/hr.
  o Toxicity can be monitored clinically by checking for decreased deep tendon reflexes and pulmonary edema.
  o Use caution with renal insufficiency (MgSO₄ is excreted by the kidneys).
- Monitor IV fluid input and urine output closely.

NAUSEA AND VOMITING OF PREGNANCY

S **Obtain general history of complaint**

Onset: *Onset* of nausea and vomiting (NVP) after 10 weeks is unusual and requires a
  workup for etiologies other than pregnancy
Duration
Frequency
Ability to "hold down" any intake

Does the pt have any associated abdominal pain, fever, or headaches?

Pain other than that associated with retching or gastric reflux from vomiting suggests an
  abdominal process independent of pregnancy.
Fever also suggests an alternate etiology.

> Pyelonephritis, which is common to pregnancy, can sometimes present initially as nausea and
> vomiting.

Headaches may suggest a central nervous system process.

Are there any specific offending agents?

Certain foul smells can cause a reflex nausea response.
Prenatal vitamins and iron preparations can also trigger nausea.

**Is the nausea and vomiting affecting daily activities with family or
employment?**

The response to this question will give the practitioner an idea of the severity of the
  problem and guide treatment.
This is also a good opportunity to invite the pt's partner to become involved in the pt's
  care by attending the prenatal visits.

> Support at home can improve outcome.

O **Does the patient have evidence of weight loss, fever, or ketonuria?**

Fever, as previously stated, should not be associated with NVP.
Weight loss (or no weight gain) and ketonuria are signs of more severe disease.

Perform PE

Neck: Check for presence of goiter.
Abdomen: More than mild tenderness is suspicious for GI process.
Neurologic: Check for mass lesion effect (focal neurologic deficits).

Obtain CBC, CMP, amylase, and lipase

A pt with nausea and vomiting of pregnancy (NVP) may exhibit several laboratory
  abnormalities that can be confused with other disease states:
  • Bilirubin can be up to 4 mg/dL.
  • Amylase can be up to 900 U/L.
  • TSH is suppressed secondary to the high levels of hCG in pregnancy.
    ○ If TSH is >2.5 μU/mL, suspect hypothyroidism.

Confirm viable intrauterine pregnancy (IUP)

Refractory or severe NVP can be associated with gestational trophoblastic disease.
  • If EGA is >10 weeks, perform Doppler tones.
  • If EGA is <10 weeks, perform U/S.

A **Nausea and vomiting of pregnancy (NVP)**

NVP is classified as mild, moderate, or severe.
Classification is based on:
    • Impact on daily life
    • Weight (lack of gain or loss of weight) and presence of ketonuria
Mild NVP: No effect on home life or employment

Moderate NVP: Some interference with home life or employment

Severe NVP or hyperemesis gravidarum: Evidence of weight loss (exceeding 5% of prepregnancy weight), ketonuria, or refractory vomiting necessitating IV hydration or hospitalization

P Mild to moderate NVP

NVP should be controlled early to avoid worsening of symptoms.

Outpatient treatment can start with conservative measures followed by various pharmacologic agents in a stepwise fashion.

Conservative measures include:

- Nibbling throughout day
- Eating bland, dry diet
- Changing positions slowly
- Convert PNV to folic acid supplements only
- Ginger capsules 250 mg QID

- Eating high-carbohydrate, low-fat meals
- Drinking between meals
- Getting frequent rest

If conservative treatment fails, initiate pharmacotherapy.

- Choice of medicine varies widely among practitioners and institutions.
- Options for oral medications include vitamin B_6, dopamine antagonists, and antihistamines:
  - First line: Vitamin B_6 10–25 mg PO tid to qid alone or with doxylamine 12.5 mg three to four times/day

Then add:

Dimenhydrinate 25–40 mg Q4–6 hours

OR

Diphenhydramine 25–50 mg PO every 4–6 hours

OR

Prochlorperazine 25 mg Q12 hours rectally

OR

Promethazine 12.5–25 mg every 4–6 hours PO or rectally

> Medicines dosed "qid" should be given 30 minutes before meals and at bedtime.

Severe NVP

Usually requires hospitalization

- NPO
- Metoclopramide 5–10 mg PO tid to qid
  - Hydroxyzine 25–50 mg PO tid to qid
- IV hydration until ketonuria has disappeared
- IV multivitamins
- IV pharmacotherapy options:
  - Promethazine 12.5–25 mg IV q4h
  - Metoclopramide 5–10 mg IV tid to qid
  - Ondansetron 8 mg IV bid
  - Methylprednisolone 16 mg IV tid for 3 days, taper to lowest dose over 2 weeks, maximum duration 6 weeks

SEVERE PREECLAMPSIA

S **Does the pt have any symptoms of severe preeclampsia (pregnancy-induced hypertension [PIH])?**

New onset of the following findings, in the presence of elevated BP, suggests severe preeclampsia:
- Persistent, severe headaches
- Visual changes: Scotoma, spots
- Abdominal pain: Epigastric or RUQ

O **What is BP?**

SBP ≥160 mm Hg or DBP ≥110 mm Hg taken on two occasions at least 6 hours apart after 20 weeks' gestation meets the diagnosis of severe PIH.

Does the pt have proteinuria? (see Mild Preeclampsia, p. 262)

Proteinuria is defined as >300 mg of protein in 24-hour urine collection, or protein/creatinine ratio > 0.3. Dipstick tests are variable in qualitative determinations and are discouraged for diagnostic use.

If a 24-hour urine collection is not an option, a dipstick reading of 1+ indicates proteinuria

What is the pt's CBC and expanded chemistry panel?

Laboratory evidence of severe PIH includes:
- Renal insufficiency (elevated serum creatinine >1.1 mg/dL or a doubling of serum creatinine)
- HELLP syndrome
  - Hemolysis: Low hemoglobin and elevated lactate dehydrogenase
  - Elevated liver enzymes: Elevated alanine aminotransferase and aspartate aminotransferase
  - Low platelets: Platelets <100,000 cell/mm^3

What is the result of the 24-hour urine protein and creatinine clearance?

A 24-hour urinary protein collection will quantify proteinuria.

Severe preeclampsia is diagnosed when proteinuria equals or exceeds 5 g in 24 hours.

A **Severe PIH**

Severe preeclampsia is diagnosed by the presence of the following:
- SBP ≥160 mm Hg or DBP is ≥110 mm Hg
  - After 20 weeks of pregnancy on two occasions more than 6 hours apart
- Proteinuria of ≥5 g in 24 hours

Thrombocytopenia (<100,000 platelets/mL)

Pulmonary edema

Additional signs and symptoms (in the presence of mild preeclampsia):

– Persistent, severe headaches	– IUGR
– Visual changes	– Oligohydramnios
– Epigastric pain	– Platelets <100,000 cells/mm^3
– Renal insufficiency/oliguria	– Elevated liver enzymes
– HELLP syndrome (Hemolysis, Elevated Liver enzymes, Low Platelets)	

P **Admit**

All pts suspected of having severe preeclampsia should be admitted.

Ultrasound

Perform U/S at time of admission to confirm estimated gestational age (EGA).

Management of severe PIH is based on EGA. Consider corticosteroids if 24 wk–33 6/7 wk EGA.

Monitor BP

Pts should have BP monitored while on bed rest to confirm diagnosis of severe preeclampsia (≥160/110).

Monitor every 15 minutes on arrival and then hourly if stable.

Treat blood pressure

Persistent SBP ≥160 mm Hg or DBP ≥110 mm Hg should be treated.

- First line: Labetalol 20 mg IV q 20–30 minutes up to 80 mg until response (not to exceed 300 mg total).
- Second: Hydralazine 5–10 mg IV q 20 minutes until response (not to exceed 20–30 mg total).
- Third: Nifedipine 10–20 mg orally, repeat in 30 minutes, then 10–20 mg every 2–6 hours.

Consider repeating labs

For pts with abnormal results on initial labs (low platelets, elevated LFTs), repeat labs in 4–6 hours to assess trend.

Plan delivery

Severe preeclampsia requires immediate delivery.

- If fetus is 24–34 weeks EGA and pt is otherwise stable, steroids may be considered before inducing labor to aid in fetal lung maturation.
  - Betamethasone 12 mg IM q 24 hours × 2 doses

Route of delivery depends on clinical scenario.

- Mode of delivery does not need to be C/S. The mode of delivery should be determined by gestational age, fetal presentation, cervical status, and maternal-fetal condition.
- Multiparous pts with stable BPs and labs can have a trial of labor.
- $MgSO_4$ while in labor (see Mild Preeclampsia, p. 262).

TWIN GESTATION

S **Is the pt getting enough nutritional support?**

Twin gestations require an additional 300 kcal/d, and 1 mg folic acid daily.
Total maternal weight gain should be 40 lbs (10 lbs more than singleton pregnancy).

Does pt have any symptoms suggesting an obstetrical complication?

Multiple gestations have a higher incidence of many obstetrical complications, which
mandates a lower threshold for working up any suspicious symptoms:
- Pyelonephritis → Dysuria, frequency, urgency, fever, back pain
- Preterm labor (PTL) → Preterm UCs
- Premature spontaneous rupture of membranes → Leaking fluid from vagina
- Pregnancy-induced hypertension (PIH) → H/A, visual changes, epigastric pain
- Previa/abruption → Vaginal bleeding

O **Review VS**

Monitor for signs of PIH:
- Elevation of BP
- Excessive maternal weight gain

Perform PE

Elicit two separate fetal heart tones.
- Detection of two different heart *rates* helps distinguish gestations.
- Inability to clearly document two viable gestations necessitates U/S.
Examine the cervix if pt has symptoms of PTL.

A **Twin gestation**

P **Counsel pt on risks of multiple gestation**

Counsel pt on symptoms of the many possible obstetrical complications associated with
twins (see above).

In the first trimester, use U/S to establish estimated gestational age (EGA)

Establishing an accurate EGA early in pregnancy will help in management of any complications that occur later in pregnancy.

In the first trimester, attempt to identify chorionicity by U/S

Identification of chorionicity is important in management of twin gestations.
- "Chorionicity" refers to the outer membrane that surrounds a pregnancy (the inner is
  called the amnion).
- Twins can have either dichorionic or monochorionic membranes.
- *Zygosity* dictates which membranes occur.
  - Twins can be monozygotic (which occurs when a conception of a single egg and a
    single sperm splits into two) or dizygotic (which occurs when two sperm fertilize
    two eggs).
    - Dizygotic twins always result in dichorionicity because each conception forms
      its own membranes.
    - Monozygotic twins have three possibilities, depending on how old the concep-
      tion is when it splits (note: the amnion splits before the chorion):
      - 0–3 days: Monochorionic, monoamniotic
      - 4–8 days: Monochorionic, diamniotic
      - 9–13 days: Dichorionic, diamniotic
      - >13 days: Conjoined twins
- Monochorionic gestations are more rare but have certain serious adverse obstetric
  outcomes associated with them:
  - Twin-twin transfusion syndrome (when placental vascular anomalies favor blood
    supply to one fetus over the other)
  - Monoamniotic twins (leading to cord entanglements and stillbirths)
  - Conjoined twins

Chorionicity can be inferred by several U/S findings.

Any of the following suggest dichorionicity:

- Two placentas
- Discordant fetal sexes
- Separating membrane thickness >4 mm (representing two amnions/two chorions)
- "Twin peak" sign (a triangular shape that is made as the two chorions come together and fuse into the separating membrane)

At 18–20 weeks, perform U/S anatomy scan

Multiple gestations have higher rates of fetal anomalies. A thorough anatomic survey should be performed.

- Dizygotic twins have increased chromosomal abnormalities.
- Monozygotic twins have increased structural anomalies.

Starting at 24 weeks, monitor fetal growth by U/S

Perform serial U/S (q 3–4 weeks) to assess fetal growth and amniotic fluid levels.

Tracking fetal growth detects complications of monochorionicity and intrauterine growth restriction (IUGR) (higher incidence in twins).

Consider AP testing

Routine AP testing of twins is not recommended.

Initiate AP testing for suspicion of IUGR, fetal growth discordance, fetal anomalies, PIH, or monoamniotic gestations.

Make plans for delivery according to presentation of twins

Twin gestation presentations at the time of delivery occur with the following frequencies:

- Vertex/vertex: 40%
- Nonvertex/first twin: 20%
- Vertex/nonvertex: 40%

For management concerns, presentations are placed into *one of the three categories*:

- Twin A vertex, Twin B vertex
- Twin A nonvertex
- Twin A vertex, Twin B nonvertex
- Management of the first two categories is straightforward: category 1 should attempt vaginal delivery, and category 2 should have a C/S.
- Management of category 3 depends on practitioner experience and preference:
  - Twin A can be delivered vaginally followed by breech extraction of twin B.
  - Twin A can be delivered vaginally followed by external version of twin B.
  - Both twins can be delivered by C/S.

URINARY TRACT INFECTION

S **Does the pt have any urethritis symptoms?**
Dribbling
Mucopurulent discharge

Does the patient have any cystitis symptoms?
The classic triad of cystitis is:
- Frequency
- Urgency
- Burning

Other symptoms include:
- Dribbling
- Hesitancy
- Suprapubic pain

Has the pt had previous urinary tract infections (UTIs)?
Pts with a history of previous infection should receive longer courses of treatment.
Previous urine cultures may be used in selecting antibiotics.

Does the patient have any symptoms more common to a pyelonephritis? (see Pyelonephritis, p. 282)
The following symptoms are more suggestive of upper GU disease:
- Fever
- Chills
- Back pain (costovertebral area)

O **Review VS**
A fever is usually not seen in uncomplicated cystitis and should alert the clinician to the possibility of pyelonephritis.
Pts with pyelonephritis can show signs of septicemia (hypotension and tachycardia).

Perform PE
Suprapubic tenderness
Back
Costovertebral angle tenderness is associated with pyelonephritis

What is the result of the office reagent strip testing (urine dip)?
An office urine dip can support a diagnosis of UTI by the presence of:
- WBCs: Indicating infectious process
- Nitrites: Representing enzymatic activity of coliforms
- Leukocyte esterase: Representing enzymatic activity of neutrophil granules

What are the results of the U/A and culture and sensitivity?
U/A will give presumptive diagnosis of infection by demonstrating some combination of bacteriuria, pyuria (>5 cells/cc urine), proteinuria, nitrites, or leukocyte esterase.
U/A with WBC casts suggest renal involvement (pyelonephritis). Urine culture will reveal specific organism.
Sensitivities should be used to guide antibiotic choice.

A **Urinary tract infection**
Acute urethritis
Acute cystitis
Asymptomatic bacteriuria
- >100,000 organisms/cc of urine
- There is an association between asymptomatic bacteriuria and preterm labor, intrauterine growth restriction, pregnancy-induced hypertension, and anemia

Obtain urine culture

Urine culture confirms the diagnosis and provides sensitivities for antibiotic selection.
- *Escherichia coli* is by far the most common etiologic agent, accounting for about 90% of cases.
- Other pathogens include *Klebsiella pneumoniae, Proteus mirabilis*, group B streptococci, and the enterococci.

A clean-catch specimen of >10,000 colonies/cc of urine is considered positive.

A catheterized specimen is considered positive for >100 Units/cc.

Treat empirically with antibiotics

Several antibiotics covering gram-negative rods are acceptable.
- Cephalexin 250 mg PO qid × 3 days
- Amoxicillin-clavulanic acid 250 mg PO tid × 3 days
    - Avoid sulfonamide drugs in the late third trimester for potential effects on protein binding of bilirubin.

- Ampicillin is best avoided for empiric treatment because 25% of *E. coli* stains are resistant.

- For urethritis, consider treatment for gonococcus and *Chlamydia*.
    - Ceftriaxone 125 mg IM × 1 day
    - Azithromycin 1 g PO × 1 day

Consider a WBC count

In cases where the suspicion of pyelonephritis is raised, an elevated WBC count supports this diagnosis.

WBCs are traditionally not elevated with uncomplicated cystitis.

Follow-up sensitivities

Drug sensitivities can be followed up to ensure that appropriate antibiotics have been given.

Perform a test of cure

All pts should have a repeat urine culture performed after treatment.

A negative repeat urine culture assures adequate treatment (test 2 weeks after treatment).

All subsequent clinic visits should include a screen for recurrent infection with a dip for urine nitrites and leukocyte esterase.

LABOR AND DELIVERY

TERM LABOR

S **Notate the time of onset of contractions, status of fetal membranes, presence of vaginal bleeding, and recent fetal activity**

Status of fetal membranes is important in the management of chorioamnionitis and group B streptococcus (GBS) status (see Third Trimester Visit, p. 244)

Does the pt use any medications or have any allergies?

These are important answers to establish up front in case of sudden obstetric emergency.

O **What are the pt's baseline vital signs?**

Preeclampsia is often picked up at the initial assessment of labor.

Baseline vitals can be compared with subsequent values in the face of an obstetric emergency.

What is the fetal presentation and position?

Fetal presentations other than vertex generally require cesarean delivery.

Position of fetus is important in assessing *labor dystocia* (see p. 278).

What is the pattern of uterine contractions?

Uterine contractions should be noted for frequency, duration, and quality.

What is the pt's cervical exam?

Cervical exam should note dilation, effacement, and station.

Cervix of multiparous pts is frequently noted to be slightly dilated before onset of labor.

Membrane's status can be noted when dilation is adequate.

Presenting part can be confirmed.

Review pt's prenatal record

Note any problem list, obstetrical history, and Rh/rubella/GBS status.

Review fetal heart rate tracing

Fetal heart rate tracings (FHRTs) are important to note upon presentation.

Abnormal patterns developing later in labor can be compared with earlier patterns to aid in evaluation and management.

The following standardized terminology should be used when describing the FHRT:

- Baseline
  - Approximate mean heart rate over a 10-minute period (round to nearest 5 beats/min)
  - Must be constant for at least a 2-minute period
    - Normal 110–160 bpm (tachycardia >160 bpm, bradycardia <110 bpm)
- Variability
  - Fluctuations in baseline with two or more cycles/minute
    - Absent, minimal ≤5 bpm, moderate 6–25 bpm, marked >25 bpm
- Accelerations
- Decelerations
  - Early: associated with head compression
    - Nadir occurs with the peak of contraction
  - Variable: associated with cord compression
    - Rapid decline from baseline to nadir
  - Late: associated with uteroplacental insufficiency
    - Gradual decline from baseline with return after the end of contraction
    - Nadir occurs after the peak of contraction
      Category I—FHR baseline is 110–160 beats per minute, moderate variability, no late or variable decelerations, with or without early decelerations and accelerations.
      Category II—FHR tracings that are not Category I or III
      Category III—absent variability and any of the following:
      Recurrent late decelerations, recurrent variable decelerations, bradycardia

Term labor

"Term" is defined as a gestation between 37 and 42 weeks.
- <37 weeks is preterm
- 41 weeks is late term
- >42 is postterm
- >40 is "post dates" but still considered term

Labor is defined as regular uterine contractions accompanied by cervical dilation or change.
- *Latent-phase labor* is defined as regular contractions with cervical dilation <4 cm.
- *Active-phase labor* is defined as regular contractions with cervical dilation >4 cm.

P **Initial evaluation**

Evaluation for labor can frequently pick up other indications for admission.
Initial evaluation for labor should include the following:
- Continuous fetal heart rate monitoring: Any nonreassuring FHRT mandates admission.
- Blood pressure: Elevated blood pressure suggests preeclampsia.
- Urine dip: New-onset proteinuria is suspicious for preeclampsia.
- Cervical exam: Obtain initial cervical exam. If cervix is dilated 4 cm or more, pt is in active labor and should be admitted.

Observe for cervical change

In pts who are in the *latent phase* upon presentation (<4 cm), observe pt for a short interval (1–2 hours), and then check cervix for change.
Absence of cervical change suggests absence of labor.

Admit

Admit pts who are in active labor.
- Start IV fluids. Standard fluids for laboring pts is D5LR at 125 cc/hr.
- Check labs. CBC, RPR, U/A, type, and screen (if TOL, crossmatch).
- Obtain prenatal records.

Assess labor pain periodically

Level of comfort during labor should be assessed periodically throughout labor.
A pain scale can be used to yield objective data.
Pharmacologic management includes:
- Narcotics: Fentanyl, morphine, nalbuphine, remifentanil or
  - Butorphanol 1–2 mg IV q2h
- Regional anesthesia (epidural)

THIRD TRIMESTER BLEEDING

S How heavy is the bleeding?

Although subjective bleeding assessment by the pt can be inaccurate, trying to distinguish amount between "a few spots" and "a gush of blood" can help guide the workup.

Does the pt feel any associated pain?

Presence or absence of pain is the primary distinguishing factor between placenta previa and placental abruption.
- Placenta previa presents with *painless* third trimester bleeding.
- Placental abruption presents with *painful* third trimester bleeding.

Has the pt had this complaint before? Any prior workup?

Some pts may have prior admissions and workup for a KNOWN placenta previa. Review these records if available.

Has the pt had a prior U/S?

If the results of a prior U/S are available, referencing the report regarding the location of the placenta can help to quickly rule out placenta previa.

Does the pt have any risk factors for placenta previa?
- Previous C/S
- Multiparity
- Previous placenta previa

Does the pt have any risk factors for placental abruption?
- Cocaine
- Trauma
- Uterine anomalies
- Smoking
- Multiple gestations
- Premature rupture of membranes
- Prior abruption
- Multiparity
- Chronic hypertension/pregnancy-induced hypertension (PIH)

O Review VS

VS should be obtained and reviewed for any signs of cardiovascular instability (tachycardia and low blood pressure).

Hypertension (as a result of PIH or cocaine use) may be evident with placental abruptions.

Review fetal heart rate tracing (FHRT)

FHRT should be reviewed for any sign of fetal distress (late decelerations, bradycardia).
- Abnormal FHRT signals decreased blood perfusion to the fetus, which can be seen with maternal hemorrhage.

- Fetal distress in the face of maternal hemorrhage mandates immediate delivery.

Perform PE

Observe *external* genitalia (labia may be separated) for signs of active or recent bleeding.

Until placenta previa is ruled out, avoid digital cervical exam in order to prevent exacerbation of hemorrhage.

Perform U/S

Placenta previa can be diagnosed with good accuracy by U/S.

Note exact relation of placenta to internal os of cervix.
- Total previa: Cervical os is completely covered by placenta.
- Partial previa: Cervical os is partially covered by placenta.
- Marginal previa: Placenta edge lies next to (but not over) cervical os.

What is the result of the CBC?

Hemoglobin result after acute blood loss may not truly reflect degree of anemia if plasma volume has not yet been replaced.

Placental abruption

Diagnosis of placental abruption is made clinically by painful third trimester bleeding.

Placenta previa

Diagnosis of placenta previa is made by U/S.

Differential diagnoses

- Bloody show
- Vasa previa

Secure blood products

If suspicion for placenta previa or placental abruption is high, secure 4 units of packed RBCs by type and cross-match.

Immediate delivery for pts with active hemorrhage

For pts who are actively hemorrhaging (caused by either *diagnosed* placenta previa or *suspected* abruption), delivery must be executed immediately via C/S.

Admission for stable pts

Admit all pts who are not currently hemorrhaging but have a diagnosis of previa (made by U/S) or clinically suspected abruption.

Further management is individualized.

- Placenta previa
  - All term pts with placenta previa should be delivered.
    - Route of delivery depends on degree of previa.
      - Pts with either a total or partial previa require delivery by C/S.
      - Pts with a marginal previa may attempt vaginal delivery if pt and fetus show no signs of distress (absence of late decelerations on FHRT).
  - If preterm, pt may be admitted for observation.
    - If estimated gestational age (EGA) is <34 weeks, administer steroids for fetal lung maturity.
      - Steroids aid in fetal lung maturity in case the fetus needs to be delivered prematurely (high likelihood in the face of a diagnosed placental previa).
        - Betamethasone 12 mg IM q 24 hours × 2 doses
    - If pt remains stable, observation may be continued until either delivery is mandated by further heavy bleeding or fetus reaches an EGA that allows it to be delivered safely.
      - Generally, once fetus reaches 35 weeks EGA, an amniocentesis may be performed to demonstrate fetal lung maturity
- Placental abruption
  - Generally requires immediate C/S.
    - Vaginal delivery may be attempted in certain clinical scenarios (multiparous pt who is actively laboring, cervix is rapidly dilating, and FHRT shows no signs of distress).

CHORIOAMNIONITIS

S **Does the pt have any symptoms of chorioamnionitis?**
Maternal symptoms include fever/chills and uterine pain.

Does the pt have any risk factors for chorioamnionitis?
Risk factors include:
- Prolonged labor
- Preexisting infection
- Internal fetal monitoring
- Young age
- Prolonged rupture of membranes
- Multiple vaginal examinations
- Nulliparity
- Low socioeconomic status

O **Review VS**
Check for the presence of fever.
Check for signs of sepsis (tachycardia, low BP, decreased urine output).

Perform PE
Comprehensive physical exam to rule out other sources of infection.
- HEENT: Evaluate for upper respiratory infection (URI) → Throat exudates, nasal congestion
- Lungs: Evaluate for pneumonia → Decreased breath sounds, rhonchi
- Abdomen: Evaluate for appendicitis/cholecystitis → Rebound, guarding, Murphy sign
- Back: Evaluate for pyelonephritis → Costovertebral angle tenderness
- Extremities: Evaluate for deep vein thrombosis (DVT) → Swelling, color changes, Homans sign

Pelvic
- Vagina: Malodorous discharge is suggestive of chorioamnionitis.
- Uterus: Uterine tenderness is suggestive of chorioamnionitis.

Is the WBC count elevated?
Elevated WBC count is consistent with infection.

Labor itself may elevate WBC count slightly.

Assess fetal heart rate tracing (FHRT)
Fetal tachycardia often accompanies maternal fever.
Review FHRT for signs of compromise (see Term Labor, p. 272).

A **Chorioamnionitis**
Escherichia coli and group B streptococcus (GBS), both colonizers of the vaginal-rectal area, are the two most common microbes involved in chorioamnionitis.
Other pathogens are anaerobic bacteria, making chorioamnionitis *a polymicrobial infection.*
Differential diagnosis includes:
- Pneumonia
- Pyelonephritis
- URI
- DVT
- Appendicitis
- Cholecystitis

P **Start antibiotics**
Broad-spectrum Abx are selected with focus on coverage of *E. coli* and GBS. Gold standard regimen:
- Ampicillin 2 g IV q6h and gentamicin 1.5 mg/kg q8h

Penicillin-allergic pts can receive alternatives:
- Clindamycin 900 mg IV q8h or vancomycin 1 g q12h

Cooling measures
Initiate cooling measures for fevers:
- Tylenol 650 mg PO/PR q 4–6 hours
- Cooling blanket

Consider workup for alternate source
Blood cultures, U/A, CXR
U/S for DVT

Consider amniocentesis if preterm
A suspected diagnosis of chorioamnionitis in a *preterm* fetus can be confirmed by evaluating the following in amniotic fluid (not used with term, laboring pts):
- Glucose: Usually lowered with infection
- Interleukin-6: Elevated levels (very sensitive test)
- Leukocyte esterase: Product of WBC action signifying infection
- Gram stain and culture: Gram stain may miss some infections

For laboring pts, assess labor curve up to this point
If labor is prolonged, consider active management to decrease time until delivery and risk of sepsis.

Watch for labor dystocia
Pts with chorioamnionitis have an increased risk of labor dystocia.
These pts also have a poor response to oxytocin.

Watch for PPH
Amnionitis places the pt at increased risk for uterine atony.

LABOR DYSTOCIA

S **What is the patient's degree of fatigue?**
Prolonged labor can lead to maternal exhaustion and inability to complete a vaginal birth successfully.

How well is the patient's pain controlled?
Uncontrolled labor pain can result in failure to progress through a normal labor.

If the pt is in the second stage of labor, does she feel her pushing efforts are effective?
Epidural anesthesia may prevent optimal pushing efforts.

O **Review the patient's labor curve up to this point**
Note general appearance of labor curve.
See definitions of abnormalities below.

What is the pt's current cervical and pelvic exam?
Cervical exam should generally be performed every 4 hours when the patient is in latent phase (<4 cm dilation) and every 2 hours in active phase (>4 cm dilation).
- It is preferable to have the same examiner for each "check" because cervical exams can be subjective, especially in noting station.
- Pelvic exam should note any overdistended bladder or firm perineal body, which can both interfere with second stage.
- Rare anatomic findings that could be contributory to dystocia are vaginal septum, fibroids, or pelvic tumors.

What is fetal presentation?
Fetal presentations should be reconfirmed to be cephalic (a.k.a. vertex). Note any of the following:
- Caput succedaneum formation (scalp edema)
- Molding (changes in the relationship of skull bones at the sutures to accommodate pelvis)
- Compound presentation
  - Fetal extremity is found alongside major fetal presenting part (head).

What is the pattern of the fetal heart rate?
Fetal well-being should be confirmed before any interventions for dystocia are initiated (see Term Labor p. 272).

A labor dystocia
Labor dystocia is "difficult" or abnormal labor.
Normal labor is divided into three stages:
- First stage is from onset of labor to complete cervical dilation.
  - This stage is further divided into two phases:
    - Latent phase: 0–4 cm dilation
    - Active phase: 4–10 cm (complete) dilation
- Second stage is from complete cervical dilation to delivery.
- Third stage is from delivery of infant to delivery of placenta.

Abnormal labor patterns can occur at any stage.
- Latent phase of labor is considered prolonged when it exceeds:
  - >20 hours for nulliparous patients
  - >14 hours for multiparous patients
- Disorders of the active phase of labor can be divided into *arrest, protraction, or combined* disorders.
  - Arrest disorders are defined as no cervical dilation for >2 hours.
  - Protraction disorders are defined as:
    - Cervical dilation <1.2 cm/hr in nulliparous patients
    - Cervical dilation <1.5 cm/hr in multiparous patients

- Disorders of the second stage of labor can be divided into arrest and protraction disorders.
  - Arrest disorders are defined as failure to descend past a given station for >2 hours.
  - Protracted second stage is defined as:
    - Descent <1 cm/hr in nulliparous patients
    - Descent <2 cm/hr in multiparous patients

P   Assess the power, the passenger, and the passage

The power refers to uterine contractility.
- Adequate uterine contractions may be assessed by frequency (>3/10 minutes) or strength (Montevideo units > 200).

- Montevideo units = Frequency of UCs per 10 minutes × Strength of UCs in mm Hg

The passenger refers to the fetus.
- Estimate fetal weight
- Position
  - Occiput anterior/posterior/transverse
- Attitude
  - Posture fetus assumes at term
    - Normal is curved spine, flexed head
    - Abnormal is some degree of head extension
- Asynclitism
  - When fetal sagittal suture is deflected away from midline or transverse axis of pelvis

The passage refers to the maternal pelvis.
- Use clinical pelvimetry to qualitatively assess architecture of pelvis.
  - Can sacral promontory be reached with the middle finger? (diagonal conjugate)
  - Is sacrum concave, flat, anterior?
  - Are ischial spines average, prominent?
  - Is subpubic arch average, narrow, wide?

Consider interventions

Protraction disorders may be considered for the following interventions:
- Nonoperative
  - Analgesics for pain relief
  - Amniotomy
  - Augmentation of labor (oxytocin)
- Operative vaginal delivery
  - Forceps
  - Vacuum

Arrest disorders generally require cesarean section.

PRETERM LABOR

 When was the onset of contractions and how intense are they?

True preterm labor (PTL) is likely to have a rapid onset with contractions similar in intensity to term labor.

Are there any other accompanying symptoms?

Additional symptoms of PTL include:
- Backache
- Vaginal spotting
- Increased vaginal discharge

Does the patient have a history of PTL or preterm birth (PTB) with previous pregnancy?

History of preterm labor puts the patient at higher risk to have a repeat problem.

O **What are the results of the U/S?**

A comprehensive U/S should be performed.
- Fetus
  o Estimated gestational age/estimated fetal weight (EFW) is the most important piece of information when forming management plans for PTL.
  o Several findings contraindicate tocolysis:
    - Intrauterine growth restriction, intrauterine fetal demise
    - Lethal fetal anomalies
    - Nonreassuring fetal status
    - Severe preeclampsia or eclampsia
    - EFW >2,500 g
    - Chorioamnionitis
  o Note presentation—transverse fetal lie is a contraindication to vaginal delivery.
- Amniotic fluid index
  o Evaluate for preterm premature rupture of membranes if oligohydramnios is present.
- Placental location
- Uterine abnormalities
  o Uterine fibroids may contribute to PTL.
- Cervix
  o Cervical length can be assessed for shortening by transvaginal U/S.
  o A length >3.5 cm places the pt at low risk for impending delivery.
  o Note any funneling (as the internal os opens, the relationship of the cervix to the lower uterus changes from a "T" to a "Y" to a "U" shape).
  o Observe any changes with pt performing Valsalva.

What is the result of the fetal fibronectin (FFN)?

FFN is a protein found between the decidua and placenta.
- It is normally absent in cervical/vaginal secretions between 24 and 34 weeks.
- Detection (by cervical/vaginal swab) during this time places the pt at increased risk for PTB.
  o Results are reported as positive or negative.

> - Swab cannot be performed if the pt had digital vaginal exam, intercourse, or vaginal bleeding in previous 24 hours.

What is the pt's cervical exam?

Cervical exam should be performed after sampling for FFN is done.
Note dilation, effacement, and station.

Is there any evidence of infection?

CBC should be assessed for possible elevated WBCs.
U/A should be assessed for possible infection.

Preterm labor

PTL is defined as the onset of labor before 37 weeks' gestation.

- PTL is not as easy to diagnose as term labor, and a diagnosis is often made retrospectively.
  - Management must proceed based on all findings, erring on the conservative side.
  - Customarily, cervical change while under observation or a cervical exam with a dilation >2 cm or 80% effacement is considered diagnostic.

Etiologies include:

- Infection
- Mechanical factors
- Uterine overdistention
- Uterine anomalies
- Intrinsic premature activation of labor by the fetus
- Cervical incompetence

 Start tocolysis

A trial of tocolysis is begun in all gestations <35 weeks to allow antenatal corticosteroid administration prior to birth. There is no evidence that tocolysis improves outcomes other than allowing administration for corticosteroids and magnesium sulfate for fetal neuroprotection.

- This gestational age is empiric because, after 35 weeks, the risk of the fetus developing respiratory distress syndrome (RDS) is minimal.

Contraindications to tocolysis include severe hypertension, hemorrhage, and cardiac disease.

Several acceptable tocolytics are available:

- Magnesium sulfate 4 g IV load and then 2 g IV qh—also used for fetal neuroprotection (reduces cerebral palsy) in gestations <32 weeks
  - Watch for respiratory depression and blunted deep tendon reflexes.
  - Consider checking level if suspicious of toxicity.
  - Reduce dose with renal insufficiency.
- Calcium channel blockers
  - Nifedipine 10 mg SL × 3 load and then 10 mg tid.
    - Avoid use with $MgSO_4$.
- β-Adrenergics
  - Terbutaline 0.25 mg SQ q 1–4 hours (max 5 mg/24 hrs).
    - Avoid with hyperthyroidism and uncontrolled diabetes mellitus.
- NSAIDs
  - Indomethacin 25 mg PR load and then 25 mg PO q 4–6 hours.
    - Potential ductus arteriosus closure and oligohydramnios

Consider steroids

All gestations <34 weeks should receive steroids to enhance fetal lung development and minimize the risk of a preterm infant developing RDS.

- Two agents and regimens are available:
  - Betamethasone 12 mg IM q 24 hours × 2 (Rec)
  - Dexamethasone 6 mg IM q 12 hours × 4 (Alt)

Caution should be exercised with diabetic pts because steroids can increase blood sugar and increase the risk of the pt developing diabetic ketoacidosis.

Culture for GBS and start antibiotics

Preterm infants are especially susceptible to early-onset group B streptococcus disease and should be cultured for this upon arrival (see Third Trimester Visit, p. 244).

While awaiting culture results, antibiotics should be started:

- Penicillin G 5 million U load and then 2.5 million U q4h (Rec)
- Ampicillin 2 g IV load and then 1 g q4h (Alt)
- Clindamycin 900 mg IV q8h (Alt)

PYELONEPHRITIS

S **Does the pt have documented fevers?**

Pts with pyelonephritis usually present with fevers.

Check for any other source of fever (see Chorioamnionitis, p. 276).

Does the pt have any nausea and vomiting (N/V)?

N/V is commonly associated with pyelonephritis.
* Assess the degree of problem by asking when was the last time the pt ate.
* Moderate to severe N/V will have associated hypokalemia.

Does the pt have any urinary tract infection (UTI) symptoms?

Check for history of classic UTI triad: Dysuria, frequency, and urgency.

Has the pt had pyelonephritis or UTI previously during this pregnancy?

Some pts will have had prior infections and been noncompliant with their suppressive therapy (see below).

Does the pt have any underlying GU pathology?

Underlying GU pathology predisposes pt to pyelonephritis.

Inquire about history of renal stones, ureteral stents, or congenital anomalies of the kidneys.

Does the pt have any allergies?

Allergy history is important in selecting antibiotic treatment.

O **Review VS**

Document fever.

Check VS for evidence of septicemia (low BP, tachycardia, oliguria).

Does the pt have costovertebral angle tenderness (CVAT)?

CVAT is usually markedly evident. May be absent in very early infection.

Perform comprehensive PE to rule out other etiologies (see Chorioamnionitis, p. 276).

Assess for contractions

UCs are common with pyelonephritis.

What are the results of the U/A, CBC, and CMP?

U/A is usually very "dirty" with the presence of bacteria, WBCs, nitrites, and leukocyte esterase.
* Note WBC level, which is commonly elevated.
* Pts with pyelonephritis frequently have emesis with resultant hypokalemia.

A **Pyelonephritis**

Pregnancy predisposes the pt to pyelonephritis by two main mechanisms:
* Via progesterone
  * Progesterone's smooth muscle effect relaxes ureters and allows ascending bacteria to infect kidney.
* Via mechanical changes
  * Uterus rests on ureters at pelvic brim.
  * Right side is more affected by this (pyelonephritis occurs more often on the right side).

P **Admit**

All pts who are pregnant with pyelonephritis need to be admitted.

Start antibiotics

Antibiotics are selected to cover the most likely organisms.
* Most common are *E. coli*, group B streptococcus, *Klebsiella,* and *Proteus*
* Cefazolin 1–2 g IV q8h (Rec)
* Gentamicin/Ampicillin (Alt)

Cooling measures

Pts with pyelonephritis can have very high fevers (>104° F).
Interventions include:
- Tylenol 650 mg PO q4h
- Cooling blanket

IV hydration

Start IV hydration with replacement fluids to ensure adequate urine output.

Replace potassium

Potassium lost with emesis should be replaced with IV fluids.

Diet depending on N/V

In pts with moderate to severe N/V, consider holding PO intake until symptoms
improve.

Monitor for signs or symptoms of fluid overload or adult respiratory distress syndrome (ARDS)

Pregnancy is a high-volume state, which makes it susceptible to fluid overload when pts
are receiving IV fluids and antibiotics.
Monitor fluid balance closely.
- Urine output should be maintained at >30 cc/hr.
- Check lung fields periodically for evidence of fluid overload.
  o Get CXR if crackles are present.
- Limit IV fluids after giving first few liters. Pregnant pts with pyelonephritis are
  susceptible to ARDS.
- Gram-negative bacteria release endotoxins when killed.
- Endotoxin damages respiratory endothelium.

Follow-up culture and sensitivity

Sensitivity to current antibiotics needs to be confirmed.
25% of *E. coli* is resistant to ampicillin.

Consider U/S of kidneys if no improvement

Pts who fail to respond within 48–72 hours of treatment should be assessed for possible
underlying pathology.
Consider perinephric abscess or kidney stones blocking ureter.

Discharge after 48 hours afebrile

Oral Abx to *complete a 10-day course* of treatment. Cephalexin 250 mg PO qid.

Long-term antibiotic prophylaxis

All pts require long-term antibiotics in prophylactic doses for the remainder of
pregnancy.
Verify sensitivities to nitrofurantoin (100 mg PO qd) or cephalexin (250 mg PO qd).

RUPTURE OF MEMBRANES

S **Obtain a detailed history of event**

What happened? How much fluid came out? Is this the first episode?

Has the pt experienced any fevers/chills? How long ago did the loss of fluid occur?

- Prolonged rupture can lead to chorioamnionitis.

Is there a possibility that the leakage was not amniotic fluid?

O **Review VS**

Tachycardia and fever can signify infection.

Verify fetal well-being

Pt should be immediately placed on continuous fetal heart monitoring.

Perform sterile speculum exam

Visualize the cervix on speculum exam for cervical dilation—do not do a cervical exam if preterm.

Check for pooling.

- Pooling is the presence of a large collection of amniotic fluid in the vagina.
  - For gestations >32 weeks, collection and analysis of amniotic fluid to assess fetal lung maturity may be helpful in management.
    - Phosphatidylglycerol can be used.
    - The lecithin/sphingomyelin ratio can be affected by contamination.

Perform nitrazine test.

- Nitrazine paper is pH sensitive and will turn dark blue in the presence of a pH > 6.
  - Amniotic fluid pH is 7.1–7.3 and will turn paper dark blue.
  - Semen and blood also have an alkaline pH, which can yield a false-positive result.

Check for ferning.

- Swab posterior vaginal fornix and smear onto slide. After drying, the slide can be examined under the microscope for fern-like pattern.
- Evaluate cervix for dilation.

> - Try to visualize cervix with sterile speculum to avoid digital exam and the introduction of infection.

Perform ultrasound

Amniotic fluid index (AFI)

- If SSE is equivocal, assess the AFI for oligohydramnios.
  - Oligohydramnios, <5 cm of fluid, provides indirect evidence of rupture of membranes (ROM).

Fetus

- Confirm estimated gestational age (EGA).
- Measure fetal weight.
- Note presentation.
  - Nonvertex presentations have a higher risk of cord prolapse.

Labs

Elevated WBC count can be noted to support a diagnosis of intra-amniotic infection but does not help in the absence of clinical evidence.

- Corticosteroids, as used in the management of preterm ROM, can elevate WBCs.

Consider indigo carmine

If the above tests cannot confirm diagnosis, indigo carmine dye can be injected into the amniotic cavity by amniocentesis.

- Pt is observed for passage of dye from vagina, which confirms diagnosis.

A **Premature rupture of membranes (PROM)**

Rupture of membranes at term (>37 weeks) before onset of labor

Preterm premature rupture of membranes (PPROM)

Rupture of membranes before 37 weeks' gestation

Differential diagnosis

- Urinary incontinence
- Vaginal douches
- Vaginal discharge
- Semen
- Cervicitis
- Bloody show

P **Manage PROM with induction**

If group B streptococcus (GBS) status is unknown and rupture occurred >18 hours prior, start the pt on antibiotics (see Preterm Labor, p. 280).

Management of PPROM depends on EGA

If <32 weeks

- Corticosteroids
- Magnesium sulfate for neuroprotection
- Broad-spectrum antibiotics
  - Increase the latency period and may decrease neonatal sepsis
    - Ampicillin 2 g and erythromycin 250 mg IV q6h for 2 days followed by amoxicillin 250 mg and erythromycin 333 mg PO q8h for 5 days
- Continuous monitoring
- Strict bed rest
- Induction for any symptoms/signs of chorioamnionitis
- Watch for abruption (increased incidence with ROM)

If between 32 and 33 6/7 weeks:

- Expectant management
- Antibiotics, single-course corticosteroids, GBS prophylaxis
- Continuous fetal monitoring
  - If vertex and well-engaged, may consider intermittent monitoring after first 48 hours.
- Strict bed rest
  - High risk of cord prolapse, especially if nonvertex presentation
- No tocolysis
- Take a GBS culture and start antibiotics (see Preterm Labor, p. 280)
- Induction for any symptoms/signs of chorioamnionitis

If 34 weeks or later:

- Start induction
- Antibiotics for GBS up to 37 weeks (if status unknown)

MATERNITY WARD

POSTPARTUM DAY 1

 Has the pt experienced any heavy bleeding or cramping?

Concern about heavy bleeding should prompt an objective assessment.

Inquiry about when the current pad was last changed will help assess recent bleeding activity.

Cramping can be associated with involution of the uterus and is sometimes noticeable with breastfeeding as oxytocin is released.

Pts requiring more than acetaminophen with codeine should be suspected of having pathologic etiologies of pain.

Has the pt ambulated?

Early ambulation reduces the risk of postpartum deep vein thrombosis (DVT) as well as postpartum bladder and bowel complications.

Has the pt eaten or had a bowel movement?

Gastrointestinal function should be confirmed.

Has the pt voided spontaneously?

Urinary function should be confirmed.

Does the pt have any questions about the delivery?

Discuss any questions the pt might have about the delivery, especially if any complications occurred.

O **Review VS**

Assess cardiovascular stability.

Assess for fever.

Review I/O.

- Adequate urine output (>30 cc/hr) should be confirmed because there is often increased capacity and decreased sensitivity in the postpartum period.
- The following factors increase the pt's risk for urinary retention:
  - Conduction anesthesia
  - Vaginal operative delivery
  - Uncontrolled pain from an episiotomy site

Perform PE

Breasts
- Examine for signs of engorgement or tenderness.

Current pad
- Assessing degree of saturation of current pad provides objective evidence of recent bleeding activity.

External genitalia
- Assess any abnormal swelling for a hematoma.
- Confirm that episiotomy is intact.

Uterus
- Palpation of the abdomen should reveal the uterine fundus.
- Confirm involution and firmness.

Monitor blood sugars in pregestational and A2 gestational diabetes mellitus pts

 Postpartum day 1 status-post normal spontaneous vaginal delivery

Other types of vaginal deliveries:
- Postpartum Day 1 status-post vacuum-assisted vaginal delivery
- Postpartum Day 1 status-post forceps delivery

P ## Dietary management

Most pts can be maintained or started on a regular diet.

Pregestational and gestational diabetics should be maintained on an ADA diet.

Encourage frequent ambulation

Risk of the following postpartum complications can be reduced with early and frequent
    ambulation:

- DVT
- GI (constipation, bloating)
- GU (retention)

Consider interventions for episiotomy pain

Pts with persistent episiotomy pain can benefit from topical anesthetic sprays, warm
    compresses, and oral analgesics.

Follow-up CBC

Hemoglobin should reflect the predelivery hemoglobin along with the estimated blood
    loss.

Leukocytosis is common after normal delivery.

Confirm rubella immunity

Pts who are rubella nonimmune should be offered and receive rubella vaccine before
    discharge.

Confirm Rh status

Pts who are Rh negative and antibody negative should have an updated antibody screen
    during their delivery admission.

Pts who have remained antibody negative should have the infant checked for Rh status.

If the infant is Rh positive, the pt is eligible for anti-D immune globulin.

- Anti-D immune globulin is given as one vial of 300 µg.
- 300 µg of anti-D IgG can suppress immunity of up to 30 cc of fetal Rh-positive blood.

Consider lactation consult

Pts who appear to have trouble breastfeeding immediately postpartum will benefit from
    an early lactation consult.

Arrange for postpartum tubal ligation (PPTL) (if applicable)

PPTL can be performed any time from immediately following delivery to postpartum
    day 1.

POSTPARTUM DAY 2

S **Has the pt experienced any heavy bleeding or cramping?**

Lochia (postpartum uterine discharge) should continue to decrease in amount by post-partum day 2.

Cramping should be minimal and not require more than acetaminophen.

Does the pt have any breast complaints?

Engorgement of the breasts (swelling from blood, lymph, and milk) usually occurs around this time and can be uncomfortable.

Any excessive discomfort raises suspicion for mastitis or plugged duct.

Is the pt planning on breastfeeding?

Discussions pertaining to breastfeeding provide an opportunity for education and help plan follow-up care in the postpartum period.

- Maternal benefits include decreased risk of postpartum hemorrhage and delayed return of fertility.
- Neonatal advantages include decreased incidence of atopic skin disorders, diarrhea, and infections (GI, respiratory, meningitis, otitis media).

Does the pt have any questions about discharge from the hospital?

Pts without complications are usually discharged on postpartum day 2.

This is a good time to discuss any questions the pt might have had about what to expect in the following weeks after delivery.

How is the pt's affect?

"Postpartum blues" (anxiety, sadness, or restlessness) can be expected in most pts at some time during the first 10 days postpartum.

Symptoms are transient and usually require only explanation and understanding. Any pt with a prior history of depressed affect should be observed closely for postpartum depression, a serious complication that warrants medical treatment.

O **Review VS**

Confirm that pt is afebrile.

In preeclamptic pts, review blood pressure.

Pts with pregnancy-induced hypertension should have normal BPs for at least 24 hours before discharge.

Perform PE

Breasts

- Firmness of breasts secondary to engorgement is common.
- Signs of inflammation (redness, heat) on nipple or skin are abnormal and must prompt evaluation for cracked nipples, mastitis, or abscess.

Abdomen

- Confirm uterine firmness.
- If the pt had a postpartum tubal ligation (PPTL), confirm that the wound is clean, dry, and intact.

Current pad

- Confirm that the degree of saturation of current pad is decreasing.

External genitalia

- Confirm that episiotomy remains intact.

Uterus

- Confirm that involution and firmness remain.

A **Postpartum day 2 status-post normal spontaneous vaginal delivery**

Other types of vaginal deliveries:

- Vacuum-assisted vaginal delivery
- Forceps delivery

P ### Discharge pt to home

Pelvic rest for 4 weeks

Pt should be instructed to avoid sexual intercourse until perineum is comfortable and bleeding has diminished.

Tampon use should be avoided in pts with perineal repairs but are acceptable otherwise (provided they are changed frequently).

Schedule follow-up visit in clinic

A 4-wk follow-up visit is customary.

- Schedule appointment sooner if there were any complications during delivery or the postpartum period.
- A 6-wk follow-up is acceptable for uncomplicated pts who are breastfeeding. (Ovulation can return by 5 weeks postpartum in pts who are not breastfeeding.)
- A 1-wk follow-up for a wound check is necessary for pts who have had a PPTL.

Instruct pt to return immediately for any signs of heavy bleeding, infection, or depression.

Prescribe iron supplementation, analgesics, and stool softeners as needed

Pts who are anemic (Hb <10.0) should be given a prescription for iron supplementation before discharge.

Pts with a PPTL usually are given an analgesic preparation containing both acetaminophen and codeine.

Pts with postpartum constipation benefit from stool softeners.

- Docusate sodium 100 mg PO bid

Consider a home health nursing visit

Any pts at high risk for complications occurring before their postpartum clinic appointment should be monitored at home.

- Pts with a history of preeclampsia and delay in resolution of high BPs in the postpartum period
- Pts at risk for postpartum depression

Consider a lactation consult before discharge

Any pts experiencing breastfeeding problems will be more successful when they receive counseling before returning home.

Consider contraception

Customarily, contraception can be offered at the postpartum visit in 4–6 weeks.

Consider offering contraception before discharge for:

- Potential noncompliant pts
- Potential fallouts
- Pts who should not get pregnant again

See individual Family Planning sections (pp. 306–317) for detail.

DYSPNEA

 Is the pt having any symptoms other than dyspnea?
Pts with pulmonary embolus can also experience pleuritic chest pain and
apprehension.

Does the pt have a history of cardiac, valvular, or vascular disease?
Underlying cardiac disease can predispose pt to pulmonary edema.
- The postpartum period may be the first presentation of such disease.
- Pts with coronary artery disease are at increased risk for myocardial infarction
  (MI).

**Does the pt have any risk factors for deep vein thrombosis (DVT)/pulmonary
embolus?**
Prior DVT/pulmonary embolus
Hypercoagulable state (familial or acquired thrombophilia)
Antiphospholipid syndrome (see Antiphospholipid Syndrome, p. 250)

O Review delivery history
Check for complications of delivery, which may predispose the pt to some of the etiolo-
gies of dyspnea.
- Pts with pregnancy-induced hypertension (PIH) are at increased risk for pulmonary
  edema.
  o These pts are usually on $MgSO_4$ in the postpartum period.
    - The hypooncotic pressures associated with PIH and the increased fluids associ-
      ated with $MgSO_4$ use place the pt at increased risk for pulmonary edema.
    - $MgSO_4$ can also directly suppress the respiratory rate.
- Pts with intrapartum infection are at risk for sepsis.
- Pts who received general (endotracheal) anesthesia are at increased risk for
  aspiration.

Review VS
Temperature: Low-grade fever may be associated with pulmonary embolus.
Check for tachypnea and cardiovascular stability.
Check I/O: A positive fluid balance suggests fluid overload.

Perform PE
Heart
- Atrial fibrillation can lead to clot formation and pulmonary embolus.
Lungs
- Check for signs of pulmonary edema or decreased breath sounds associated with
  pulmonary embolus or infiltrate.
Extremities
- Check for signs in the lower extremities that could signal DVT:
  o Swelling
  o Tenderness
  o Homans sign (calf pain upon dorsiflexion of the ankle)

Obtain stat pulse ox
Pulse oximetry can be used to rapidly assess blood oxygenation.
Saturation values <90% imply inadequate oxygenation.

A A Dyspnea
Differential diagnosis:

– Pulmonary embolus	– Pulmonary edema
– Aspiration	– Adult respiratory distress syndrome (ARDS)
– Pneumonia	– Sepsis
– MI	– Pneumothorax

P

Obtain ABG
PE findings include decreased O_2 and CO_2 and respiratory alkalosis.
pO_2 value >90 mm Hg essentially rules out pulmonary embolus.

Obtain CXR
Check for infiltrate or edema.
Usually normal with pulmonary embolus but may have radiolucent area.

Obtain ECG
Check for ischemia or MI.
PE findings inconsistent but can have nonspecific T-wave inversions or triad of S1Q3T3.

Obtain CBC
Elevated WBCs are consistent with infection.

Consider D-dimer level
D-dimer level <0.25 mg/L is very sensitive for ruling out DVT.

Consider MgSO₄ level
If pt is on $MgSO_4$, consider checking level for toxicity.
$MgSO_4$ toxicity (>15 mg/dL) can lead to respiratory depression.

Consider imaging workup for DVT or pulmonary embolus
U/S: U/S can be used to assess DVT with a sensitivity >90%.
Spiral CT scan: Detects pulmonary embolus with a high degree of sensitivity.

Consider empiric treatment of pulmonary embolus
Baseline PT/PTT.
Load with 7,500 U heparin (70–80 U/kg) followed by 1,500 U/hr (20 U/kg/hr).
Follow PTT values every 4 hours and titrate to 1.5–2.5 times control (60–80 sec).

Treat underlying etiology
Diuresis for evidence of fluid overload
Antibiotics for evidence of pneumonia

Consultation
Early consultation for management of pulmonary embolus, MI, ARDS, or pneumothorax.

POSTPARTUM FEVER

S **Does the pt have any symptoms that may localize the source of infection?**
HEENT/lung complaints: Upper respiratory infection (URI), pneumonia
Breast complaints: Abscess, mastitis
Wound pain: Infection
Extremities: Deep vein thrombosis (DVT)
GU complaints: Urinary tract infection, pyelonephritis

Does the pt have any risk factors for postpartum endometritis?
Risk factors include:
- Cesarean section
- Prolonged rupture of membranes
- Low socioeconomic status
- Prolonged labor
- Preexisting infection
- Multiple vaginal examinations

O **Check VS**
Mild fever is common in the first 24 hours postop and of no clinical significance.
  Cardiovascular stability should be confirmed by BP and heart rate. Document all I/O.
Urine output should be >30 cc/hr.

Perform PE
Comprehensive PE to rule out other sources of infection
- HEENT
  ○ Evaluate for URI → Throat exudates, nasal congestion
- Lungs
  ○ Evaluate for pneumonia → Decreased breath sounds, rhonchi
- Abdomen
  ○ Evaluate for appendicitis/cholecystitis → Rebound, guarding, Murphy sign
  ○ Evaluate for wound infection (for C/S) → Skin color changes, wound discharge
- Back
  ○ Evaluate for pyelonephritis → Costovertebral angle tenderness
- Extremities
  ○ Evaluate for DVT → Swelling, color changes, Homans sign
Pelvic
- Vagina
  ○ Malodorous discharge is consistent with endomyometritis
- Uterus
  ○ Check for presence of uterine tenderness, which is suggestive of
    endomyometritis
    • Very subjective finding if pt had C/S (secondary to incision tenderness)

What is the result of the CBC?
Hemoglobin should reflect intraoperative estimated blood loss.
Elevated WBCs can be a result of surgery.

A **Endomyometritis**
Polymicrobial infection with same pathogens as chorioamnionitis (see
  Chorioamnionitis, p. 276)
Anaerobic bacteria are especially predominant after C/S
Differential diagnosis
- Enterococcal infection
- Septic pelvic thrombophlebitis
- Septic shock

Start antibiotics

Broad-spectrum antibiotics are selected, including coverage of anaerobic bacteria.
Gold standard regimen:
Gentamicin 1.5 mg/kg IV q8h and clindamycin 900 mg IV q8h.

Cooling measures

Initiate cooling measures for fevers:
- Tylenol 650 mg PO/PR q 4–6 hours
- Cooling blanket

Consider workup for other sources

CXR
Blood cultures
U/S for DVT

Consider monitoring gentamicin levels

Peak and trough levels should be evaluated for the following:
- Bacteremic pts
- >5 days of treatment
- Obese pts
- Pts with renal insufficiency

Evaluate response to treatment

Response to treatment is evaluated by defervescence.
Response should be evident within 48–72 hours.

Consider enterococcal coverage

Enterococcus is not sensitive to the gentamicin/clindamycin regimen and can occasion-
ally be a contributory pathogen to endomyometritis.
For pts who do not defervesce in 48–72 hours, add ampicillin for enterococcal coverage.
- Ampicillin 2 g IV q6h

Consider septic vein thrombophlebitis

If pts continue to spike fevers, consider septic vein thrombophlebitis.
- Diagnosis is usually one of exclusion, and therapy consists of empiric heparin.
  - Load with 7,500 U heparin (70–80 U/kg) followed by 1,500 U/hr (20 U/kg/hr).
  - Follow PTT values every 4 hours and titrate to 1.5–2.5 times control (60–80 sec).
  - Continue IV heparin until defervescence.
- CT scan may provide imaging evidence of thrombus.

POSTPARTUM HEMORRHAGE

S **Is the pt responsive?**
An initial observation of the pt's state gives you an idea of cardiovascular status.

Does the pt feel dizzy?
Dizziness is another subjective indicator of severity of blood loss.

Obtain history from Nursing
Nursing will be able to review the *immediate* bleeding history, pad counts, and timing to give you an idea of the degree of bleeding.

O **Review delivery history**
Look for a history of lacerations or difficult placental delivery that might focus exam regarding etiology.
The following are risk factors for postpartum hemorrhage (PPH):
- Oxytocin use
- Macrosomia
- High parity
- Distention of uterine cavity (multiples, polyhydramnios)
- Tocolytic use
- Chorioamnionitis
- Rapid or prolonged labor

Review VS
Stat VS should be reviewed for cardiovascular stability.
Urine output is the primary indicator of fluid volume status.
Oliguria is urine output <30 cc/hr.

Perform PE
Adequate inspection and palpation is key to finding the etiology of hemorrhage.
If bedside exposure is not adequate, consider transferring pt from maternity to a labor and delivery room.
This also allows for the pt to be ready in case a D&C or surgical exploration is required. Use a flashlight or good lighting source for inspection.
External genitalia and vagina
• Note any lacerations.
Bimanual exam
• Evacuate all blood clots.
  o Blood clots can cause a blockage at the cervix and prevent the uterus from involuting.
• Note firmness of uterus.
  o A large, boggy uterus is consistent with uterine atony.

What are the results of the pt's CBC?
Noting the Hb/Hct result (from before delivery) will give you an idea of the pt's reserves. Consider PT/PTT.

Consider U/S
If PE does not yield etiology, consider a U/S to search for fragments of retained placenta.
Retained products are seen ultrasonographically as echogenic foci along the endometrial lining (stripe).

A **Postpartum Hemorrhage**
Defined as a 10% change in Hct from admission to postpartum period or need for transfusion.
• Average estimated blood loss (EBL) for vaginal delivery is 500 mL and for C/S 1,000 mL.
• Subjective assessment of EBL is notoriously inaccurate.

The differential diagnosis for PPH in the immediate postpartum setting includes:

- Uterine atony
- Genital laceration
- Retained placental products
- Uterine inversion
- Uterine rupture
- Placenta accreta

P Secure venous access

Stat fluid bolus for hypovolemia

Secure blood products

Type and screen if not already done
- Cross-match packed RBCs if anticipating a transfusion.
- Transfusion criteria based on individual picture:
  - Considered for *symptomatic pts* or *Hb <8 g/dL*

Treat underlying etiology

Atony
- Uterine massage and evacuation of any blood clots
- Pharmacologic treatments:
  - Oxytocin
    - 20–30 U in 1 L of IV fluids with continuous infusion
  - Prostaglandins
- E^1 analogue 400–100 µg PR
- E^2 dinoprostone 20 mg PR q2h (may cause hypotension)
- $F2\alpha$ 0.25 mg IM or IMM q 15 minutes (contraindicated with asthmatics)
  - Methylergonovine 0.2 mg IM q2h (may cause or worsen hypertension)

Genital laceration
- Surgically repaired

Retained products
- Requires D&C (useful to have ultrasound available for guidance)

Uterine inversion
- IMMEDIATE manual replacement (may be aided by halothane for uterine relaxation)

Consider surgical exploration (laparotomy)

For unclear etiology or persistent bleeding from the uterus (suspected uterine rupture or accreta), consider laparotomy.

Intraoperative interventions to stop hemorrhage include ligation of uterine or ovarian arteries, repair of ruptured uterus, or hysterectomy.

Consider selective artery embolization

Performed in angiography suite by interventional radiologist

Works by catheterization of femoral artery followed by identification of bleeding artery (by fluoroscopy) and embolization

GYNECOLOGY CLINIC

WELL-WOMAN EXAM

S **When was the pt's last menstrual period, and what is her recent menstrual history?**

Review menstrual history for complaints that require a workup:
- Abnormal uterine bleeding, oligomenorrhea, and amenorrhea
- Noting day in current cycle will help interpret findings on PE

Review PMH, PSH, medications, allergies, and social history

Notate any possible drug-contraceptive interactions.

Previous gynecologic surgeries should be noted in relation to any current complaints and PE.

Review family history

Special attention should be paid to gynecologic or breast cancers.

O **Perform PE**

Breasts
- The clinical breast examination allows for early detection of breast cancer and other breast diseases (see Breast Mass, p. 300).
- Optimally performed in first half of menstrual cycle.

Pelvis
- Vulva
  - Inspect
  - Palpate
    - Skene glands empty into the urethra at the meatus, which can be found anterior to opening of vagina.
    - Bartholin glands can be palpated just inside vaginal opening on the posterior lateral portion (5 o'clock and 7 o'clock position).

Insert speculum to expose vagina and cervix.

- Vagina
  - Multiple rugae or folds are visible.
  - Check for presence of discharge (see Vulvovaginitis, p. 336).
- Cervix
  - External os (opening to endometrial cavity) is visible on inspection.
  - May visualize ectropion and normal amount of cervical mucus.
  - Small, white "pimples" are nabothian cysts.
  - Nulliparous cervix is smaller, multiparous larger.
  - Inspect for gross lesions or any abnormal discharge.
  - Perform Pap smear.
    - Rotate spatula twice at the external os to sample the transformation zone.
    - Rotate cytobrush once inside the os to sample the endocervix.
  - Offer STD screening.
    - For pts desiring STD screening, *Neisseria gonorrhoeae* and *Chlamydia* cultures may be run by polymerase chain reaction off the Pap sampling.

Remove speculum and perform bimanual examination.

- Uterus
  - Palpated on bimanual examination, check for mobility, size, tenderness, contour, and masses.
  - Nulliparous women have smaller uteri than multiparous women.
- Adnexa
  - Palpated on bimanual examination, check for size, consistency, and presence of any masses.
  - Note cycle day in the presence of ovarian enlargement.
    - Functional cysts can enlarge up to 3.5 cm.

- Rectum
  - Begin digital rectal exam at age 35.
  - Check for uterosacral ligament nodularity, which may indicate endometriosis.

Review past Paps and mammograms

Annual exam provides a good time to pick up any ongoing problems.

A P Well-woman exam

Annual tests

Starting at the age of 21, all women should have a Pap smear every 3 years.

Women >30 y/o should have HPV with Pap smear every 5 years.

Women >40 should have a mammogram every 1–2 years.

Women >50 should have a mammogram every year and a colonoscopy.

Contraceptive counseling

Annual exam provides opportunity to reinforce continued use in current contraception users.

Pts not currently on contraception (or abstinent) should be counseled and offered some form of birth control.

STD counseling

Provide information on protection, partner selection, and sexual practices.

Educate pt about specific diseases, risk factors, and screening tests.

Fertility counseling

Annual examination is a good opportunity to review future childbearing plans.

Fertility declines rapidly at age 35–37, and efforts should be made to promote childbearing accordingly.

Women planning to conceive after age 35 need to be counseled about their increased risk of trisomies.

Dietary counseling

All women of reproduction age should be taking:
- Folate 0.4 mg daily
- Calcium 1,000 mg total intake daily

Gynecologic cancer counseling

Provide information on all gynecologic cancers with emphasis on risk factors and prevention.
- Uterine cancer is the most common type of gynecologic malignancy
  - Risk factors: Hypertension, obesity, estrogen excess
- Cervical cancer
  - Risk factors: Multiple sexual partners, early coitarche, human papilloma virus exposure, low socioeconomic status
- Ovarian cancer
  - Risk factors: Family history, nulliparity, environmental, breast or GI cancers

ABNORMAL UTERINE BLEEDING

S **Obtain a detailed menstrual history**
Normal cycle
  • Length: Normal cycle length is 21–35 days.
  • Menstruation characteristics: Normal menstruation lasts 4–7 days and has an average flow of 30 cc.
Features of complaint
  • Cycle changes, flow changes, intermenstrual bleeding
  • Duration of problem
  • Dysmenorrhea symptoms confirm presence of ovulation

Is the pt currently using any contraception or medicines?
Contraceptive hormones, IUDs, numerous medications, and herbs can cause abnormal uterine bleeding (AUB).

Does the pt smoke?
Smoking can be an independent etiology of AUB.

Does the pt have any risk factors for endometrial cancer?
AUB is the most common presentation of uterine cancer.
The following are risk factors for uterine cancer:

  – Hypertension
  – Nulligravidas
  – Diabetes

  – Obesity
  – Long history of anovulation
  – Tamoxifen use

Does the pt have a history of easy bleeding or bruising?
Consider a coagulopathy as the etiology.

Does the pt have any history that precludes estrogen therapy?
Estrogen therapy plays an important role in the medical treatment of AUB.
Smokers >35 y/o or pts with a history of deep vein thrombosis should not use estrogen therapy.

O **Perform PE**
General: Note obesity (BMI >30).
Neck: Check thyroid for presence of goiter.
Skin: Examine for bruising, hirsutism, or acanthosis nigricans.
Abdomen: Check for hepatosplenomegaly, which can suggest systemic disease as the underlying cause.
Pelvis: Inspect and palpate for evident pathology and possible foreign bodies.

Check labs
  – β-hCG (rule out pregnancy)
  – TSH
  – PT/PTT and Von Willebrand disease (if coagulopathy is suggested)
  – Pap, gonococcus, and *Chlamydia* testing (if not current)

  – CBC (check for anemia)
  – Prolactin

Consider transvaginal U/S
U/S may detect intracavitary lesion such as polyp or fibroid.

Consider endometrial biopsy (EMB)
Rule out cancer with EMB in *any pt >35 y/o* or with risk factors.

A **Abnormal uterine bleeding**
This is the general diagnosis given to these pts while a workup attempts to find a definitive etiology. Possible etiologies include:

PALM-COEIN:

PALM: Structural Causes	**COEIN: Nonstructural Causes**
Polyp	Coagulopathy
Adenomyosis	Ovulatory disorders (PCOS)
Leiomyoma	Endometrial
Malignancy or hyperplasia	Iatrogenic (anticoagulants)
	Not yet classified

Many times, a definite etiology is not found, and a diagnosis of exclusion is made.
- If no apparent etiology can be found and the pt has evidence of ovulation, the diagnosis can further be specified as ovulatory AUB.
- If no apparent etiology can be found and the pt does not have evidence of ovulation, the diagnosis can further be specified as anovulatory AUB-O.

P Identify and treat any underlying (organic) disease

Treat any etiology identified during the above workup.

If no organic etiology can be found, treat according to the diagnosis of exclusion.

Treat ovulatory AUB with hormones, NSAIDs, antifibrinolytic agents, progesterone IUD, or tranexamic acid

Oral contraceptives (numerous formulations available)

NSAIDs (Motrin 400 mg PO tid for first 3–4 days of period)

Antifibrinolytic agents (tranexamic acid 1 g PO qid for 1st 3–4 days of period)

Progesterone (levonorgestrel) IUD

Treat DUB with hormones

Oral contraceptives

Progestins (medroxyprogesterone acetate 10 mg PO for 10 days each month)

Consider surgery

AUB refractory to medical treatment may require surgical therapy.

Options include:
- Hysteroscopy to remove endometrial polyps or myomas
- Hysterectomy
- Ablation: The use of heat or electrical energy to "burn" endometrial lining

BREAST MASS

S **Does the pt feel a lump?**
Pts frequently present with having "felt a lump" on breast self-examination.
Masses appreciated by patient and not clinician still warrant complete workup.

How long has the mass been present?
New masses are more suspicious for malignancy.
Consider fibroadenoma in an established mass. Fibroadenoma is a benign, slow-growing
tumor common in the reproductive years (onset usually before 20 y/o).

Has the mass increased in size?
Any rapidly growing mass should be excised, even if previous biopsy has documented
it as benign.

Does pt have any symptoms associated with her menstrual cycle?
Consider fibrocystic breast disease in pts who complain of multiple, bilateral lumps that
increase in size and become tender or "burn" before menstruation.

Is pt experiencing any breast discharge?
Unilateral bloody or serous nipple discharge may indicate malignancy.

Is pt having screening mammograms?
Mammograms are recommended every 1–2 years (begin screening at age 40 or 10 years
before the pt reaches the age a first-degree relative was diagnosed with cancer).

Does the pt have any risk factors for breast cancer?
Risk factors for breast cancer should be reviewed; however, all palpable masses must be
worked up regardless of risk factors.
- History of breast cancer
- History of ductal carcinoma in situ
- First-degree relatives with breast cancer, family members with brca1 or 2
- History of atypical hyperplasia

O **Perform breast exam**
Best timing is shortly after menstruation (document where pt is in menstrual cycle).
General
- Sitting exam
  - Inspection: Note any area of skin thickening or nipple retraction.
  - Palpation: Assess axillae for lymph node enlargement.
- Supine exam
  - Arms lifted above head.
  - Palpate lightly, medium, and deeply to assess tissue at various depths.
  - Use the pads of three fingers with circular, coin-sized movement.
  - Examine a large area (from the sternum to the midaxillary line and from the clavi-cle to the bra line) in vertical, overlapping rows.
  - Squeeze areola to extract any nipple discharge.
Mass
- Size
- Consistency → Fibroadenomas are rubbery
- Mobility → Fixed masses are suspicious for malignancy
- Contour → Smooth (likely benign) versus irregular (suspicious)
- Skin changes → Peau d'orange (interstitial fibrosis secondary to edema)

A **Palpable breast mass**
Differential diagnosis includes fibroadenoma, simple cyst, fibrocystic changes, benign
lesions with or without atypia, cancer, fat necrosis, and metastasis to breast.

P **Perform fine-needle aspiration (FNA) or ultrasonography**
If mass is readily palpable by clinician, the first step is differentiation between a solid
(potentially malignant) and cystic (probably benign) mass.

Both FNA and U/S help qualify a palpable breast mass as cystic or solid.

- FNA uses a 21- to 24-gauge needle to aspirate tissue or fluid from a palpable mass.
  o If clear or dark fluid returns, the mass is a simple cyst.
  o If tissue or sanguineous fluid (bright blood) is obtained, the specimen is submitted to a pathologist for cytologic examination for malignancy.
  o Lack of any aspirate suggests a solid mass and mandates further workup.
- Ultrasonography directly characterizes size, border, and echogenicity (solid versus cystic) of mass.
- Once detected on U/S, simple cysts may be either followed up routinely or aspirated to alleviate pt symptoms or anxiety.

Consider diagnostic mammogram

If FNA or U/S is inconclusive or *clinician* cannot palpate a mass that is apparent to *patient*, perform a diagnostic mammogram (in women <30 y/o, U/S is preferred over mammography because cysts are expected and radiation is avoided).

A diagnostic mammogram differs from a screening mammogram in that the former requires the presence of a radiologist for immediate review and planning of further workup.

The following classification system is used in reporting mammogram results:

- Bi-Rads 1: no abnormality detected, routine follow-up
- Bi-Rads 2: benign findings, resume screening mammography
- Bi-Rads 3: most likely benign, but follow-up imaging recommended in ≤6 months
- Bi-Rads 4: suspicious appearance, biopsy recommended (see below)
- Bi-Rads 5: almost certainly a malignancy, biopsy/excision required (see below)
- Bi-Rads 0: used by radiologists to define an examination as inconclusive and further studies needed or old films necessary for comparison

Consider core-needle biopsy

Core-needle biopsy is performed under U/S guidance or using a stereotactic device (digital x-ray and computer-aided positioning of a biopsy gun loaded with a 14- to 18-gauge needle).

Consider open biopsy

Used for further workup of positive mammogram findings when core-needle biopsy is not available or when a breast abnormality is thought to exist, but mammogram and U/S do not detect lesion.

- MALIGNANCY IS NOT EXCLUDED with negative imaging studies.
- Up to 15% of mammograms are falsely negative, and open biopsy is needed for tissue diagnosis in the presence of suspected pathology.

CHRONIC PELVIC PAIN

S **Obtain a detailed chronologic history of the pain**
- Where exactly is the pain?
- What is the timing of the pain?
- Associated life events?
- Are there any other sites of pain, such as the back or H/A?
- Any previous medical evaluations?
- Any interventions?
- Any GI or GU complaints?

Obtain a detailed menstrual history
What is the cycle length and regularity? Any cyclic pain?
- Pain during menses suggests endometriosis.
- Pain midcycle suggests ovulatory pain. Is there any abnormal uterine bleeding?

Does the pt have a history of pelvic or abdominal infections or procedures?
Pelvic adhesions could be a possible etiology.

Is the pt currently suffering from any emotional or psychological distress?
Educating pts on psychological contributions to pain makes them more willing to discuss this issue.

What is the pt's social history?
- What are the pt's work and leisure habits like?
- Any major stresses as child, teenager, or adult?
- Is there current family support?
- Is the pt married? With children?
- How is the family functioning?
- Any history of sexual abuse?

Obtain a sexual history
Does the patient have a history of dyspareunia? At what age did the patient become sexually active? Has she ever been sexually abused?

O **Perform generalized PE**
Assess HEENT for any neurologic source of pain.
Assess thyroid for contributory lethargy or anxiety.
Assess CVAT to rule out pyelonephritis.

Have the pt identify source of pain
Have the pt point to spot with one finger.
- Tender spots outside of the pelvis need to be evaluated.
  ○ Multiple focal tender points on trunk and extremities can suggest fibromyalgia.

Perform abdominal exam
Start with palpation of upper quadrants, looking for any hepatosplenomegaly.
Tenderness elicited from the abdominal wall can be differentiated from visceral pain by asking the pt to contract abdominal wall muscles. This will increase pain originating from the abdominal wall.
Examine any previous surgical scars for possible nerve entrapment.

Perform pelvic examination
Begin with external genitalia, inspecting vulva, labia, clitoral and perianal areas. A cotton-tipped applicator can be useful in testing focal points of tenderness.
Pts experiencing vaginismus during speculum may be relieved after contracting and relaxing perineal muscles.
Rectal exam may suggest proctitis, colitis, or endometriosis.

Obtain appropriate lab studies
WBC should be checked for possibility of infection, especially if pain has been worsening recently.
N. gonorrhoeae and *Chlamydia* cultures should be obtained to rule out pelvic inflammatory disease.

U/A can rule out GU involvement.

Consider erythrocyte sedimentation rate as a marker when following pts over a period of time.

Consider using standardized psychological testing

Minnesota Multiphasic Personality Inventory

Beck Depression Inventory

A   Chronic pelvic pain

Chronic pelvic pain (CPP) is defined as pain causing a functional disability and

- \>3 months in duration and unrelated to menses **or**
- \>6 months in duration and related to menses

Remember, this is a symptom, not a disease. Endometriosis is the leading gynecologic diagnosis.

- Other etiologies include:
  - Severe dysmenorrhea
  - Fibromyalgia
  - Hernia
  - Urethral syndrome
  - Irritable bowel syndrome
  - Interstitial cystitis
  - Arthritis
  - Depression/somatization

P   Rule out nongynecologic sources of CPP

Efforts are first made to rule out nongynecologic causes of CPP.

Systems: Psychological (anxiety, depression, PTSD, abuse, fibromyalgia)

Musculoskeletal: Spine injuries, muscle spasms, nerve disorders (Sciatic nerve)

GI: IBS, Crohn disease, ulcerative colitis, celiac

GU: Interstitial cystitis, chronic UTIs

If no nongynecologic source is found, treatment is usually begun empirically for endometriosis.

Begin empiric treatment for endometriosis

Suspected endometriosis is initially managed with empiric medical treatment.

- Oral contraceptives
  - 3-month trial (response to them is usually mediocre)
- NSAIDs—it is recommended to start OCPs and NSAIDs simultaneously
  - Ibuprofen up to 800 mg PO q6h
- Gonadotropin-releasing hormone agonist
  - Depot leuprolide acetate 3.75 mg IM q month up to 6 months
    - This medication works by shutting down the hypothalamic-pituitary-ovarian axis in order to decrease serum estrogen, the source of endometrial implant stimulation.
    - Sometimes given with low-dose estrogen replacement to counter the hypoestrogenic side effects of vasomotor symptoms and bone loss.

Consider surgical intervention

Consider surgery to aid in the diagnosis of CPP.

Surgery can also be used to treat documented endometriosis (usually resection of implants).

Consider a multidisciplinary team approach for optimal outcome

Team might include psychological and nutritional experts.

DYSMENORRHEA

S **What is the pt's menstrual history?**

Degree of dysmenorrhea is correlated to amount of flow, duration of flow, and time of menarche.

- Scant flow with symptoms throughout period is consistent with cervical stenosis.
- Primary dysmenorrhea usually starts a few months after menarche when the pt becomes ovulatory.

Does the pt have any accompanying symptoms?

Nausea, vomiting, diarrhea, headache, and dizziness can all accompany dysmenorrhea.

Symptoms should be recorded and tracked during management. Dyspareunia and a history of infertility suggest endometriosis.

Does the pt have a history of pelvic surgery or pelvic infections?

Adhesions and healed areas of inflammation can cause pain during menstruation.

Does the patient have a family history of dysmenorrhea?

Strong family histories can condition an individual's pain response.

What is the pt's current and past social history?

Stress and tension can play a large part in the etiology of dysmenorrhea.

Pain is usually gradual in onset and generally worse at specific times of stress. Lack of sleep and caffeine consumption can intensify symptoms.

Is the pt currently using an intrauterine device (IUD)?

The IUD is a potential cause of dysmenorrhea.

Does the pt have any medical conditions contraindicating NSAIDs?

NSAIDs play a major role in the management of dysmenorrhea.

Medical conditions contraindicating their use include:

- Ulcers or inflammation of the GI tract
- Chronic renal disease
- Aspirin allergy (nasal polyps, angioedema, and bronchospasm)

O **Perform pelvic exam**

A scarred or disfigured cervix should be probed to make sure os is patent.

Uterosacral ligament nodularity should raise suspicion for endometriosis.

Uterus may contain fibroids.

Adnexal exam may reveal masses.

Does the pt have up-to-date *Chlamydia* and gonococcus cultures?

Pelvic infection can lead to dysmenorrhea symptoms.

Pts should have cultures obtained if no recent results are available or if history discloses possible exposure.

Consider complementary imaging studies

The following studies may help elicit causes of secondary dysmenorrhea:

- Pelvic ultrasound
  - Hydrosonography
- Hysterosalpingography
- Hysteroscopy
- Laparoscopy

A **Dysmenorrhea**

Primary dysmenorrhea is pain without organic disease.

- Typically found in adolescents with onset shortly after menarche.

Secondary dysmenorrhea is pain as a result of organic disease.

- Typical onset is after age 20 and is associated with some identifiable organic disease.

- The following are causes:
  - Cervical stenosis or Mullerian malformations
  - Intrauterine adhesions
  - Adenomyosis/endometriosis
  - Small ovarian cysts
  - Pelvic congestion
  - Uterine retroversion
  - IUD
  - Fibroids
  - Polyps

P Primary dysmenorrhea

Treatment is selected depending on the pt's current sexual activity status.

- Sexually active: There are two first-line agents
  - Oral contraceptives provide contraception and are effective in 90% of patients suffering from dysmenorrhea.
  - The progesterone-containing IUDs are also effective in treating symptoms.
- Currently abstinent
  - NSAIDs
    - Ibuprofen 600 mg PO q6h PRN
    - Naproxen 250 PO q6h PRN
  - COX-2 specific inhibitors
    - Valdecoxib 20 mg PO q12h PRN
- Oral contraceptives or NSAIDs can be added to the primary treatment as needed for nonresponders

Secondary dysmenorrhea

Treatment is focused on underlying etiology.

- Cervical stenosis
  - Dilation of the cervical os
    - Dilation and curettage
    - Laminaria or Cytotec
- Endometriosis
  - Medical and surgical managements (see Chronic Pelvic Pain, p. 302)
- Intrauterine adhesions, fibroids, and polyps
  - Hysteroscopic resection

Consider alternative treatments

Stress reduction, behavioral modification, bio-feedback, pelvic floor physical therapy techniques might be useful.

FAMILY PLANNING—BARRIER METHOD

S ### What are pt's future childbearing plans?
Pts who are interested in long-term contraception should consider hormone contraception because barrier methods are difficult to use consistently for long periods.
If the pt has an absolute contraindication to pregnancy (coexisting medical condition), a barrier method should be used in addition to a primary method of contraception.

Is the pt in a new or nonmonogamous relationship at present?
Barrier methods are the preferred contraceptive method for new or nonmonogamous relationships.

Does the pt have a history of STDs or pelvic inflammatory disease (PID)?
Pts with a history of infection with gonococcus, *Chlamydia*, or PID should use condoms to prevent recurrence.
Transmission of viral STDs, such as HIV, HPV, and HSV, is decreased with condoms.

Does the pt have a history of toxic shock syndrome (TSS)?
Pts with a history of TSS should avoid barrier methods other than condoms.

Does the pt have an allergy to latex?
Latex allergy may be life-threatening.
Alternative materials such as polyurethane should be used.

Is the pt comfortable with inserting and removing a barrier device?
This is prerequisite to their use.

O ### Physical exam
An annual well-woman exam should be encouraged and updated when prescribing contraceptive counseling but is not necessarily a prerequisite to using barrier methods.

A ### Contraceptive counseling, desires barrier method
P ### Prescribe method
Cervical cap
 • Requires fitting and spermicide co-use.
 • Place <6 hours before use.
 • Can be used for up to 48 hours.
 • Typical failure rates is 20%–40%.
Diaphragm
 • Requires fitting and spermicide co-use.
 • Place <6 hours before use.
 • Can be used for up to 24 hours.
 • Typical failure rate is 12%.
Condoms
 • Types include male condom and female condom.
 • Materials include latex, polyurethane, silicone rubber, and lamb skin.
  o Lamb skin condoms do not protect against STDs.
 • Need to apply before genital contact and remove before loss of erection.
 • Usually use with spermicide.
  o Use water-based lubricants (oil-based lubricants can cause condom breakage).
 • Typical failure rate is 14%–20%.

Prescribe emergency contraception
Every pt on a barrier method should be prescribed emergency contraception for use as a backup in case of slippage, breakage, or retention in vagina (see Emergency Contraception, p. 310).

FAMILY PLANNING—DEPOT MPA

S **Has the pt ever used injectable contraception before?**
Pts who have had a good experience previously should do well.
Pts with previous complaints should consider an alternative.

What is the pt's recent menstrual and intercourse history?
If there is a possibility the pt could be pregnant, she will have to wait until this can be ruled out before starting injectable contraception.

Does pt have a history of irregular periods?
Irregular menses needs a workup before starting injectable contraception.

Does the pt have any of the following that might contraindicate using depot medroxyprogesterone acetate (MPA) injectable?
History of depression or other mood disorder. Depot MPA may exacerbate depression, anxiety, or PMS symptoms.
Obesity or concern about weight gain. May worsen with depot MPA use.
Liver disease
Breast cancer
Aminoglutethimide use. Reduces depot MPA efficacy.
Chest pain, cardiovascular disease, myocardial infarction, stroke

Does the pt have a history of gestational diabetes?
Such pts are at increased risk for diabetes if using depot MPA and should select alternative contraception.

What are the pt's future childbearing plans?
Depot MPA use can delay a return to fertility for an average of 10 months after cessation. Should be avoided in pts desiring immediate fertility upon cessation.

Is the pt aware of the noncontraceptive benefits of depot MPA?
Knowledge of the following noncontraceptive benefits increase pt compliance:
• Decreases menstrual blood loss (reduces risk of anemia)
• Diminishes dysmenorrhea symptoms (cramps and pain)
• May improve endometriosis symptoms
• Reduces risk of PID and ectopic pregnancy
• Reduces risk of endometrial (and possibly ovarian) cancer

O **Perform pregnancy test depending on recent menstrual and intercourse history**
Pts exempt from pregnancy test include those:
• Currently on a regular menses
• Currently using an alternative and reliable method of contraception
• Practicing abstinence since last period

A **Contraceptive counseling, desires depot MPA**
Depot MPA consists of a depot of 150 mg of medroxyprogesterone acetate and provides 13 weeks of protection
Mechanisms of action:
• Thickens cervical mucus (blocks sperm passage)
• Inhibits LH surge (prevents ovulation)
• Alters tubal motility
• May alter endometrium

P **Start injectable contraception**
If none of the above contraindications are present, start the pt on depot MPA.
• Pts can start any time during first 5 days of menses.
• If there is any possibility of current pregnancy, the pt has two choices:
  o Wait until next menses to start.

  o Use a barrier method for 2 weeks, establish a negative pregnancy test, and then start.
- First-time users should be monitored for 15 minutes for allergic or vasovagal reaction.

Counsel pt on side effects

Depot MPA can cause weight gain.

Depot MPA can cause mood changes:

- Depression
- Anxiety
- Fatigue
- PMS

Depot MPA may cause a hypoestrogenic state, which can lead to:

- Bone loss
  o Encourage pt to take supplemental calcium and vitamin D.
  o Teens should take 1,300 mg and adults 1,000 mg supplemental calcium daily.
- Hot flashes
- Decreased libido
- Vaginal dryness, dyspareunia

Counsel pt on possible menstrual changes

Users of depot MPA will encounter irregular bleeding that usually decreases over time. 50% of women achieve amenorrhea by 1 year.

Schedule next shot

Follow-up depot MPA in 11–13 weeks

FAMILY PLANNING—EMERGENCY CONTRACEPTION

S ### What is the pt's recent menstrual and intercourse history?
Last menstrual period
Previous period
Any prior unprotected intercourse in current cycle?

When was the last act of unprotected intercourse?
Date and time of last unprotected intercourse should be reviewed.
  • General rule is to initiate emergency contraception (EC) within 72 hours.
  • Can be started after 72 hours up to 5 days after unprotected intercourse; however, works better closer to the time of intercourse.

Has the pt used EC or oral contraceptives before?
Review with pt use and tolerance of any previous EC or oral contraceptives.
Pt may have a preference for a particular regimen if it was used before and tolerated well.

Does pt have any contraindications to using EC?
History of any of the following contraindicates EC use:
  • Undiagnosed abnormal uterine bleeding
  • Hypersensitivity to estrogen or progesterone
The following contraindicate estrogen-containing EC:
  • Current migraine headache
  • History of deep vein thrombosis or pulmonary embolus
  • Smoker over the age of 35

Is the pt currently breastfeeding?
Pts who are breastfeeding should use progesterone-only pills.

Will the pt be driving or operating machinery while using the EC?
Antiemetics, traditionally prescribed with EC to minimize the side effect of nausea and vomiting, can cause drowsiness.

O ### Consider pregnancy test
If intercourse history raises suspicion for conception before last intercourse, perform pregnancy test.
EC will not work as an abortifacient in pts who are already pregnant.

Physical exam

BP and PE is not necessary before prescribing EC.

A
P ### Unprotected intercourse, desires emergency contraception
Educate pt about possible side effects
Nausea/vomiting
Breast tenderness
Mood changes
Change in timing of next menses
  • Early menses if EC taken in the first half of cycle
  • Delayed menses if EC taken in the second half of cycle

Prescribe emergency contraception
EC is available in one of two forms:
  • Combined (estrogen and progesterone) pills
  • Progesterone-only pills
Multiple formulations can be used.
  • Selection of regimen is based upon:
    ○ Practitioner preference/experience
    ○ Cost

       o Pt preference
       o Availability
         • Not all prepackaged kits are available (see below).
- EC using *combined pills* is available in prepackaged kit, which contains 4 pills.
  o Each pill contains ethinyl estradiol 50 µg and levonorgestrel 0.25 mg.
  o Take 2 pills immediately and 2 pills 12 hours later.
  o If prepackaged kit is not available, *almost ANY oral contraceptives can be used.*
     • Use multiple pills so that each dose contains at least 100 µg ethinyl estradiol and either 1 mg of norgestrel or 0.50 mg of levonorgestrel.
     • Take one dose immediately and one dose 12 hours later.
- EC using the *progesterone-only pill* is available in a prepackaged kit, which contains two 0.75 mg tabs or one 1.5 mg tab levonorgestrel. This is over the counter, no ID necessary to purchase.
  o Take 1 pill immediately and 1 pill 12 hours later for the two tabs.

If not using prepackaged kit, show pt *in detail* how to use oral contraceptives.

- The copper IUD is the most effective method of emergency contraception. Place within 5–10 days after unprotected intercourse.

Plan regular contraceptive use (see individual Family Planning sections, pp. 306–317)

Pills can be resumed immediately after EC use. Use 7-day backup (condoms) if new start.

Depot medroxyprogesterone acetate can be given immediately.

Follow-up instructions

Pregnancy test is necessary if menses has not occurred by 3 weeks.

FAMILY PLANNING—INTRAUTERINE DEVICE

S **What is the pt's recent menstrual and intercourse history?**

If there is a possibility the pt is currently pregnant, contraception needs to be withheld until nonpregnant state can be confirmed.

Insertion of intrauterine device (IUD) while on menses is associated with a higher risk of expulsion.

Does the pt have a history of irregular periods?

Abnormal uterine bleeding (AUB) needs a workup before starting intrauterine contraception (see Abnormal Uterine Bleeding, p. 298).

Does the pt have heavy or crampy periods?

The levonorgestrel IUD improves dysmenorrhea and menorrhagia.

The copper IUD may *increase* dysmenorrhea and menorrhagia.

What are the pt's future childbearing plans?

Because of the cost, IUDs are generally used for pts who would like a prolonged (>2 years) period of contraception.
- Pts wanting to conceive sooner should use an alternative contraceptive method.
- The copper IUD is effective for 10 years.
- The levonorgestrel IUD is effective for 5 years.

Does the pt have multiple partners or a history of pelvic inflammatory disease (PID)?

These pts are generally not considered candidates for IUD use.

PID during IUD use can lead to a higher chance of infertility.

Does the pt have any complaints of vaginal discharge?

Pts infected with bacterial vaginosis are at increased risk for PID with IUD use.

Are the pt's Pap smear and STD tests up-to-date?

All tests should be confirmed to be normal and up-to-date before IUD use.

Does the pt have any general questions about IUD use?

Several misperceptions exist about IUD use (e.g., mode of action, etc.).

Does the pt have any contraindications to copper usage?

Wilson disease or allergy to copper contraindicates the copper IUD.

O **Perform "wet mount" for any undiagnosed vaginal discharge**

See Vaginitis, p. 336

Perform pregnancy test depending on recent menstrual and intercourse history

Pts exempt from a pregnancy test include those:
- Currently on a regular menses
- Currently using an alternative and reliable method of contraception
- Practicing abstinence since last period

Perform pelvic exam

Cervix
- Inspect for any discharge that might indicate cervicitis.

Uterus
- Verify uterine position.
  - Anterior/mid/posterior.
- Assess for any abnormal contour.
  - Fibroids can distort the uterine cavity and increase the rate of expulsion.

A **Contraceptive counseling, desires copper IUD**

The copper IUD is a T-shaped polyethylene device with two flexible arms for insertion.
- Each arm is wrapped with sleeves of copper.
- Effects contraception by working as a functional spermicide.
- Effective for 10 years.

Contraceptive counseling, desires levonorgestrel IUD

The levonorgestrel IUD is a T-shaped device that releases 20 µg of levonorgestrel per day.
- Effect on contraception is by thickening cervical mucus, altering uterotubal fluid and sperm migration.
- May prevent implantation and ovulation.
- Effective for 5 years.

P

Counsel pt on risks of insertion

Uterine perforation
- Increased risk when uterine position is not established before insertion

Infection
- Usually occurs within first 3 weeks after insertion
- Increased risk with current bacterial vaginosis or active cervical infection

Vasovagal reaction
- Increased risk with low pain threshold or stenotic os

Counsel the pt on risks of use

Possible failure: Increased ectopic rate if failure occurs.
Possible tubal damage/infertility: PID during IUD use increases the risk of tube scarring and secondary infertility.

Counsel the pt on possible menstrual changes

Users of the copper IUD will encounter irregular bleeding that usually decreases over first weeks. 50% of women achieve amenorrhea by 1 year.
Users of the levonorgestrel IUD may have spotting for up to 6 months. 20% of women have amenorrhea at 1 year.

Insert the copper IUD or levonorgestrel IUD. Schedule follow-up

Customary follow-up is made in *1 month* to verify IUD remains in place.

Counsel the pt on "warning" signs

Pts with any of the following should return to the clinic immediately:
- Pain, vaginal bleeding: May signal perforation.
- Missed period: May signal pregnancy (failed contraception).
- Fever, chills: May signal infection.
- Missing strings: May signal expulsion or migrating IUD.

FAMILY PLANNING—ORAL CONTRACEPTIVES

S **Has the pt ever used the pill before?**

Some pts have a specific brand in mind that works well for them.

How did the pill work for the pt in past?

What is the pt's last menstrual period and intercourse history?

If there is a possibility the pt could be pregnant, she will have to wait until this can be ruled out before starting oral contraceptives.

Does the pt have a history of irregular periods?

Irregular menses needs a workup before starting the pill.

Does the pt smoke?

Smokers over 35 y/o should not use the pill.

Does the pt have any medical problems that might contraindicate using a pill that contains estrogen?

- Uncontrolled hypertension
- Biliary disease
- Uncontrolled diabetes
- Breast cancer
- Liver disease
- Seizures, migraine headaches, blurry vision
- Blood clots
- Chest pain, cardiovascular disease

Is the pt currently taking any medications?

Many anticonvulsants and some antibiotics decrease steroid levels in women taking oral contraceptives, rendering them subtherapeutic. Strongly consider IUDs.

Exercise caution with concurrent use of the following:

- Barbiturates
- Carbamazepine
- Topiramate
- Rifampin
- Phenytoin
- Felbamate
- Vigabatrin
- Griseofulvin

Is the pt currently breastfeeding? If so, for how much longer?

Combined oral contraceptives lower breast milk volume.

These pts are candidates for the progestin-only pill until they complete breastfeeding.

O **Measure blood pressure**

Estrogen can exacerbate hypertension.

Perform pregnancy test depending on recent menstrual and intercourse history

Pts exempt from pregnancy test include those:

- Currently on a regular menses
- Currently using an alternative and reliable method of contraception
- Practicing abstinence since their last period

A **Contraceptive counseling, desires oral contraceptives**

P **Rule out pregnancy**

If there is any possibility of current pregnancy, the pt has two choices:

- Wait until next menses to start pill.
- Use a barrier method for 2 weeks and then establish a negative pregnancy test.

Start pt on an oral contraceptive

If none of the above contraindications are present, start the pt on an oral contraceptive. Start date will be based primarily on current day of menstrual cycle and recent intercourse history and secondarily on pt preference. Pelvic exams/physical exams and Pap smears are not required before initiating hormonal contraception.

- Pts currently on menses can start on any day of the first week of cycle (customarily Sunday). Barrier protection should be used for 1 week.
- Pts who are not currently on menses and not using an alternate method of contraception need to rule out pregnancy first (see above).

Become familiar with a few formulations of varying strengths and choose from these

The following are examples of oral contraceptive formulations:
- Monophasic (the progesterone dose always stays the same)
  - 20 μg ethinyl estradiol/0.1 mg levonorgestrel
  - 30 μg ethinyl estradiol/1.5 mg norethindrone acetate
  - 30 μg ethinyl estradiol/0.15 mg desogestrel
  - 35 μg ethinyl estradiol/0.4 mg norethindrone
- Triphasic (the progesterone dose changes during the cycle)
  - 35 μg ethinyl estradiol/0.18- 0.215- 0.25 mg norgestimate
- Progestin-only
  - 0.35 mg norethindrone

If a pt has had a good experience previously with a particular formulation, try the same formulation again.

Breastfeeding women and those with contraindications to estrogen should use the progestin-only pill.

Become familiar with common problems regarding missing pills

If pt misses 1 pill:
- Take missed pill immediately and the following pill as scheduled.

If pt misses 2 pills:
- During first half of cycle: Take 2 pills/d for next 2 days and use barrier method until menses.
- During third week of cycle (or 3 pills at anytime): Start new cycle and use barrier protection for 1 week.

Consider emergency contraception (EC)
- An alternative to "making up" for missed pills is to take EC.
- Especially useful if intercourse has occurred in last 3–5 days.
- If pt uses EC, *skip any missed pills* and resume taking the remaining pills the day after completing EC (see Emergency Contraception, p. 310).

FAMILY PLANNING—STERILIZATION

S **What are the pt's future childbearing plans?**

Only pts who are certain they have completed childbearing are candidates for sterilization. Patients younger than 30 years have a high risk of regret and should be given counseling on LARC options.

Does the pt know that there are alternatives to sterilization?

Explanation of long-term alternatives and their typical failure rates as compared to sterilization should be explained to the pt.
- IUD
  o Efficacy up to 10 years
  o Failure rate comparable to tubal sterilization
- Vasectomy
  o Efficacy and failure rate similar to tubal sterilization
  o Lower morbidity and mortality compared with tubal sterilization

Does the pt understand that sterilization is permanent?

Tubal reanastomosis is the surgical repair of fallopian tubes to make them functional again.
- Although this procedure is available, its *success is highly variable*, and it should not be relied on as a way for pts to regain their fertility if they later "change their mind." Sterilization should be considered as permanent.

Does the pt understand the risks of this procedure?

Provide counseling regarding general risks of having a surgery:
- Bleeding
- Infection
- Surgical damage to organs adjacent to fallopian tubes
- Anesthesia risks

Does the pt understand the possibility of failure?

Every sterilization procedure carries a risk of failure (see below).
- The younger the pt is at time of sterilization, the higher the failure rate.
- Tubal sterilization failures have an increased risk of ectopic pregnancy.

- One-third of failures are associated with ectopic pregnancy.

Does the pt understand that sterilization does not protect against STDs?

Pts should be counseled that sterilization does not protect against STDs and that a barrier method is required for such protection.

Is the pt's partner in agreement with this method?

Inquiry should be made into partner's views on the procedure.
- Opposition from partner, or conversely, pressure from partner is not uncommon.
- Discordance between partners may affect the relationship after sterilization and be a source of pt regret.

How is the pt's relationship in general?

Pts who are likely to regret sterilization have unstable relationships.

O **How old is the pt?**

Sterilization should be avoided in young pts because they tend to have more time in their reproductive lives to change their minds.

What is the pt's weight?

Obese pts are poor surgical candidates because of technical difficulties associated with their habitus.

A Desires permanent sterilization

P Plan timing of procedure

Pregnancy must be ruled out before procedure.

A negative pregnancy test is reliable if pt reports a history of abstinence or consistent use of contraception for the preceding 2 weeks.

Choose procedure

Sterilization can be performed by three different methods:

- Ligation
  - Usually performed for postpartum pts.
  - Involves occlusion of the tubes with suture followed by transection.
  - A piece of each tube is removed and sent to pathology for identification.
    - Because of removal and identification of a segment of tube, this procedure has lower failure rates than electrocautery or mechanical procedures.
  - Failure rate = 0.7%.
- Pomeroy technique
  - Traction on tube upward to form loop, ligation at base and transection
- The Irving
  - Segmental resection, proximal end buried in the uterus, distal in mesosalpinx
- The Uchida
  - Dissection of tube from serosal covering and burying proximal end in mesosalpinx
- Electrocoagulation procedures
  - Performed for interval procedures (pt not postpartum)
  - Done through laparoscopy
  - Failure rate = 1%–2%
    - Unipolar coagulation
    - Bipolar coagulation
- Mechanical occlusion
  - Performed for interval procedures (pt not postpartum)
  - Uses rings and clips to occlude tube
  - Greater success rates of tubal reanastomosis (if the pt regrets sterilization in future)
  - Failure rate = 1%–3.5%
    - Silastic ring
    - Spring clip

Counsel the pt on long-term follow-up

Sterilization becomes effective immediately.

Because of increased risk of ectopic pregnancy associated with sterilization failures, the pt needs to have pregnancy test performed if menses is ever missed.

If pregnancy test is positive, ectopic must be ruled out.

GALACTORRHEA

 What color is the discharge?

Lactation is usually clear or white.

Yellow or green discharge should raise suspicion for local breast disease.

Does the pt have any bloody discharge?

This is more suspicious for cancer.

Does the pt have abnormal periods?

Abnormal periods or amenorrhea may represent a hypoestrogenic state that will need to be addressed in management plans.

One-third of pts with galactorrhea will have normal menses.

Did the pt recently deliver?

In the absence of breastfeeding, galactorrhea beyond 12 months postpartum deserves workup.

Does the pt use any medications or street drugs?

Several phenothiazine-like compounds, antidepressants, antihypertensives, opioids, and amphetamines can induce galactorrhea.

Has the pt had any recent trauma, surgical procedures, or anesthesia?

All of these can lead to increased prolactin secretion.

Does the pt have excessive stress or a history of prolonged suckling?

Both can be the cause of elevated prolactin.

 Perform a detailed breast exam

Examine all quadrants of the breast, starting at the base and moving toward the nipple.

- Secretions should be discharged from multiple ducts when a hormone imbalance is the etiology.
- Single-duct discharge is more suspicious for serious pathology.

Does the pt have hirsutism?

Anovulation secondary to hyperprolactinemia can cause hirsutism.

What is the result of the prolactin test?

Blood should be drawn in the morning.

Normal prolactin levels are 1–20 ng/mL. Prolactin levels <50 ng/mL are usually physiologic.

Prolactin levels >100 ng/mL require special attention (see radiologic workup).

What is the result of the thyroid-stimulating hormone (TSH) test?

All pts with galactorrhea should have a TSH level checked.

Hypothyroidism (diagnosed by an elevated TSH) results in increases in thyroid-releasing hormone, which directly stimulates prolactin release from the pituitary.

What are the results of the radiologic workup?

All pts with galactorrhea should have a MRI coned-down view of the sella turcica. The primary purpose of this procedure is to rule out a prolactinoma that is large enough to cause anatomic distortion in the cranium.

All pts with an abnormal sella turcica or prolactin >100 ng/mL should have an MRI evaluation.

The cutoff value of 100 ng/mL is empiric based on the fact that most large tumors will have values above this level. However, if a repeat level remains elevated, even if below 100 ng/mL, then an MRI should be performed. When repeating a prolactin level, make sure she is fasting, in her follicular phase, avoiding exercise, nipple stimulation, and intercourse.

Rule out systemic disease with the following

CBC

Serum chemistries

U/A (liver and renal disease can cause elevated prolactin)

Galactorrhea

> All hormonal etiologies of galactorrhea lead back to the final common pathway of *elevated prolactin levels.*

- Most cases of nonphysiologic hyperprolactinemia can be attributed to prolactin-secreting adenomas of the anterior pituitary.
  - These tumors are classified into one of two groups based on size:
    - Microadenomas <10 mm in size
    - Macroadenomas ≥10 mm in size
- The differential diagnosis of hyperprolactinemia includes:
  - Medications: Anticonvulsants, antidepressants, neuroleptics, antihistamines, antihypertensives
  - Physiologic: Stress, exercise, sleep, sex, pregnancy, breast feeding
  - Systemic: chest wall injury—herpes zoster, seizures, renal failure, cirrhosis
  - Pituitary: Prolactinoma, acromegaly, parasellar mass, idiopathic
  - Pathological: Hypothalamic stalk damage, granulomas, infiltration, metastasis, Rathke cyst

P   **Consider treatment for microadenomas**

Treament for a prolactin-secreting microadenoma is not always necessary and is based on:
- Pt's desire for fertility
- Degree of breast discomfort from lactation
- Presence of amenorrhea (hypoestrogenic state)

Start bromocriptine or cabergoline for pts who desire to get pregnant or have a significant breast discomfort from galactorrhea.
- Bromocriptine is a dopamine agonist that binds to the dopamine receptor in the pituitary and blocks the release of prolactin.
  - Starting dose is bromocriptine 2.5 mg PO qd.
  - Increase to 2.5 mg bid as needed.
- Has significant nausea side effects compared with cabergoline. Rare risk of valvular cardiac disease for cabergoline.

If the pt has amenorrhea (and fertility is not desired and lactation is not a major problem), estrogen replacement in the form of birth control pills can be the sole treatment.

Microadenomas should undergo radiologic surveillance and prolactin levels annually for 2 years.

If stable, pt can be followed subsequently with annual prolactin levels.

Treat all macroadenomas

Treat all macroadenomas for shrinkage of tumor and maintenance.

A prolactin level >500 µg/L is diagnostic of macroprolactinoma.
- Start with medication.
  - Macroadenomas might require bromocriptine up to 10 mg/d. Monitor prolactin levels for response every 3 months and repeat MRI after 1 year.
  - Surgery for medical nonresponders (tumor extension), very large tumors, persistent visual symptoms, or bromocriptine side effects. Transsphenoidal neurosurgery.

HIRSUTISM

S **How long has the pt noticed the hirsutism?**

A rapid onset of symptoms is suspicious for an androgen-secreting tumor. Polycystic ovary syndrome (PCOS) usually has a gradual onset of hirsutism beginning in the late teens or early 20s. Hirsutism is present in 70% of women with PCOS.

Does the pt have abnormal periods?

Anovulation is strongly associated with hirsutism.

Pts who are anovulatory and hirsute should be tested for insulin resistance.

Is the pt taking any medications or over-the-counter supplements?

- Phenytoin-minoxidil   – Cyclosporine   – Diazoxide
- Exogenous androgens (dehydroepiandrosterone sulfate [DHEAS], an androgen, is a popular food supplement)

Does the pt have any signs of hyperandrogenism other than hirsutism?

Other clinical features include acne, increased libido, and virilization.

Family history

Certain ethnic groups and familial patterns are associated with hirsutism (idiopathic hirsutism) and adrenal hyperplasia.

Social history

Review lifestyle for possible drugs or environmental factors associated with hirsutism.

Is the pt pregnant?

Luteomas and theca lutein cysts can arise secondary to human chorionic gonadotropin.

Is the pt peripubertal?

These pts are more likely to suffer from nonclassical adrenal hyperplasia.

O **Perform physical exam**

General
- Moon facies and buffalo hump suggest Cushing syndrome.
- Generalized obesity is associated with PCOS, and truncal obesity suggests Cushing syndrome.

Skin
- Note type of hair growth and distribution.
  - Vellus hair is unpigmented and soft, whereas terminal hair is dark and coarse.
- Acne
  - Acne is a sign of hyperandrogenism.
- Acanthosis nigricans is a sign of insulin resistance
  - Darkened areas of skin around axilla, neck, and groin secondary to hyperinsulinemia.
- Skin signs of Cushing syndrome
  - Purple abdominal striae, thin and bruised skin.

Extremities
- Thin extremities and muscle wasting are associated with Cushing syndrome.

A **Hirsutism**

Hirsutism can be described as a change from vellus to terminal hairs.

Hirsutism represents a hyperandrogenic state from an underlying metabolic abnormality.

There are three "compartments" in which androgens are produced, each with a *specific* androgen:
- The ovaries → Testosterone
- The adrenal glands → DHEAS
- The peripheral tissues → 3α-diol G

The differential diagnosis includes:

- Anovulatory, hyperandrogenic state   – Cushing syndrome
- Idiopathic (familial) hirsutism   – Nonclassical (late-onset) CAH
- Androgen-producing tumor (ovarian or adrenal) adrenal hyperplasia

Rule out ovarian and adrenal tumors

The most important part of the hirsute workup is ruling out ovarian and adrenal tumors.

- Tumors originating from the ovary that cause hyperandrogenism can be expected to produce excess testosterone. A total testosterone level >200 ng/dL raises suspicion for a tumor.
- Androgen-producing tumors originating from the adrenal gland can be expected to have elevated levels of DHEAS. DHEAS >800 µg/dL indicates adrenal pathology.

Rule out nonclassical (late-onset) adrenal hyperplasia
Measuring a 17α-hydroxyprogesterone level tests for nonclassical adrenal hyperplasia
A level <200 ng/dL rules out the disease

Rule out cushing syndrome
Cushing syndrome should be considered in all hirsute pts and screened for when history and PE suggest the diagnosis.
Screening is performed with an overnight dexamethasone suppression test.
- Dexamethasone 1 mg PO is given at 11 PM; plasma cortisol is drawn at 8 AM.
  - Cortisol >10 µg/dL suggests Cushing syndrome.
  - Cortisol <5 µg/dL is normal.

Consider testing for hyperinsulinemia
Pts with PCOS or anovulation and hirsutism should have insulin resistance checked with a 2-hour glucose tolerance test.

Start low-dose oral contraceptives (primary treatment)
Oral contraceptives treat hirsutism by several mechanisms:
- The progesterone component suppresses LH, which lowers testosterone production.
- The estrogen component induces sex hormone–binding globulin, which increases testosterone binding and decreases free testosterone.
Treatment effects will take at least 6 months to notice, because of the lifespan of the hair follicles.
Old hairs will not be affected and need to be removed mechanically.

Consider adding antiandrogen (secondary treatment)
Spironolactone treats hirsutism by several mechanisms:
- Inhibition of androgen production in the adrenals and ovaries
- Competition for the androgen receptor in the hair follicle and inhibition of 5α-reductase
Finasteride inhibits 5α-reductase activity.

INFERTILITY

S **What is the pt's age?**

Age is the single most important factor in assessing fertility.
Fertility drops markedly after age 35.

How long has the pt been trying to get pregnant? Is the couple having regular, unprotected intercourse?

Review intercourse history, such as frequency and technique, presence of dyspareunia, possible use of spermicidal lubricants.

Has the pt been previously pregnant? Has the male partner sired any children (without current partner)?

Previous conception by either partner can help focus workup.

Has the pt had any previous workup?

Note previous tests and treatments.

Does the pt or partner have a history of STDs?

STDs place the pt at risk for reproductive organ scarring, which can cause infertility.

Does the pt have normal (monthly) periods?

Regular, monthly periods is the easiest sign to confirm monthly ovulation.
Mittelschmerz (midpain), premenstrual symptoms, and cervical mucus change also suggest ovulation.

Does the pt have a history of gynecologic problems?

History of pelvic pain, prior gynecologic surgery, and intrauterine device use raises suspicion for anatomic abnormalities.

O **Perform physical exam**

General: Hirsutism? (polycystic ovary syndrome) Acanthosis nigricans? (insulin resistance)
Neck: Thyroid (abnormalities are associated with infertility)
Pelvic: Anatomic abnormalities? Pain?

Is there evidence of ovulation?

Ovulation can be inferred or confirmed by the following:
- History of normal menstrual cycles
- Elevated progesterone in midsecretory phase
- Gross evidence of ovulation on U/S

What is the result of the semen analysis?

Normal semen analysis is:

– Volume	2 mL or more
– Concentration	15 million/mL or more
– Motility	40% or more with forward progression
– Morphology	60% or more normal forms
	4% by Strict Kruger

What is the result of the hysterosalpingogram?

A hysterosalpingogram is a radiographic image of the pelvic anatomy.
- Performed by injecting radio-opaque dye into the uterine cavity and tubes.
- Images are assessed for any structural abnormalities (fibroids, polyps, tubal distortion).
- The "spill" of dye from the fallopian tubes into the peritoneal cavity indicates tubal patency.

Consider U/S

U/S can help survey pelvic organs beyond the PE.

Consider hysterosonogram or hysteroscopy

Hysterosonogram is an U/S survey of the uterus after its cavity has been distended with water (by catheter).

Hysteroscopy involves direct visualization of the uterine cavity and tubal ostia (tube openings to uterus).

 Infertility

Failure to conceive despite regular unprotected intercourse for 1 year if <35 years old, 6 months if 35 and older.

- Primary infertility: no previous pregnancies
- Secondary infertility: at least one previous pregnancy

Etiology

– Anatomic (tubal or pelvic)	35%
– Male factor	35%
– Anovulation	15%
– Unexplained	10%
– Other (including cervical)	5%

 Treat anovulation with ovulatory induction agents

Two main classes of induction agents:

- Clomiphene citrate
  - Works centrally to antagonize estrogen receptors and "trick" body into thinking it is deficient in estrogen.
  - In response, natural gonadotropins are increased in order to stimulate ovaries to produce an egg.
  - Starting dose is 50 mg (max. up to 250 mg) daily on menstrual cycle days 3–7.
- Gonadotropins
  - Injectable medications that directly stimulate ovaries to produce eggs.
  - Examples include FSH only or FSH/LH/hCG preparations.

Treat male factor infertility with intrauterine insemination (IUI) or intracytoplasmic sperm injection (ICSI)

IUI uses a catheter to bypass the cervix and introduce sperm directly into the uterine cavity.

- Indications include oligospermia, antisperm antibodies, and cervical factor. ICSI has revolutionized the treatment of male factor infertility.
- ICSI is performed in laboratory; process of injecting a single sperm into egg.

Treat anatomic problems with surgical correction

Surgically correctable defects include fibroids, polyps, and adhesions.

Surgery is performed with hysteroscopy or laparoscopy.

Treat unexplained infertility with in-vitro fertilization (IVF)

Multistep process whereby gametes are retrieved from both partners, the egg is fertilized in laboratory, and embryo is placed directly into the uterus.

Eggs are surgically retrieved from the female after stimulation of ovaries with gonadotropins.

MENOPAUSE

S **When was the pt's last menstrual period?**
This information provides the practitioner with an idea of how long the pt has been in menopause and guides treatments.

Is the pt currently experiencing any symptoms?
Hot flashes, day sweats, night sweats; insomnia (secondary to night symptoms)
Decreased libido
Genital dryness (secondary dyspareunia)
Urinary incontinence

Does the pt smoke?
Smoking exacerbates the symptoms of menopause and adds to osteoporosis risk.

Does the pt have any risk factors for depression?
Menopause does not cause depression, but women with a history of depression (including postpartum depression and PMS) are susceptible to recurrence during this time of physical and emotional stress.

Does the pt have any risk factors for osteoporosis?
Osteoporosis is a leading cause of morbidity for postmenopausal women.
Risk factors include:

- Smoking
- Low body weight
- Menopause without estrogen replacement
- Sedentary lifestyle

O **Perform physical exam**
Weight and blood pressure
Breasts
Pelvic
- External genitalia: Atrophy, signs of inflammation
- Speculum: Perform PAP smear
- Bimanual: Abnormalities in uterus, pelvic masses

Consider follicle-stimulating hormone (FSH)
Menopause can be confirmed with FSH >30–40 IU/L

Review results of the most recent mammogram
The annual postmenopausal exam provides a good time to review previous mammogram; results encourage continued surveillance.

A **Menopause**
12 months of amenorrhea after age 40
Average age is 51 years

P **Provide symptom relief**
Most symptoms of menopause can be relieved with hormone (estrogen) replacement. In women with an intact uterus, a progesterone must also be given to protect the endometrium from unopposed estrogen. Use the lowest dose for the shortest amount of time.
- Examples of combination hormone replacement therapy (HRT):
  - 0.625 mg conjugated equine estrogens/2.5 mg medroxyprogesterone acetate
  - 1 mg estradiol/0.5 mg norethindrone acetate
  - 5 µg ethinyl estradiol/1 mg norethindrone acetate
  - Alternatives—nonhormonal therapy: SERMs, Wellbutrin, Gabapentin

Provide counseling on short- and long-term use of HRT:
- Much debate in the literature is currently surrounding the use of HRT.
- Appropriate counseling in terms of interpreting the current literature and relative risks should be provided to all HRT new-starts.

Other treatments
- Hot flushes: Remove triggers, dress in layers
- Vaginal dryness: Lubricants, moisturizers
- Depression: SSRIs

Provide osteoporosis-preventive counseling

Osteoporosis/fractures
- Nonpharmacologic therapy
  - Weight-bearing exercise   – Fall-prevention counseling
  - Alcohol limits   – Smoking cessation
- Pharmacologic treatments for the prevention of osteoporosis and fractures
  - Bisphosphonates: Alendronate 5–10 mg PO qd or 35–70 mg PO weekly
  - SERMs: Raloxifene 60 mg PO qd
  - Calcitonin: Calcitonin-salmon 1 spray (200 units) in alternating nostrils daily
  - Calcium/vitamin D
    - Total daily intake of calcium (diet and supplement) should be at least 1,500 mg without HRT and 1,000 mg with HRT.
    - Consider vitamin D supplementation for pts at risk for low levels.
- Consider dual-energy x-ray absorptiometry (DEXA) scan. Use the FRAX calculator to identify risk of osteoporosis.
  - The DEXA scan is used to diagnose osteopenia and osteoporosis and guide treatment and prevention.
  - Results are reported as "a score."
  - A "T score" compares the pt's bone mineral density (BMD) with the mean BMD value of a young adult:
    - Normal   Less than −1.0 SD of the young adult mean
    - Osteopenia   Between −1.0 and −2.5
    - Osteoporosis   More than −2.5

PERIMENOPAUSE

 What is the pt's menstrual history?

Menstrual cycles normally range from 21–35 days.
- As menopause approaches, cycles become irregular.
- Large variability between consecutive cycles is common.

Does the pt have a sense that she is entering perimenopause?

Pt perception can be predictive of menopausal onset.

Is the pt experiencing any of the following symptoms of perimenopause?

Hot flashes, night sweats

Vaginal dryness

Urinary incontinence

Is the pt experiencing any sexual dysfunction?

Sexual dysfunction is a common problem among perimenopausal women.

Symptoms can be secondary to physical or hormonal changes of perimenopause.

Does the pt have a history of depression?

Although perimenopause does not cause depression, women with a history of depression are susceptible to recurrence during this time of physical and emotional stress.

Has the pt had a hysterectomy?

An ovarian-sparing hysterectomy is associated with an earlier menopause secondary to altered ovarian blood flow.

Does the pt smoke?

Smokers experience earlier menopause than nonsmokers and tend to have a shorter transition.

O **What is the pt's age?**

Age is one of the most important factors in determining perimenopausal state. Median age of perimenopause is 46–47 y/o.

Perform PE

Weight and blood pressure

Thyroid
- Hypothyroidism is a common disease of women in their 40s and can mimic perimenopausal symptoms.
  o Should be screened for in the presence of menstrual irregularities and suspicion on PE.

Breasts

Pelvic
- External genitalia: Atrophy, signs of inflammation
- Speculum: Perform Pap smear
- Bimanual: Abnormalities in uterus, pelvic masses

Is the vaginal pH elevated?

Elevated vaginal pH in the absence of pathogens is associated with a hypoestrogenic state.

Consider follicle-stimulating hormone (FSH) and inhibin B levels

Changes in these hormones may signal perimenopause; however, these hormones can fluctuate markedly.

Perimenopause is associated with elevated FSH (>24 IU/L) and low inhibin B (<30 ng/L).

Estradiol is highly variable, especially in early perimenopause, where it can actually be elevated.

Perimenopause

Time between regular periods and cessation of menses when periods become irregular in length and often heavier.
- Early perimenopause: Cycle irregularity with <3 months of amenorrhea.
- Late perimenopause: Cycle irregularity with 3–11 months of amenorrhea. Average age of onset is 46 years of age; average duration is 5 years.

P **Provide symptom relief**

Most symptoms of perimenopause can be relieved with oral contraceptives (OCs).
- OCs regulate periods, relieve vasomotor symptoms or genitourinary atrophy, and provide contraception.
- Start with low-dose OC
  - Formulations containing 20 µg of ethinyl estradiol
  - Avoid with smokers (>15 cigarettes/d)

Consider antidepressants for depressive symptoms

Consider endometrial biopsy (EMB)

All perimenopausal-age pts with irregular bleeding need an EMB.

Provide lifestyle counseling

Perimenopause is the start of a major change in a woman's life and provides an excellent opportunity for education and promotion of general healthy living.
- Diet
  - Review healthy dietary habits with an emphasis on calcium intake for the prevention of osteoporosis.
    - Reproductive-age women should be taking a total of 1,000 mg calcium/d.
    - Consider vitamin D supplementation for pts at risk for low levels.
- Exercise
  - Aerobic exercise promotes a healthy cardiovascular system.
  - Weight-bearing exercise maintains bone health.
- Smoking
  - Contributes to worsening of many perimenopausal issues such as vaginal dryness, cardiovascular disease, and osteoporosis.

Offer screening tests

Mammogram
- Every 1–2 years beginning at age 40
- Annually after age 50

Cholesterol
- Beginning at age 45, cholesterol testing every 5 years

Diabetes and thyroid
- Beginning at age 45, fasting glucose and TSH every 3 years

PREMENSTRUAL SYNDROME

S **Obtain a detailed history of complaints**

Premenstrual syndrome (PMS) symptoms can vary widely, including:

– Bloating
– Breast discomfort
– Headaches
– Irritability
– Crying
– Fatigue
– Thirst

– Feeling of weight gain
– Pelvic pain
– Hot flushes
– Depression
– Decreased libido
– Insomnia
– Hunger

Review PMH

It is important to verify that the symptoms are not attributable to any other medical problem. All of the following can worsen in the premenstrual period.

• Depression
• Intestinal problems
• Migraines
• Arthritis

O **Physical exam**

A compete PE should be performed to rule out any medical problems as the etiology.

A **Premenstrual syndrome**

A group of symptoms, both physical and behavioral, that occur in the second half of the menstrual cycle

They are followed by a period that is entirely free of symptoms, and they often interfere with work and personal relationships.

Up to 50%–75% of women experience some combination of PMS symptoms.

Premenstrual dysmorphic disorder

A psychiatric term to diagnose a "severe" form of PMS characterized by a marked interference with daily activities and relationships.

Only about 5% of pts meet this criterion.

P **Symptom diary**

A symptom diary is the most effective way to manage PMS.

• Symptoms are recorded daily and rated on a severity scale of 1–4.
  ○ Stress the importance of documentation of the top three to four symptoms that most affect the pt's quality of life.
  ○ Document menstrual period days.

Keeping a diary helps target treatments to symptom specifics.

• Documents symptoms over time with patterns and associations.
• Avoids underestimation of symptoms.

Initiate treatment

Medical approaches to therapy

• NSAIDs
  ○ Good if principal symptom is cramping, heat intolerance, or diarrhea
  ○ Generally very safe
  ○ Use intermittently (as needed during symptoms)
• Anti-anxiety drugs
  ○ Benzodiazepines
  ○ Good for symptoms that predominate around anxiety
  ○ Not good for long-term use
• Diuretics
  ○ Good if main symptom is feeling of bloating or weight gain
• Birth control pills—first line
• Gonadotropin-releasing hormone agonists
  ○ Dangerous potential for side effects: osteoporosis

- Selective serotonin reuptake inhibitors (SSRIs)
  - Serotonin plays a role in PMS through an unclear relationship with estrogen.
    - Estrogen appears to promote serotonin production and prevents its degradation.
    - Three regimens to take SSRIs for PMS:
      - Continuous
      - Intermittent
        - Taking SSRI only during last 2 weeks of cycle
      - As needed
  - Side effects include interrupted sleep and sexual dysfunction.

Complementary and alternative medicine
- Nutritional approaches (diet)
- Botanical medicines
- Vitamins
  - Magnesium: 200–400 mg/d
  - Vitamin B_6: Can damage nerves >100 mg/d
  - Calcium: 1,200–1,600 mg/d
    - Added benefit of osteoporosis prevention
- Mind-body approaches
  - Relaxation
  - Guided imagery
  - Group therapy
  - Yoga
  - Aerobic exercise
  - Light therapy
  - Massage

RECURRENT PREGNANCY LOSS

S **Obtain a detailed history of all pregnancies and losses**

The fetal *gestational age* at the time of loss is important to note.
- Etiologies of recurrent loss tend to cluster in groups according to gestational age.
  - Second trimester losses should raise suspicion for anatomic problems.
    - Antiphospholipid syndrome (APS) is associated with pregnancy loss after 10 weeks' gestation and recurrent first trimester loss.
- Age estimates by last menstrual period are not always accurate because fetal death often occurs "silently" several weeks earlier.
- Age estimates by measuring the fetal size on U/S are more accurate.

Elicit any history of genetic diseases or anomalies

Familial reproductive problems suggest possible genetic etiologies.

Is the pt taking any medications or drugs, smoking or using alcohol, or have any occupational exposures to teratogenic substances?

All of these factors have been associated with early pregnancy loss.
Lead, mercury, solvents, and ionizing radiation are all teratogens.

Has the pt had any previous pelvic infections, uterine instrumentation, or diethylstilbestrol (DES) exposure?

This history can suggest anatomic distortion leading to pregnancy loss.
- Synechiae are scars in the uterine cavity usually secondary to instrumentation.
- DES is a synthetic estrogen used in the 1970s for threatened abortions and has been associated with early pregnancy losses.

Is history compatible with cervical incompetence?

Cervical incompetence follows a classic pattern:
- Painless dilation
- Leakage of fluid (rupture of membranes)
- Delivery of a live fetus

Does the pt have any chronic medical illnesses or galactorrhea?

Uncontrolled diabetes, thyroid disease, and thrombophilias are all associated with recurrent pregnancy loss (RPL).
Hyperprolactinemia is also associated with pregnancy losses.

Any prior workup or treatments?

Note any prior studies and treatments in order to focus the workup.
Karyotyping of previous losses provides important information on possible chromosomal problems.

O **Height, weight, body habitus, and blood pressure. Perform PE**

Breasts
- Galactorrhea

Cervix
- Evidence of trauma
- Malformation

Uterus
- Note size and shape

Does the pt have any signs of diabetes or hyperandrogenism?

Signs of diabetes mellitus (DM) mandate a workup for glucose intolerance.
Acne and hirsutism are signs of hyperandrogenism.

A **Recurrent pregnancy loss**

RPL is classically defined as the loss of three first trimester pregnancies, but evaluation should begin after two first consecutive first trimester losses. (A single second trimester loss is not RPL—it's an adverse fetal outcome in APS.)

The cause of RPL is elicited in only 60% of cases. That's a high quote—ASRM PB 2012 says 75% of RPL cases will not have a cause.

Proposed causes of RPL and their incidences are as follows:
- Genetic (5%): aneuploidy is 60%
- Anatomic (12%)
- Infectious (5%): not a cause of RPL
- Endocrine (17%): thyroid, prolactin, diabetes, obesity
- Autoimmune (50%): APS incidence is 5%–20%
- Other (10%): anatomic factors, lifestyle (cigarette smoking, EtOH, caffeine, cocaine)

P Rule out anatomic etiologies

Hysterosalpingogram: Plain x-ray film of *uterine cavity and tubes* after filling with radio-opaque dye

Hydrosonogram: Instillation of saline into uterine cavity followed by visualization by U/S

Hysteroscope (the gold standard): Instrumentation used to directly visualize the uterine cavity and tubal ostia

Rule out APS

The two most common laboratory tests to rule out APS (see Antiphospholipid Syndrome, p. 250) are:
- Anticardiolipin antibodies
- Lupus anticoagulant

Obtain karyotype of both partners

Most common abnormality found is balanced translocations:
- Two-thirds reciprocal
- One-third Robertsonian

Consider other endocrine or metabolic disorders
- TSH
- Obesity
- DM
- Prolactin

Treat anatomic defects

Treat anatomic defects according to the obstetric history:
- Cervical incompetence
  o Cervical length surveillance and IM 17 OHP4 therapy
- Cerclage
- Septated uterus, submucosal myomas, and synechiae
  o Hysteroscopic resection

Treat APS

Daily low-dose aspirin (80 mg)
Subcutaneous heparin 7,500 U q12h

Treat chromosomal abnormalities

Preconceptional counseling
Genetic counseling early in pregnancy

Treat endocrine causes

Thyroid disorders—treat hypothyroidism with levothyroxine
Hyperprolactinemia—treat with cabergoline
Control diabetes
Obesity—reduce BMI to <30 with diet and exercise

SECONDARY AMENORRHEA

S **Is there a possibility the pt is currently pregnant?**
Always consider pregnancy first when the pt complains of amenorrhea.

Obtain a detailed menstrual and contraceptive history
Last menstrual period
Previous cycle lengths

Is the pt taking any hormone contraception?
Hormone contraception such as the levonorgestrel IUD or the depot medroxyprogesterone acetate injection can cause amenorrhea.

Is the pt currently suffering from any stress?
Emotional or psychological distress can cause hypothalamic dysfunction.

What is the pt's diet?
Dietary restriction resulting in a low BMI can lead to hypothalamic dysfunction.

What are the pt's exercise habits?
Excessive exercise can lead to hypothalamic dysfunction.

Does the pt have a family history of premature menopause?
Review family history for potential genetic inheritance of ovarian failure, such as Fragile X

Does the pt have a recent history of uterine curettage?
Asherman syndrome (uterine synechiae) is more likely after uterine curettage.

O **Check the pt's age**
Pts older than 45 should be considered for perimenopause or menopause.

Perform PE
General: Obesity (BMI >30) is associated with excessive cortisol production and polycystic ovary syndrome (PCOS).
Skin: Check for evidence of hirsutism and acanthosis nigricans, which are seen in PCOS.
Pelvic: Vaginal atrophy or dryness suggests hypoestrogenic state.

Perform pregnancy test
This is the single most important test in the workup of secondary amenorrhea.

Draw the following labs to assess hormonal status
- TSH
- FSH
- Estradiol
- Prolactin

Rule out systemic disease with the following
CBC
Serum chemistries
U/A

A **Secondary amenorrhea**
Secondary amenorrhea is defined as 6 months without menses or a time equivalent to three of the previous cycle intervals without menses. A workup can be initiated upon pt presentation regardless of duration.
A general diagnosis of "secondary amenorrhea" is given to these pts while a workup attempts to find a definitive etiology.
Most patients will have secondary amenorrhea caused by anovulation.
Other possible etiologies include:
- Asherman syndrome
- Prolactin tumors
- Excess cortisol
- Ovarian failure
- Hypothyroidism
- Excess androgens (PCOS)
- Hypothalamic suppression caused by stress, diet, or exercise
- History of using depot medroxyprogesterone acetate

P Perform progesterone challenge test

Management of secondary amenorrhea consists of a series of tests designed to locate where in the hypothalamic-pituitary-ovarian-uterine axis the dysfunction lies.
The first step is to perform a progestational challenge test.

- This test confirms a functional ovary (capable of making estrogen) and a functional uterus (outflow tract).
- The test is performed by administering medroxyprogesterone acetate 10 mg PO q day for 5 days.
  o If a period results, the uterus and ovaries have been confirmed to be working and a diagnosis of anovulation can be made.

If progestational challenge test is negative, administer estrogen followed by progesterone

Administration of estrogen and progesterone mimics a normal hormonal cycle as produced by a normally functioning hypothalamus, pituitary, and ovary.

- If a period ensues, the problem lies in the ovaries or in the central nervous system.
- If withdrawal bleed is absent, suspect Asherman syndrome or other outflow tract issues, such as Mullerian anomalies (no cervix, vaginal septum)

If period ensues with estrogen and progesterone, check gonadotropin levels

Gonadotrophs (FSH and LH) are released from the pituitary in response to gonadotropin-releasing hormone released from the hypothalamus. Their target organ is the ovary.

- Therefore, high levels of gonadotrophs indicate an unresponsiveness of the ovary (ovarian failure).
- Low or normal levels indicate a pituitary or hypothalamic problem.

If gonadotrophs are low, perform a coned-down view MRI of sella turcica

The sella turcica is the cranial bone in which the pituitary lies.

- A pituitary tumor affecting gonadotroph secretion would visibly distort the cranial anatomy on MRI.
  o A normal MRI implies that amenorrhea is the result of hypothalamic dysfunction.

The following is a description of an encounter for pts requesting *screening* for STDs. Refer to individual SOAPs (vulvar ulcers, vulvovaginitis, PID) for treatment of *current* infection.

URINARY INCONTINENCE

S   Obtain a detailed history

How many times a day does the pt urinate? (>8 times/d is considered excessive)
Does she lose urine when coughing, laughing, or sneezing? How often?
Does she have nocturia? How many times a night does she get up?
Does she experience urgency or frequency?
Does she lose urine before "making it to the bathroom"? (symptom of urge incontinence)
Does she wear a pad for the incontinence?

Does the pt have pain?

Pain may indicate interstitial cystitis or urinary tract infection (UTI).

Has the pt had a previous surgery for urinary incontinence? Previous pharmacologic treatment?

Pts with previous treatment require more detailed evaluation.
A record of prior medicine used can help tailor recommendations.

Does the pt have glaucoma, gastroesophageal reflux disease, or dementia?

These medical problems can be exacerbated by anticholinergics, the drugs of choice in
   treatment of overactive bladder.

Does the pt have diabetes?

Can lead to urinary frequency
Can be a risk factor for neurogenic bladder (paresis)

Is the pt taking any medicines?

Antihypertensives, cholinergic agents, neuroleptics, and xanthines can all cause
   incontinence.

Is the pt postmenopausal?

Hypoestrogenic states can lead to urogenital atrophy and irritative symptoms.
Urogenital tissue is responsive to replacement estrogen cream.

O   Perform detailed PE

Urethra: Check pain associated with diverticula
Bladder
Signs of pelvic floor relaxation (cystocele, rectocele, enterocele)
Evidence of loss of urine under Valsalva (supine, sitting, and standing)

What are the findings on simple cytometric evaluation?

Simple cytometrics are performed as a way of defining the etiology of the problem.
- Direct visualization of the genitourinary anatomy (urethra and bladder) with a
  cystoscope.
- Simulation of bladder filling with CO_2 gas or water and observation for signs of blad-
  der (detrusor muscle) contractions and bladder capacity (hyperdistention).
- "The Q-tip test"
  - A cotton-tipped applicator is inserted into the urethra.
  - The angle the cotton-tipped applicator makes with the floor represents the angle of
    the urethral-vesicular junction (UVJ).
  - Test is considered positive if, under Valsalva pressure, this angle can be observed
    to change>30 degrees.

What is the result of the U/A and culture?

Always rule out a UTI in the workup of the incontinent pt.

A   Urinary incontinence

Common diagnoses are:
- Stress urinary incontinence (SUI)
- Mixed urinary incontinence (MUI)
- Urgency UI (commonly known as irritable bladder)

Less common etiologies include (the new terms are): overactive bladder, insensible urinary incontinence, chronic urinary retention, coital urinary incontinence, continuous urinary incontinence, extraurethral urinary incontinence, functional urinary incontinence, nocturnal enuresis, occult stress incontinence, postmicturition leakage, sui, urgency urinary incontinence

– Overflow incontinence   – Interstitial cystitis
– Overactive bladder   – Intrinsic sphincter deficiency

P   **UI is treated with pharmacologic agents and behavioral modifications**

Common pharmacologic agents are:
- Anticholinergics and antispasmodics
  - Work by blocking muscarinic activity, thereby avoiding bladder stimulation.
  - Counsel pts on common side effects such as xerostomia and blurry vision.
    - Propantheline 15 mg PO bid
    - Oxybutynin hydrochloride 5 mg PO tid/oxybutynin ER 5–10 mg PO qd
    - Tolterodine tartrate 1–2 mg PO bid/tolterodine tartrate ER 4 mg qd
- Adrenergics
  - Work by relaxing detrusor muscle with β-adrenergic stimulation and stimulating the urethral sphincter via α-adrenergic receptors
    - Imipramine 25 mg PO tid
    - Amitriptyline 50 mg PO tid

Behavioral modifications include:
- Maintaining normal amounts of fluid intake during day (5–6 glasses of water)
- Avoiding fluid intake at night
- Avoiding alcohol and caffeinated beverages, which increase urine production
- Bladder "training"
  - This involves gradually increasing the time interval between voiding episodes in hopes of establishing a new higher threshold at which urge incontinence occurs.
- Kegel exercises
  - Contraction and relaxation of the pubococcygeal muscles

SUI is treated with surgery

More than 300 procedures for SUI have been described.

Gold standard is a midurethral polypropylene sling.

Other options include:

Retropubic urethropexy:
- Involves "restoring" the UVJ to its original angle.
- Sutures are placed in tissues surrounding the UVJ and used to pull it up and anchor it.
  - Burch procedure: UVJ anchored to iliopectineal (Cooper) ligament.
  - Marshall-Marchetti-Krantz: UVJ anchored to pubic symphysis.

VULVOVAGINITIS

S **Obtain a detailed history of the current complaint**

Discharge
- Duration
- Consistency
- Factors related to onset
- Color
- Previous over-the-counter treatments

Pruritus

Odor: Pts with bacterial vaginosis (BV) may experience an increase in odor after sexual intercourse secondary to semen-triggered release of amines from anaerobic bacteria.

Does the pt give a history of anything that could upset the normal vaginal environment?

- Any recent antibiotic use?
- Douches?
- Changes of partners?
- Foreign body/tampon use?
- Hormone/contraceptive use?
- Increase in sexual intercourse?

Is the complaint limited to the vulva?

Symptoms limited to only the external genitalia should prompt an allergy review:
- Deodorant soaps?
- Laundry detergents?
- Perfumed or dyed toilet paper?
- Swimming pool chemicals?
- Synthetic clothing?

O **Perform PE**

External genitalia
- Inspect for any of the following:
  - Erythema
  - Edema
  - Ulcers
  - Pallor
  - Excoriations
  - Blisters

Vagina
- Inspect for any discharge:
  - *Candida* is curdy, white, cottage cheese–like.
  - Bacterial vaginosis is thin, dark, and homogenous.
  - *Trichomonas* is yellow-gray or green and frothy.
- Test vaginal pH
  - Test vaginal pH by touching nitrazine paper to the lateral wall of the vagina.
  - Vaginal pH is normally acidic (pH = 3.8–4.2) secondary to the predominant flora, lactobacillus.
  - An alkaline pH (>4.5), as indicated by the paper turning dark blue, is abnormal and consistent with BV or trichomonas vaginitis.

Perform wet mount and "whiff test"

Collect a specimen of discharge with a cotton-tipped applicator and place into 1–2 cc normal saline (NS) in a test tube.

Perform wet prep by placing a drop of NS onto one-half of a microscope slide and a drop of 10% potassium hydroxide (KOH) onto the other side.
- To each of these, add a drop of the vaginal discharge prep.
- Examine NS side for clue cells (consistent with BV) and trichomonads (flagellated protozoa).
  - Presence of many leukocytes in this prep is also consistent with trichomoniasis.
- Examine KOH side for hyphae (evidence of yeast).

Perform "whiff test" by adding a drop of KOH to the vaginal discharge.
- Release of a strong, fishy odor (amines) can be appreciated in the presence of BV and *Trichomonas* infection.

Consider a Gram stain and culture

Consider culture for a yeast infection that has failed over-the-counter or prior medical treatment.

Culture is also more sensitive than wet mount for diagnosis of *Trichomonas*.

Gram stain is more useful for BV because culture is not specific.

A **Vulvovaginitis**

Most causes of vulvovaginitis are infectious.

The three major etiologies are:
- Candida vulvovaginitis
- Bacterial vaginosis
- Trichomonas vaginitis

Less common causes are noninfectious:
- Irritant/chemical
- Atrophic
- Dermatitis (contact, seborrheic, atopic)
- Dermatoses (lichen simplex, lichen sclerosus)
- Systemic dermatoses (eczema, psoriasis)

P **Treat vulvovaginal candidiasis with antifungals**

Numerous intravaginal preparations are available:
- Miconazole 2% cream 5 mg intravaginally for 7 days
- Terconazole 0.8% cream 5 g intravaginally for 3 days
- Clotrimazole 500-mg vaginal tablet for one dose

One available oral treatment:
- Fluconazole 150 mg PO × 1

Treat bacterial vaginosis with metronidazole

Metronidazole gel 0.75%, 5 g per vagina qd for 5 days (Rec)

Metronidazole 500 mg PO bid for 7 days (Rec)

Metronidazole 2 g PO in a single dose (Alt)
- Avoid alcohol while taking medication.

- Metronidazole can give a disulfiram-like reaction.

Treat trichomonas vaginitis with metronidazole
- Metronidazole 2 g PO in a single dose (Rec)
- Metronidazole 500 mg PO bid for 7 days (Alt)
- Only *oral* metronidazole is effective against *Trichomonas*.
- *Trichomonas* infection is considered a sexually transmitted disease.
  ○ Arrange for treatment of the pt's partner.

EMERGENCY ROOM AND CONSULTATIONS
FIRST TRIMESTER BLEEDING—ABORTION

S **Obtain a detailed menstrual history**
Describe onset and duration of bleeding.
Number of pads used and degree of saturation (heavy, medium, or light).

Are there any associated cramps?
The answer to this question can help differentiate between threatened and complete
 abortion; cramping is often felt as the products of conception (POC) are passed
 through the uterus in a complete abortion.
Intense pain should always raise suspicion for a possible ectopic pregnancy.

O **Review VS**
Check for signs of cardiovascular instability.

Check CBC
Elevated WBCs may indicate infection; low hematocrit may reflect a hemoperitoneum.

Check β-hCG level
This level is important in interpreting U/S findings.

Check Rh status
All pts with first trimester bleeding should have their Rh D status checked.
 • Administer 50 µg anti-D immune globulin to pts with Rh D–negative blood.

Perform pelvic exam
Is the cervical os open or closed?
 • An open os is consistent with inevitable abortion.
 • A closed os is consistent with threatened or complete abortion.
Is there active bleeding?
Is there any POC visible inside the os that can be manually removed?
What is the size and position of uterus?
 • This information may be important if surgical therapy is required.
Any adnexal tenderness or masses?
Always consider the possibility of an ectopic pregnancy.

Obtain U/S
U/S directly surveys the contents of the uterus.
 • The first embryonic structure to develop that is identifiable by U/S is the gestational
  sac, followed by the yolk sac, and, finally, the fetal pole.
  ○ Abdominal U/S is able to detect a gestational sac when the β-hCG level is >6,000
   IU/L.
  ○ Transvaginal U/S is able to detect a gestational sac when the β-hCG level is
   >1,000–1,500 IU/L.

 • The absence of a gestational sac in the presence of β-hCG levels above these cutoff values
  means that the pt has either a completed abortion or an ectopic pregnancy.

 • The following findings on U/S support a diagnosis of inevitable or missed abortion:
  ○ Collapsed gestational sac
  ○ Absence of the yolk sac when the gestational sac is 8 mm
  ○ Absence of the fetal pole when the gestational sac is 16–18 mm
  ○ Absence of cardiac motion when the embryo is 4–5 mm in length

A **Spontaneous abortion**
This is a general diagnosis that can be further specified as follows:
 • Blighted ovum (a.k.a. anembryonic gestation)
  ○ A gestational sac is >17–18 mm without an embryo visualized

- Complete abortion
  - Spontaneous and complete expulsion of all POC from uterus
  - Diagnosis supported by closed os, history of cramping, and an endometrial thickness <15 mm
- Incomplete abortion
  - Partial expulsion of all POC from uterus
  - Endometrial thickness >15 mm and/or continued active bleeding
- Inevitable abortion
  - Cervical dilation and uterine bleeding before expulsion of POC
- Missed abortion
  - Fetal death before 20 weeks of pregnancy without expulsion of POC
- Septic abortion
  - Intrauterine infection accompanying abortion

P **Therapeutic options for abortion include surgical, medical, and expectant management**

Treatment choice depends on:
- Condition of pt at the time of assessment
- Pt preference

Surgical management
- Dilation and curettage (D&C)
  - Requires an operating room
- Manual vacuum aspiration (MVA)
  - Can be done in the ER or clinic

Medical management
- Vaginal delivery of 800 µg misoprostol (dose may be repeated once in 24 hours as needed) and waiting up to 2–3 days

Complete abortion
No intervention necessary

Incomplete abortion
D&C or MVA

Inevitable abortion
D&C, MVA, or expectant management

Missed abortion
D&C, misoprostol, or expectant management

Septic abortion
IV antibiotics
D&C after antibiotics are on-board

FIRST TRIMESTER BLEEDING—ECTOPIC PREGNANCY

S **Obtain a detailed menstrual history**

When was the pt's last menstrual period?

Has there been any irregular bleeding?

Bleeding associated with ectopic pregnancy is generally less than with abortion.

Obtain a detailed description of the pain

Characteristic of the pain
- Pain before rupture is usually colicky or vague; after rupture, pain intensifies.

Where is the pain located?
- Site of pain usually corresponds to ectopic site but can be bilateral.
- Shoulder pain can represent diaphragmatic irritation seen with hemoperitoneum.

Assess pt's desire to maintain future fertility

Future childbearing plans often are taken into account when making treatment decisions
in the management of ectopic pregnancy.

O **Check VS first**

Check for signs of cardiovascular instability (hypotension and tachycardia).

Consider orthostatics.

Perform abdominal and pelvic exam

Are there signs of peritonitis?

Adnexal tenderness or masses present?

Be careful not to rupture ectopic pregnancy by applying too much pressure.

Check CBC

Hematocrit will give you an idea of the pt's stability.

Check β-hCG level

β-hCG level, along with U/S, forms the basis of management decisions.

Check Rh status

Rh-negative pts with negative antibody screen need anti-D immune globulin before
discharge.

Obtain U/S

Attempts to directly visualize the earliest evidence of a pregnancy: the gestational sac (GS).
- Based on the principle that when the β-hCG level reaches a certain point, the GS
should be able to be visualized (in the uterus) by U/S.
- This level is called the "discriminatory level."
  o Abdominal U/S is able to detect a GS when the β-hCG level is >6,000 IU/L.
  o Transvaginal ultrasound is able to detect a GS when the β-hCG level is
  >1,500 IU/L.
- If the β-hCG level is above these "discriminatory levels" and a pregnancy cannot be
visualized, a diagnosis of "an abnormal pregnancy" can be made.
  o If the clinical assessment is highly suspicious for ectopic, the pregnancy can be
  treated as such.

An ectopic pregnancy can often be *directly visualized* by U/S.
- Findings range from a complex or cystic adnexal mass to visualization of an actual
embryo.

Free fluid on U/S is suggestive of hemoperitoneum.

A **Ectopic pregnancy**

The differential diagnosis includes:

- Abortion
- Ruptured corpus luteum/hemorrhagic cyst
- Dysfunctional uterine bleeding
- Endometriosis

- Salpingitis
- Appendicitis
- Adnexal torsion
- Degenerating fibroid

P **Observation for unclear clinical picture**

If the pt's condition worsens, surgical exploration is necessary.

If the pt's condition remains stable, perform serial CBCs, abdominal exams, and, in 48 hours, a repeat β-hCG.

If β-hCG level is not doubled, the diagnosis can be specified as an *abnormal pregnancy* and managed as an ectopic if the clinical picture matches.

Surgical management

The following clinical scenarios mandate surgical exploration:
- Unstable pts
- Pts with ruptured ectopics
- Pts who have completed childbearing
- Pts with contraindications to medical management (see below)

Immediate surgical exploration after stabilization:
- Two large-bore IVs, copious fluids, type and cross-match blood, arrange for operative management via laparotomy

Medical management (methotrexate)

Medical management may be considered for pts who are stable and desire future fertility.

Absolute contraindications to usage include:

– Hemodynamic instability	– Intrauterine Pregnancy
– Immunodeficiency	– Breastfeeding
– Noncompliant pt	– Elevated liver function tests
– Ruptured ectopic	– Clinically important hepatic dysfunction
– Thrombocytopenia, severe anemia, or leukopenia	– Renal insufficiency
– Active peptic ulcer	– Active pulmonary disease

Relative contraindications:

Fetal cardiac activity detected on TVUS

High initial hCG concentration or >6,500 hCG level

Ectopic pregnancy greater than 4 cm

Refusal to accept blood transfusion

Dosing is 50 mg/m^2 based on body surface area.

Close follow-up of declining β-hCG levels is necessary.
- Check β-hCG level on day 4 and day 7.
  - β-hCG level should decline by 15% between days 4 and 7.
    - If level declines, follow with β-hCG levels qwk.
    - If not, repeat methotrexate or perform surgery.

Follow up all pts after treatment until β-hCG is negative with a weekly β-hCG!

ACUTE PELVIC PAIN

 Obtain a detailed history of complaint

Nature of pain
- Hollow organs such as bowel or fallopian tubes are associated with crampy pain.
- Ovarian etiologies are associated with constant, sharp pain.

Location of pain
- Unilateral, lower quadrant pain is suspicious for adnexal problem.
- Bilateral lower quadrant pain can be pelvic inflammatory disease (PID).
- Gynecologic etiologies may present with symptoms and signs referred to the upper quadrants.

Is there bleeding present?

Cramping associated with vaginal bleeding raises suspicion for spontaneous or inevitable abortion or ectopic pregnancy.

Is nausea and vomiting (N/V) present?

N/V is associated with adnexal torsion.

Does the pt have any risk factors for infectious process?

Recent gynecologic procedures

Review PMH

Reproductive-age or postmenopausal women may have history of a medical problem (diverticulitis, PUD) that might focus the workup.

O **Age**

Prepubertal or adolescent pts have a higher incidence of ovarian torsion.

Vital signs

Verify that the pt is stable.
Presence of fever raises suspicion for infectious process.

Perform PE

Pelvic
- Abdomen
  - Rebound, tenderness
  - Bowel sounds
  - Distention
- Cervix
  - Discharge
  - Cervical motion tenderness
- Uterus
  - Enlargement: Associated with fibroids
  - Tenderness: Associated with endometritis
- Adnexa
  - Tenderness
  - Masses
- Rectal
  - Information complements bimanual exam

 Acute pelvic pain

The differential diagnosis can be divided into gynecologic and nongynecologic.
Problems of gynecologic origin can further be classified according to pregnancy status:
- Gynecologic—Pregnancy-related
  - Ectopic
  - Abortion
- Nongynecologic
  - Appendicitis
  - Bowel obstruction
  - Pancreatitis

- ○ GU infections
- ○ Diverticulitis
- • Gynecologic—Nonpregnancy-related
  - ○ Cervicitis
  - ○ Torsion
  - ○ PID (including tubo-ovarian abscess)
  - ○ Degenerating fibroid
  - ○ Endometritis

P   Perform pregnancy test

A pregnancy test is the single most important evaluation in the workup of acute pelvic pain.

A positive test dramatically focuses the differential diagnosis and places ectopic pregnancy at the top of the list.

Obtain other laboratories

CBC: Elevated WBCs can indicate an infectious process.

Comprehensive metabolic panel: Hepatic or biliary abnormalities may focus the differential diagnosis.

Amylase/lipase: Consider with pancreatitis.

Consider imaging studies

Imaging studies may complement the PE in narrowing the diagnosis.

- • U/S
  - ○ Gold standard imaging test of the pelvic viscera
  - ○ Able to assess organ size, masses, and free fluid
  - ○ May be able to directly visualize ectopic pregnancy
- • CT
  - ○ Useful when etiology cannot clearly be distinguished between abdominal and pelvic origin
- • MRI
  - ○ Generally not used in the acute gynecologic setting, but may have a role in the presence of acute pain with a normal pregnancy

GESTATIONAL TROPHOBLASTIC DISEASE

 What is the pt's menstrual history?

Molar pts usually present with painless vaginal bleeding following a missed menses. Pt may report passage of grape-like vesicles.

Most pts are considered to be pregnant at the time of bleeding presentation.

Does the pt have any recent obstetrical history?

Partial moles frequently have been given antecedent diagnosis of missed or incomplete abortion.

Some gestational trophoblastic diseases (GTDs) can occur after a term pregnancy.

Does the pt have any excessive nausea or vomiting?

Molar pregnancies frequently have nausea and vomiting symptoms.

Does the pt have any symptoms of hyperthyroidism?

The high hCG level associated with molar pregnancy can stimulate thyroid hormone production, leading to hyperthyroidism.

O **Check VS first**

Cardiovascular instability (hypotension and tachycardia): Emboli from the molar tissue can occur.

Elevated blood pressure: Early preeclampsia (<20 weeks) has been associated with GTD.

Perform PE

Cervix may be open and expulsing hydropic villi.

Uterus may be larger than dates in some complete moles (50%).

Ovaries can be enlarged secondary to hormonal stimulation.

Check CBC

Massive bleeding can occur with moles.

Check β-hCG level

β-hCG level is frequently highly elevated.
 • β-hCG can be >1 million IU/L with complete molar pregnancies.

> • In normal pregnancy, β-hCG peaks at 100,000 IU/L at about 10 weeks.

Thyroid-stimulating hormone (TSH)

High levels of β-hCG can cause stimulation of the thyroid gland and symptoms of hyperthyroidism.

> β-hCG and TSH are similar hormones that share the same "alpha subunit."

Check Rh status

Rh-negative pts with no antibodies require anti-D immune globulin before discharge.

What are the results of the U/S?

Complete molar pregnancies are often diagnosed before treatment. The classic appearance of a complete mole is a "snowstorm" pattern on U/S.

U/S may also pick up theca lutein cysts, which result from high levels of β-hCG.

> β-hCG and luteinizing hormone (LH) are similar hormones that share the same "alpha subunit."

What is the result of the CXR?

A CXR should be performed to look for metastatic disease or trophoblastic emboli.

Gestational trophoblastic disease

Benign GTD
- Molar pregnancies can be qualified as *complete* moles or *partial* moles.
  - A complete mole results from the fertilization of an *empty egg* by a single sperm, resulting in a haploid set of chromosomes.
    - Complete moles are more common in general and more frequently present with enlarged uteri, very high β-hCG levels (and its systemic sequelae as described above), and a clear diagnosis on U/S.
  - A partial mole results from the fertilization of a normal, haploid egg with *two sperm*, resulting in a triploid pregnancy.
    - A partial mole is a pathologic diagnosis made after examining tissue retrieved from a missed or incomplete abortion.

Malignant GTD
- Invasive mole
- Choriocarcinoma
- Placental site trophoblastic tumor

 Dilation and evacuation

Mainstay of treatment of molar pregnancy is evacuation of the uterine contents.
- Cervix must be dilated.
- Suction is followed by sharp curettage and oxytocin administration.
- Blood products must be available because these pts can have massive intraoperative hemorrhage.
- Laparotomy must be prepared for in case a hysterotomy is needed to control bleeding.

Long-term follow-up

All molar pregnancies have the potential to transform into malignant disease (see below).

This can occur as a delay from the time of treatment.

Therefore, all pts need to be followed for a period of 1 year with negative β-hCG determinations.
- Start with β-hCG every 1–2 weeks until negative twice, then monthly for 6–12 months.
- Pts with a slow fall in β-hCG should be followed for 2 years.
- Perform physical exams every 2 weeks until β-hCG is negative and then every 3 months.

Prescribe contraception during the follow-up period.
- Oral contraceptives are customary.

Evaluate for malignant GTD

Pts with any of the following need evaluation for malignant GTD:
- Metastatic disease (positive findings on CXR)
- Choriocarcinoma
- β-hCG >20,000 IU/L more than 4 weeks after initial treatment
- β-hCG increases at any point in surveillance
- β-hCG plateaus over 3 weeks
- Persistently detectable β-hCG 4–6 months after evacuation

Treat malignant GTD

A variety of single and multiagent chemotherapy regimens are available.

PELVIC INFLAMMATORY DISEASE

S **What symptoms is the pt. experiencing?**

Symptoms for pelvic inflammatory disease (PID) vary widely from none to severe peritonitis.

Abdominal pain is the most consistent complaint.

Right upper quadrant complaints may signal Fitz-Hugh-Curtis syndrome (PID with perihepatic involvement).

What is the timing of complaints?

Duration of symptoms is usually short (<2 weeks).

Pain secondary to *Neisseria gonorrhoeae* infection has acute onset during or just after menses.

Is the pt at high risk for STDs?

The following are considered high-risk factors:

- Prior history of STD   - Prior PID
- New partner   - Multiple partners
- Symptomatic partner   - Young age
- No contraception

Does pt have a history of recent instrumentation?

Any procedure that breaks the mucus plug of the cervix increases the chances of ascending infection:

- Endometrial biopsy   - D&C
- Intrauterine device placement - Hysteroscopy

Does pt appear reliable and compliant?

Consideration of pt compliance should be made when prescribing outpatient therapy (see below).

O **What is the pt's age?**

Younger pts have a higher risk for PID.

Obtain VS

Fever is sometimes present but not necessary for the diagnosis.

Perform PE

Cervix: Assess for presence of mucopurulent discharge and cervical motion tenderness (CMT).

Uterus: Assess for the presence of tenderness.

Adnexa: Assess for tenderness and masses.

Rule out ectopic pregnancy

Obtain pregnancy test.

What is the result of the CBC?

WBCs may be elevated but not consistently.

Obtain cultures and consider Gram stain

Cultures

• Obtain cultures for *Chlamydia trachomatis* and *N. gonorrhoeae*.

Gram stain

• May be useful in the presence of gross cervical pus.

• Perform saline prep of the discharge.

  ○ Presence of many WBCs suggests PID.

Pelvic inflammatory disease

Diagnosis must be met by the presence of ALL of the following (and absence of another diagnosis):

- Lower abdominal pain and tenderness
- Adnexal tenderness
- CMT

With one additional sign indicating the presence of infection:

- Fever >38.3°C
- Cervical mucopurulent discharge
- Elevated erythrocyte sedimentation rate
- Elevated C-reactive protein
- Documented infection with *C. trachomatis* or *N. gonorrhoeae*

Most likely pathogens are *N. gonorrhoeae, C. trachomatis,* anaerobes, gram-negative facultative bacteria, and streptococci.

 Assess severity of disease

Pts with PID can be treated as outpatients or inpatients.

- Certain criteria have been put forth to guide practitioners in making this decision.
  - The following clinical scenarios mandate inpatient treatment:
    - Pt noncompliance
    - Fever >38°C
    - Uncertain diagnosis
    - Oral treatment failure
    - Suspected tubo-ovarian abscess
    - Pregnancy
    - Nausea and vomiting (unable to take oral meds)

Start antibiotics

Outpatient

- Recommended
  - Ofloxacin 400 mg PO bid × 14 days **and**
  - Metronidazole 500 mg PO bid × 14 days
- Alternative
  - Ceftriaxone 250 mg IM × 1 **and**
  - Doxycycline 100 mg PO bid × 14 days

Inpatient

- Recommended
  - Cefotetan 2 g q12h **and**
  - Doxycycline 100 mg IV q12h
- Alternative
  - Clindamycin 900 mg IV q8h **and**
  - Gentamicin load 2 mg/kg then 1.5 mg/kg q8h

Monitor response

IV antibiotics can be stopped 24 hours after clinical response.

Complete a 14-day course of treatment with PO antibiotics (doxycycline 100 mg bid).

Treat or refer partner

PELVIC MASS

S **Obtain complete gynecologic history**

Include all past infections, operations, and diagnoses.

Is the pt experiencing symptoms because of the mass?

Torsion should be considered in the presence of pain and requires emergent surgery.

Functional cysts do not usually cause pain.

GI symptoms should prompt evaluation of colon.

How long has the mass been diagnosed?

Any mass that is unresolved for more than one cycle needs surgical evaluation.

A simple, cystic mobile unilateral mass that is <8 cm in a reproductive-age woman can be followed for 6–8 weeks.

Family history

Inquire about possible hereditary ovarian cancer.

O **What is the pt's age?**

Age is the single most important factor for predicting possible malignancy.

Any size adnexal mass in the premenarche or postmenopausal age group needs surgical evaluation.

Perform PE

Abdomen
- Palpate for any masses.
- Advanced-stage ovarian cancer can produce a rigid abdomen.
  - This is a result of massive tumor infiltration of the omentum, making it a solid organ (a.k.a. "omental caking").

Pelvic (have pts empty bladder and rectum before exam)
- External genitalia: Inspect and palpate for any evidence of a mass externally.
- Vault: Inspect and palpate for a mass.
- Cervix: Inspect the cervix grossly for any lesions.
- Corpus
  - Palpate during bimanual exam.
  - Note uterine size, contour, tenderness, and mobility.
- Adnexa
  - Note mass.
  - Describe size (in cm), contour, consistency, and mobility.
- Rectal
  - A rectovaginal exam provides the best information about the nature of any adnexal mass.
  - It is a mandatory part of any evaluation.

Obtain CBC

Elevated WBCs focuses the workup on an infectious etiology such as tubo-ovarian abscess (TOA).

A **Pelvic mass**

Gynecologic etiologies
- Uterus
  - Fibroids

Nongynecologic etiologies
- Bowel
  - Abscess, irritable bowel disorder, CA
- Tubes
  - Salpingitis, paraovarian cyst, CA
- Retroperitoneal
  - Lymphoma

- Ovaries
  - Nonneoplastic
    - Functional cyst, theca lutein cyst, endometrioma, TOA
  - Neoplastic
    - Mature teratoma (dermoid), cystadenoma, fibroma, CA

P Rule out ectopic pregnancy

Ectopic pregnancy is a common cause of an adnexal mass in the reproductive age.

Obtain U/S to complement PE

U/S is the gold standard test in evaluation of the pt with a pelvic mass.
The following findings on U/S of an adnexal mass raise suspicion for ovarian CA:

- – Solid components
- – Internal papillations
- – Presence of ascites
- – Bilateral cysts

Order CA125

CA125 is a tumor-associated surface antigen.

- It is found on most nonmucinous epithelial ovarian cancers but can also be found in association with many benign conditions.
- For this reason, it is not used as a screening test but should be obtained in the presence of a pelvic mass.

Consider further radiologic studies for evaluation

CT can help evaluate masses in the retroperitoneal area.
Barium enema or colonoscopy can help distinguish a GI lesion.

Observation for masses <8 cm in the reproductive-age pt

Use of oral contraceptives is thought to speed resolution of functional cysts.
Persistence beyond 6–8 weeks mandates surgical evaluation.

Surgical exploration of all suspicious masses in the reproductive-age pt

This includes:

- Mass >10 cm
- Presence of ascites
- Presence of internal papillations or solid component on U/S

Surgical exploration of all masses in the premenarche or postmenopausal pt

Because these age groups do not have functioning ovaries, all masses are suspicious for CA.

IV
SURGERY AND EMERGENCY MEDICINE

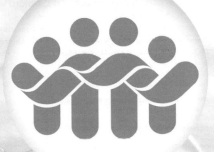

CARDIOLOGY

AORTIC DISSECTION

S **Determine the onset of the pt's symptoms**

What are the pt's current symptoms?
Pts typically complain of acute onset of tearing chest pain that radiates to the back.
Approximately 10% of cases may be asymptomatic.
Other symptoms include hoarseness, syncope, nausea/vomiting, abdominal pain, and paralysis.

Does the pt have any neurologic symptoms?
Weakness, numbness, or cerebrovascular accident (CVA) symptoms may represent an extension of the dissection into the carotid arteries, causing ischemia.
Pts with a CVA are less likely to be able to report their pain, so it should remain part of your differential.

Does the pt have any risk factors for aortic dissection?
- Hypertension (most common)
- Aortic coarctation
- Connective tissue disorders (Marfan syndrome, Ehlers-Danlos syndrome, etc.)
- Cocaine abuse
- Recent cardiac catheterization or cardiac surgery
- Male sex (10 times more likely to suffer a dissection)
- Pregnancy
- Smoking
- Diabetes
- Atherosclerosis
- Tertiary syphilis

Obtain a past medical history

Obtain a list of the pt's current medications
Have they changed, missed, or stopped any of their current medications? This may result in uncontrolled or rebound hypertension (HTN) leading to dissection.
Is the pt taking any herbal supplements? Several herbs (e.g., licorice in apparent mineralocorticoid excess and ephedra) can cause HTN.

Perform a general review of symptoms
There are many mimics of aortic dissection: Esophageal spasm, gastroesophageal reflux disease, biliary colic, peptic ulcer disease, and pericarditis.

O **Check vital signs**
Hypertension and/or tachycardia can exacerbate the dissection.

Perform a physical exam
Cardiac: Note aortic heart sounds. Is there a murmur suggesting aortic insufficiency (classically diastolic, although can be systolic)? Pericardial rub? A new murmur may signify that the dissection has compromised the aortic valve.
Neck: Listen for carotid bruits, which may indicate turbulent flow caused by vessel wall abnormalities.
Neurologic: Check for focal deficits and mental status changes.

Obtain an ECG
Used to exclude myocardial infarction from the diagnosis, although the dissection can extend into the coronary arteries, causing myocardial ischemia.
Signs of left ventricular hypertrophy may support the diagnosis of long-term HTN.

Obtain a CXR
CXR is 90% sensitive for aortic dissection. May see a widened mediastinum, blurred aortic knob, an aortic double density, deviation of trachea, or pleural effusion.

Obtain a diagnostic study

Chest CT scan, MRI, and transesophageal echocardiogram (TEE) all approach 100% in sensitivity and specificity for dissection.

Choice of exam depends on availability and expertise at your individual hospital.

- Chest CT requires IV contrast and will require premedication if pt has an iodine allergy.
- TEE, although invasive, is ideal for the critically ill pt because it can be done at bedside.
- MRI, when available, is less invasive. However, it may be difficult to obtain in the critically ill pt.
- If suspicion is high, two negative diagnostic studies are needed to exclude the diagnosis.

 Aortic dissection

Aortic dissection is a tear in the aortic intima, where blood passes into the aortic media, thereby separating (dissecting) the intima from the surrounding media and/or adventitia, and creating a false lumen.

Differential diagnosis

- Myocardial infarction
- Acute pericarditis
- Peptic ulcer disease
- Pancreatitis
- Pulmonary embolus
- Pneumothorax
- Esophageal spasm
- Biliary colic

P **Immediate blood pressure lowering and control of heart rate is needed**

An elevated blood pressure and tachycardia increase the shear forces on the aorta.

A goal of a systolic blood pressure less than 120 mm Hg should be achieved.

Initial therapy consists of β-blockers or Ca channel blockers.

Add vasodilators (e.g., nitroprusside, hydralazine) if blood pressure remains elevated. Monitor heart rate closely because reflex tachycardia may result from the use of vasodilators.

Provide pain relief

Narcotics are preferred.

Diagnostic study will dictate whether operative intervention is needed

Stanford type A

- All dissections involving the proximal (ascending) aorta
- 70% of aortic dissections
- Has a greater risk for complication with extension into carotid/coronary arteries
- Requires surgical repair. Consult cardiothoracic surgeon
- Mortality rate increases 1% per hour during the first 48 hours
- Worse prognosis than type B

Stanford type B

- Dissection involving the distal (descending) aorta only
- 30% of dissections
- Greater likelihood of being successfully managed medically
- Surgical repair needed if there is evidence of extension into the renal or mesenteric arteries as seen by renal failure and/or mesenteric ischemia

Admit the pt to the ICU

BRADYCARDIA/COMPLETE HEART BLOCK

 Determine whether the pt has any symptoms

Some pts have no symptoms and are only found to have complete heart block or brady-cardia on a routine physical exam or ECG.

Pts may complain of lightheadedness, palpitations, dyspnea, chest pain, syncope, or mental status changes.

Has the pt been started on any new medications or were any doses increased?

β-Blockers, Ca channel blockers, tricyclic antidepressants (TCAs), and digoxin may all cause atrioventricular (AV) node block and lead to bradycardia.

Amiodarone and clonidine toxicity can present with bradycardia.

Determine if the pt may have taken too much medication.

Does the pt have a history of coronary atherosclerotic disease (CAD) or myocardial infarction (MI)?

Progression of CAD and MI can cause complete heart block.

Has the pt fallen, had a recent stroke, or suffered a head injury?

Increased intracranial pressure due to intracerebral hemorrhage, cerebrovascular accident, or subarachnoid hemorrhage can cause heart block (Cushing triad: bradycardia, hypertension, bradypnea).

Does the pt have any history of amyloidosis or sarcoidosis?

This disease can infiltrate the conduction system, notably the sinoatrial (SA), AV nodes, leading to heart block.

Has the pt traveled or been outdoors recently?

Chagas disease and Lyme disease cause heart block.

Perform a general review of symptoms

This may help elicit any potential medical problems complicating the heart block.

Weight gain and/or cold intolerance may suggest hypothyroidism, a potentially reversible cause of heart block.

 Perform a physical exam

Thyroid: Check for masses or thyromegaly.

Neck: Measure jugular venous distention. Cannon A waves can be seen in complete heart block (atrial contraction against a closed tricuspid valve due to atrioventricular dyssynchrony).

Cardiac: Listen for murmurs, irregular pulse, S3 or S4 as signs of congestive heart failure.

Lungs: Listen for rales, a sign of heart failure.

Neurologic: Check for focal deficits or mental status changes.

Check orthostatics

Evaluate whether the pt is able to compensate with a faster heart rate.

Use caution if pt is hypotensive or has had a syncopal episode.

Check the ECG

Pay particular attention to the P waves and PR interval.
- First-degree heart block: PR interval constant but >200 ms.
- Second-degree heart block:
    o (Mobitz I—Wenckebach): Progressively prolonged PR interval with an intermittent nonconducted P wave.
    o (Mobitz II): Constant PR interval with intermittent nonconducted P waves.
- Third-degree (complete) heart block: P waves are not conducted and not related to the QRS complex.

Attempt to differentiate whether the pt has sinus bradycardia, first-, second-, or third-degree heart block.

Evaluate for left bundle branch or right bundle branch blocks.

Check the following labs

Cardiac enzymes to rule out recent myocardial ischemia or infarction.

Thyroid function tests to rule out hypothyroidism.

Digoxin level and/or urine drug screen to check for TCA use.

A ### Sinus bradycardia

Heart rate <60 bpm.

First-degree heart block

An atrioventricular conduction delay with PR duration (time from the end of the P wave to the beginning of the QRS complex) >200 ms (1 large box on ECG paper)

Second-degree heart block

An atrioventricular block where an occasional impulse from the atria does not propagate to the ventricles, resulting in a nonconducted beat

Third-degree heart block (complete heart block)

Complete electrical dissociation between the atrium and the ventricles

P ### If the pt is asymptomatic, observation and discontinuation of any agents that may block the AV node (e.g., β-blockers, Ca channel blockers, digoxin, TCAs) is all that is needed

If the pt is symptomatic, consider the following

Administer atropine.
* Increases SA and AV nodal conduction.
* Not effective if the pt has had a heart transplant.

Administer epinephrine.
* Used if the pt is in asystole or has continued symptomatic bradycardia despite atropine use.

Place transcutaneous pacemaker leads on the pt and start pacing if medical management fails.

Place transvenous pacemaker if above measures fail.

If bradycardia is caused by a medication overdose and pt is symptomatic, administer

IM or IV glucagon for β-blocker overdose

IV Ca salts (calcium gluconate or chloride) for Ca channel blocker overdose

Digoxin-specific antibody fragments for digoxin overdose (typically restricted to life-threatening toxicity only)

Arrange admission to a monitored nursing floor or coronary care unit

CARDIAC ARREST

S **Determine how long the pt has been in cardiac arrest**

Determine how long the pt was unconscious before CPR was initiated

A delay of more than 5 minutes is generally associated with major neurologic injury.

Witnessed arrest with immediate initiation of CPR improves outcomes.

Obtain a quick past medical history

Does the pt have a history of sudden cardiac death or arrhythmias?
  • Recurrent arrhythmia
Has the pt had a myocardial infarction (MI) in the past or a coronary artery bypass graft
  or percutaneous coronary intervention (PCI)?
  • Possible acute myocardial infarction
Does the pt have a history of depression or suicide attempts?
  • Hints at a possible overdose and repeat suicide attempt

Does the pt have a known code status?

What was the pt doing before arresting?

If eating, the pt may have choked and had a primary respiratory arrest.
If the pt was working on his or her house or car, he or she might have been electrocuted.

Did the the pt complain of any pain or other symptoms before arresting?

Lightheadedness, palpitations, or a racing heartbeat suggests an arrhythmia as cause.
Chest pain may be seen with MI or pulmonary embolism (PE).
Shortness of breath is also associated with MI and PE.

Is the pt a victim of a recent trauma?

Internal injuries and exsanguination need to be ruled out.

Does the pt have any risk factor for PE?

See Pulmonary Embolism, p. 376.

O **Ventilate the pt with a bag-valve-mask or intubate**

Quickly place the pt on a monitor and determine the underlying rhythm

Pts in ventricular fibrillation or ventricular tachycardia have the greatest survival rate if
  they are defibrillated early.
Follow the appropriate advanced cardiac life support (ACLS) algorithm.
If the pt has a normal rhythm on the monitor, think of potential treatable causes for
  pulseless electrical activity:

– Hypovolemia	– Acidosis	– Cardiac tamponade
– Hypo-/hyperkalemia	– Hypothermia	– Pulmonary embolism
– Hypoxemia	– Overdose	– Tension pneumothorax

Initiate chest compressions and check frequently for a spontaneous pulse

Perform a physical exam

Look closely for signs of trauma or drug use.
Ensure that the pt has equal breath sounds bilaterally.
Note any tracheal deviation as a sign of tension pneumothorax.

If concerned about hypothermia, check a core body temperature

Establish venous access to administer medications

If unable to obtain venous access, the following medications can be administered down
  the endotracheal tube:

– Epinephrine	– Lidocaine
– Atropine	– Narcan

Obtain a CXR

Look for signs of pneumothorax, enlarged cardiac silhouette as a surrogate marker for cardiac tamponade, and any rib fractures or other signs of trauma.

Obtain an ECG

If signs of an acute MI are present, the pt needs to be taken to cardiac catheterization lab ASAP. Thrombolytics are contraindicated with prolonged chest compressions.

Check the following labs

Cardiac enzymes to rule out ischemia

Full set of electrolytes to exclude any major electrolyte disturbance

CBC to exclude anemia

ABG to demonstrate whether the pt has been oxygenated and ventilated well and if the patient has a normal pH

Cardiopulmonary arrest -or-

Myocardial infarction -or-

Pulmonary embolism

Differential diagnosis

   – Overdose   – Cerebrovascular accident

Follow ACLS protocols

Treat underlying disorders

Replace electrolytes immediately.

If the pt has hyperkalemia, you may administer:

   – Ca gluconate   – Albuterol

   – IV insulin (with dextrose)   – Kayexalate

   – Furosemide (loop diuretic)

If overdose, treat accordingly.

If hypovolemic or hemorrhaging, treat aggressively with IV hydration and/or administer blood products (packed red blood cells, fresh frozen plasma, platelets, etc.).

If the pt is having a myocardial infarction

If possible, make arrangements for immediate PCI.

Again, thrombolytics (tPA) are typically contraindicated because of the risk of bleeding post-CPR.

If unable to establish a perfusable rhythm within 30–60 minutes, the pt is typically pronounced dead

Follow local guidelines concerning the notification of your local coroner or medical examiner.

Arrange for admission to the coronary care unit

If normal circulation is restored.

ENDOCARDITIS

S **What are the pt's current symptoms?**

Common presenting symptoms include:

– Fever	– Malaise	– Sweats
– Myalgias	– Arthralgias	– Weight loss
– Shortness of breath	– Chest pain	– Rash

Common complications of endocarditis that pts may present with include:
- – Cerebrovascular accident – Renal failure
- – Myocardial infarction – Chest pain from pulmonary infarction
- – Heart block – Congestive heart failure

Does the pt have any risk factors for endocarditis?

Indwelling venous catheter
History of endocarditis
Poor dentition
Intravenous drug abuse (IVDA)
Diabetes
Recent surgical procedure
Valvular heart disease
- • Mitral valve prolapse
- • Bicuspid aortic valve
- • Prosthetic heart valve

Has the pt been on antibiotics recently?

May affect sensitivity of blood cultures.

Obtain a good review of symptoms

May elicit other causes of fever and/or infection source.

O **Perform a physical exam**

Look for physical signs of endocarditis:
- • *Osler nodes:* Painful nodular lesions normally seen on the extremities
- • *Janeway lesions:* Painless microhemorrhages typically seen on the palms or soles of feet
- • *Splinter hemorrhages:* Microhemorrhages under fingernails or toenails
- • *Roth spots:* Retinal hemorrhages with central clearing
- • *Petechiae:* Can be seen on mucosal membranes, conjunctiva, and hard palate
- • New-onset murmur

Obtain an ECG

A heart block may be seen with extension of the infection into the atrioventricular node or conduction system.
Ischemic changes can be seen if the vegetations embolize down a coronary artery.

Obtain a CXR

May demonstrate pulmonary infarctions or pneumonia.

Obtain blood cultures

Two to three sets taken over several hours maximize isolation of the causative agent.

Obtain CBC, electrolytes, and renal function tests

An elevated WBC may be seen.
Anemia is associated with subacute endocarditis.
May see renal failure from embolization to renal arteries.

Consider an echocardiogram

Evaluates heart valves and may notice vegetations.
TTE may miss 20% of vegetations. Consider TEE if clinical suspicion is high.

Endocarditis -or-

Noninfective endocarditis

Duke criteria are used to make diagnosis. Need two major **or** one major and two minor **or** five minor criteria to make diagnosis.

- Major criteria
  - ○ Positive blood culture for typical organisms (HACEK, viridans streptococci, *Streptococcus bovis*) in two different blood cultures
  - ○ Evidence of endocardial involvement
    - Oscillating intracardiac mass on valve or supporting structures, in the path of regurgitant jets, or on implanted material in the absence of an alternative anatomic explanation or
    - Abscess or
    - New partial dehiscence of prosthetic valve
- Minor criteria
  - ○ Predisposition: Predisposing heart condition or IVDA
  - ○ Fever: temperature >38.0°C (100.4°F)
  - ○ *Vascular phenomena:* Major arterial emboli, septic pulmonary infarcts, mycotic aneurysm, intracranial hemorrhage, conjunctival hemorrhages, and Janeway lesions
  - ○ *Immunologic phenomena:* Glomerulonephritis, Osler nodes, Roth spots, and rheumatoid factor
  - ○ *Microbiologic evidence:* Positive blood culture but does not meet a major criterion, as noted above, or serologic evidence of active infection with organism consistent with infective endocarditis (IE)
  - ○ *Echocardiographic findings:* Consistent with IE but does not meet a major criterion, as noted above

Differential diagnosis

Systemic vasculitis

Rheumatologic disease

 Start empiric antibiotics

Consider vancomycin, gentamicin, and rifampin.

Consider surgical intervention for

Signs of congestive heart failure or hemodynamic compromise caused by valvular heart disease

Evidence of paravalvular abscess

Progressive heart block

Persistent bacteremia despite appropriate antibiotics

Infection of a prosthetic heart valve

Admit to monitored nursing floor or ICU

Need to monitor for progressive heart block and hemodynamic instability.

HYPERTENSIVE CRISIS

S **What are the pt's current symptoms?**

Most pts with hypertension (HTN) are asymptomatic.

Symptoms that correlate with end-organ damage:

- Neurologic symptoms
  - Headache
  - Seizure
  - Confusion
  - Focal deficits
  - Coma
- Cardiac symptoms
  - Chest pain
  - Palpitations
  - Congestive heart failure (CHF)
- Renal symptoms
  - Hematuria
  - Oliguria
  - Proteinuria

Does the pt have a history of HTN?

If this is an initial presentation, need to exclude secondary causes of hypertension:

- Pheochromocytoma
- Primary hyperaldosteronism
- Cocaine and illicit drug use
- Coarctation of the aorta
- Renal artery stenosis

What medications is the pt taking?

Inquire about herbal supplements, especially ephedra and licorice.

Has the pt missed any doses? Can see rebound HTN with missed doses of clonidine.

Obtain a detailed social history

Inquire about illicit drug use, alcohol use, and tobacco use.

Perform a review of symptoms

May reveal a secondary cause of HTN.

O **Perform a physical exam**

Fundoscopic exam: Evaluate for retinal hemorrhage and papillary edema, signs of end-organ damage.

Lungs: May hear rales as a sign of CHF.

Cardiac:
- Evaluate point of maximum impulse for a prominent apical impulse.
- Palpate for right ventricle heave.
- Make note of any murmur or S4.

Abdomen: Listen for renal bruits, sign of renal artery stenosis.

Neurologic: Ensure that there are no focal deficits or signs of a cerebrovascular accident (CVA).

Obtain an ECG

Evaluate for cardiac ischemia.

May see left ventricular hypertrophy as a sign of long-standing HTN.

Consider CT scan of head if there are any neurologic signs

Rule out intracranial hemorrhage (ICH) or subarachnoid hemorrhage (SAH).

Obtain electrolytes, renal function tests, cardiac enzymes, and urinalysis

Rule out renal insufficiency.

May see hematuria and proteinuria.

Cardiac enzymes may be elevated as a result of cardiac injury and strain.

Obtain a urine drug screen if drug abuse is suspected

Obtain a CXR

May see signs of pulmonary congestion and cardiomegaly.

Evaluate mediastinum for widening, which may be associated with aortic dissection.

Hypertension

If pt's blood pressure is elevated, but there is no evidence of end-organ damage

Hypertensive urgency

Severe HTN where there is a pending risk for end-organ damage.

Blood pressure needs to be lowered over the next 24 hours in order to prevent end-organ injury.

Hypertensive crisis/emergency

Severely elevated blood pressure with evidence of end-organ damage.

Blood pressure needs to be lowered immediately in order to prevent continued end-organ damage.

Differential diagnosis

- Pheochromocytoma
- CVA
- Brain tumor
- Cocaine or amphetamine use
- Aortic dissection
- ICH or SAH

P Control the blood pressure

If asymptomatic and the pt has not taken his or her home medications, you can give the usual home dosing and follow closely.

If asymptomatic, can give oral medications. Consider:

- Clonidine
- Nitroglycerin
- β-Blockers
- Hydralazine
- Ca channel blockers
- ACE-inhibitors

If there is evidence of end-organ damage, immediate control of blood pressure warrants starting an IV medication for titratable control.

- Common medications used include:
  - Nitroprusside
  - Esmolol
- Goal drop in blood pressure is 20%–25% of starting blood pressure over the first 60 minutes.
- Because of compensatory measures in the brain and kidneys, dropping the blood pressure too quickly can lead to CVA and hypoperfusion of the kidneys.
- Place arterial line for accurate and constant blood pressure measurement.

Admit to ICU if there is evidence of end-organ damage

Admit to monitored nursing floor for hypertensive urgency

Discharge home

If the pt is asymptomatic, responded to treatment in the ED, and will have close follow-up with a primary care provider in the a.m., you can discharge home.

MYOCARDIAL INFARCTION

S **Determine the PQRST of the pain (see Chest Pain, p. 170)**

When inquiring about pain, ask if pts are having any discomfort, because some pts will deny pain but report intense pressure, heaviness, or a discomfort in their chest.

Have they had similar pain in the past? Does the pain change with exertion or stress?

Suggests prior history of angina

Does the pt have any risk factors for myocardial infarction (MI)?

Risk factors include a history of cigarette smoking, hypercholesterolemia, hypertension, diabetes, obesity, prior MI, male gender, prior angioplasty or percutaneous coronary intervention (PCI), or family history of MI.

Diabetics frequently present without typical signs and symptoms of MI, and typically will not experience pain.

Does the pt have any associated symptoms?

Diaphoresis, shortness of breath, nausea, or vomiting

Has any treatment been initiated before your evaluation?

Have paramedics given nitroglycerin? Was there any improvement with treatment rendered?

Has the pt received aspirin or take aspirin daily?

Has the pt tried self-treatment with antacids? Did it help?

Obtain a medication list

Inquire if any medications have been missed or if there have been any recent changes.

Obtain a past medical history

Particular attention needs to be paid to any history of coronary artery bypass graft or PCI.
• When, which vessels, and were there any complications postprocedure?
• Has there been any recent cardiac catheterization or stress testing?

O **Evaluate vital signs**

Ensure that the pt is hemodynamically stable.

Perform a physical exam

Cardiac: May hear an S3 or a new murmur.

Lungs: Typically normal exam. Listen for egophony, or pleural rub, which suggests an alternative diagnosis. Rales may indicate acute heart failure from infarction.

Often, the exam is normal and not very informative.

Obtain an ECG within 10 minutes of arrival

ST elevation in two or more contiguous leads or new left bundle branch block warrants emergent revascularization.

May also see hyperacute T-waves, inverted T-waves, or ST depression (reciprocal changes).

Consider a right-side ECG if there are peripheral signs of heart failure.

Approximately 20% of initial ECGs do not show any ischemic changes; serial ECGs may be needed.

Obtain cardiac enzymes

CK, CKMB, and Trop-I may be elevated as early as 4 hours after the onset of pain.
• Trop-I can remain elevated for up to 2 weeks (cleared by kidneys).

Myoglobin may be elevated as early as 2 hours but lacks significant specificity.

Trop-I is the most specific enzyme available.

Several sets of enzymes over an 8- to 12-hour period are needed to completely rule out MI.

Obtain a CXR

May exclude other causes of chest pain.

 Myocardial infarction

Sudden interruption or insufficiency of the supply of blood to the heart.

Differential diagnosis

- Unstable angina
- Chest pain
- Congestive heart failure
- Pleurisy
- Pneumonia
- Gastroesophageal reflux disease

Initiate anti-ischemia therapy immediately. Pts should receive

Aspirin: 325 mg or four 81-mg aspirins. If on chronic aspirin therapy, this does not need to be repeated.
- Administer clopidogrel if the pt is aspirin intolerant or PCI is planned.

Nitroglycerin: Sublingual tablets, topical paste, or IV formulations are available.
- Titrate nitroglycerin for pain relief while ensuring that SBP remains greater than 90.

Morphine: Provides pain relief, decreases the preload, and reduces the pt's anxiety. The resulting effect is a decrease in overall myocardial oxygen demand and decrease in myocardial ischemia.

Heparin: Unfractionated or low-molecular-weight heparin; helps prevent extension of the thrombus.

β-Blocker: Avoid if the pt is hypotensive, bradycardic, or has severe lung disease.
- Decreases myocardial oxygen demand
- Has been shown to improve mortality if given within 12 hours

Arrange for emergent revascularization

Primary PCI has been associated with improved outcomes if done within 2 hours.
- If the pt is going for primary PCI, consider giving clopidogrel and/or a glycoprotein IIb/IZIa. Shown to decrease the rate of premature closure of the PCI site.

Thrombolytics should be given if pain has been present for <12 hours, and primary PCI cannot be done within 2 hours.
- Major contraindications to thrombolytic therapy include:
  o Active bleeding
  o Major surgery or trauma in the past 3 weeks
  o Neurosurgery or stroke in the past 3 months
  o Prolonged (>10 minutes) or traumatic CPR

Monitor for reperfusion arrhythmias

Typically occur within the first hour after revascularization. V-Tach and an accelerated idioventricular tachycardia are most common. May see sinus bradycardia or complete heart block.

Admit to coronary care unit

PALPITATIONS

S **What symptoms did the pt experience?**
Pts may complain of a racing heartbeat or a feeling of their heart skipping a beat.

Was there associated lightheadedness or syncope?
Seen with arrhythmias that cause hemodynamic compromise. Requires a more thorough workup because it may be a warning sign for sudden cardiac death.

What was the pt doing when the palpitations started?
Exercise and psychological stress may induce arrhythmias.

Inquire about recent caffeine, alcohol, tobacco, or cocaine/amphetamine use
These agents can cause myocardial irritation and excitation, causing arrhythmias.

How long did the palpitations last and are they still present?

Does the pt have a history of palpitations, coronary atherosclerotic disease (CAD), or congestive heart failure (CHF)?
Palpitations may be a sign of ischemia or CHF exacerbation.
If they have had palpitations before, do they know what arrhythmia they had and how it was treated? May help direct your current treatment.

What has the pt done to try to stop the palpitations?
Some pts know to try a Valsalva maneuver by bearing down, cough, or perform carotid massage, which increase vagal tone.

Obtain a thorough past medical history
History of chronic obstructive pulmonary disease (COPD) or pulmonary disorders is associated with atrial flutter, atrial fibrillation, and multifocal atrial tachycardia.
History of CHF or CAD is associated with V-Tach, heart block, and premature ventricular contractions (PVCs).

O **Perform a physical exam**
Look for signs of a CHF or COPD exacerbation. Generally, the exam is normal and not very helpful in determining the cause of the arrhythmia.

Obtain an ECG
Look for signs of ischemia, heart block, or an arrhythmia.
Atrial flutter will show flutter waves, which are organized, rapid (300 bpm, "sawtooth pattern" on ECG) depolarizations of the atrium with variable conduction to the ventricles.
Atrial fibrillation will have an absence of P waves because atrial activity is disorganized, with irregular conduction to the ventricles.
V-Tach will typically show a regular ventricular response with a widened QRS complex. Ventricular response is independent of any atrial activity.
Look for delta waves: A shortened PR interval with a slurring of the initial portion of the QRS complex. Diagnostic of Wolfe-Parkinson-White syndrome and represents a bypass tract between the atrium and the ventricles.

Place pt on a cardiac monitor

Obtain a CXR
May show signs of pneumonia or CHF exacerbation

Check electrolytes and/or thyroid-stimulating hormone (TSH)
Hypo-/hyperthyroidism and electrolyte imbalances of potassium, calcium, or magnesium may cause arrhythmias.

If suspicious for cardiac ischemia (e.g., chest pain), check cardiac enzymes

A Atrial fibrillation/flutter –or–

Supraventricular tachycardia/PSVT –or–

Ventricular tachycardia –or–

Premature ventricular contractions (PVCs)

P Consider an adenosine challenge

If unable to determine rhythm because of a rapid rate, consider an adenosine challenge.

Administer 6, 12, or 18 mg of adenosine rapid IV push. Causes transient block of the atrioventricular (AV) node, allowing you to see the atrial activity. Can be associated with a brief period of asystole.

May correct palpitations caused by AV nodal reentrant tachycardia.

Consider cardioversion

If the pt becomes hemodynamically unstable as per advanced cardiac life support (ACLS) protocols

Premature ventricular contractions do not require any treatment if there is no evidence of hemodynamic compromise

If the pt had lightheadedness or syncope, need to rule out undiagnosed ventricular tachycardia.

Atrial fibrillation/flutter

Typically require admission for cardiac monitoring, anticoagulation, and workup to consist of TSH and echocardiogram.

Cardioversion should not be attempted in the ED until after the pt has been fully evaluated because of the risk of CVA.

Treat any underlying pulmonary disorder that may be exacerbating the cardiac arrhythmia.

Control rate with calcium channel blockers, β-blockers, and/or digoxin (uncommon).

If concerned about Wolff-Parkinson-White syndrome, rate can be controlled with procainamide. Avoid digoxin, calcium channel blockers, and β-blockers.

Supraventricular tachycardia/PSVT

May be associated with tobacco, alcohol, caffeine, and drug use.

Typically transient in nature, and treatment is to discontinue the causative agent.

Can obtain rate control with β-blockers, calcium channel blockers.

If recurrent or evidence of an accessory pathway, the pt may require an electrophysiology (EP) study.

Ventricular tachycardia

If stable, can attempt to convert by administering lidocaine or amiodarone.

- Amiodarone will affect your ability to perform an EP study, although it is considered the first-line agent according to ACLS protocols.

Admit to MNF or ICU

Consider discharge home

If the pt's symptoms were mild, workup in ED was negative, and there is good follow-up, consider sending the pt home with a Holter monitor.

SYNCOPE

S **Did the pt truly lose consciousness? Was the event witnessed?**

If witnessed, determine how long the pt was unconscious and if there were any symptoms leading up to the event.

Ask about seizure activity or incontinence. Some pts can have jerking movement of their limbs that are believed to be seizures by the lay bystander.

How long did it take for the pt to begin to think and act normally? Syncope should have a quick return to baseline, where a seizure may have a prolonged postictal phase.

What was the pt doing before the syncopal episode?

Prolonged standing, standing up quickly, and emotional upset can all trigger a vasovagal episode, leading to syncope.

Defecating and micturition can trigger a syncopal episode by activating hypersensitive peripheral receptors.

Has the pt been eating or drinking appropriately?

Does the pt have a history of syncope?

Determine circumstances around prior episodes. Has the pt had any testing done to determine the etiology?

Where there any symptoms before the episode?

Lightheadedness, chest pain, palpitations, and a racing heartbeat all suggest a cardiac cause of syncope.

Headache, confusion, focal weakness, or numbness suggests a neurologic cause.

Does the pt have a history of diabetes, seizures, coronary atherosclerotic disease, hypertension, congestive heart failure, or arrhythmias?

Prior cardiac history increases risk for myocardial infarction (MI) and arrhythmias.

Is there a history of hypoglycemia?

Has the pt started any new medications? What medications are being taken?

New hypertensive agents may be causing postural hypotension and syncope, such as alpha blockers for BPH.

O **Evaluate the pt's vital signs**

Perform orthostatics, which will help determine if postural (orthostatic) hypotension is the cause.

Perform a physical exam

Look for signs of trauma or injury.

Evaluate mental status, and ensure that there are no neurologic deficits.

Perform a rectal exam to rule out occult GI bleeding.

Generally, the physical exam is completely normal.

Obtain an ECG

Evaluate for signs of ischemia or arrhythmia.

Check the pt's blood sugar

New-onset diabetes with dehydration may present with syncope.

If history suggests or pt has risk factors for MI, obtain cardiac enzymes

If there were any neurologic symptoms preceding the event, obtain a CT scan of the head

Exclude intracranial hemorrhage, subarachnoid hemorrhage, or space-occupying mass as cause.

Consider a CT if the pt has fallen and there is evidence of a head injury.

If there is a possibility of pregnancy, check β-hCG

If the pt has a seizure disorder, consider checking levels of any antiseizure medications

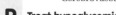 **A** Syncope

In most cases, a cause for the syncopal episode cannot be determined. A good history is your best weapon in determining the cause.

Most clinical studies are normal and nondiagnostic.

Differential diagnosis

- Seizure
- Cerebrovascular accident
- Hypoglycemia
- Anxiety or panic attack

P Treat hypoglycemia with intravenous fluids (IVFs) and D50

Treat arrhythmias as indicated

If orthostatic or signs of dehydration present, administer IVFs

Recheck orthostatics after fluid resuscitation to ensure that symptoms have resolved.

If pt has suffered an injury, further inpatient workup is warranted

Generally, suggests that there was no warning or preceding symptoms that indicated a sudden cardiac arrhythmia as cause.

Consider obtaining an echocardiogram

If valvular heart disease is suspected

Admit pts to a monitored nursing floor or the ICU with any of the following

- Syncope while supine
- Old age
- Trauma
- Recurrent syncope
- Prolonged loss of consciousness
- Headache or focal neurologic signs
- Young pt with exertional syncope

Consider discharge home

Pts who have classic vasovagal syncope where the precipitating factor is identified (e.g., prolonged standing in church) and no cardiac symptoms or significant risk factors can be discharged home.

UNSTABLE ANGINA

S Determine the PQRST of the pain (see Chest Pain, p. 170)

Does the pt have a known history of angina?

Has there been a change in the amount of exercise the pt can perform before getting short of breath or developing chest pain?

Has the pt experienced chest pain at rest?

All initial diagnoses of angina are considered unstable by definition, as they are undifferentiated.

Do any specific actions exacerbate the chest pain?

Walking, stair climbing, or aerobic exercise is more consistent with cardiac ischemia.

What makes the pain or symptoms resolve?

Pain that resolves quickly with rest or nitroglycerin is consistent with angina.

Nitroglycerin can relieve esophageal pain and spasm; therefore, relief with nitroglycerin is not diagnostic of angina.

Does the pt have any associated symptoms?

Shortness of breath, nausea, vomiting, and diaphoresis. Diaphoresis is not a common symptom and should increase your suspicion for true pain/ischemia.

Has the pt undergone any coronary revascularization procedures in the past?

Symptoms following coronary artery bypass graft (CABG) or percutaneous coronary intervention (PCI) can he caused by subacute closure of the grafts, stents, or angioplasty site.

What are the pt's risk factors for coronary atherosclerosis?

See Myocardial Infarction, p. 362.

Ask about any new medications or whether the pt has missed any doses

Recurrence of angina may be caused by pt noncompliance with medical management.

Perform a general review of systems

This may help elicit any potential medical problems complicating the chest pain.

O Perform a physical exam

Lungs: Typically normal, may hear rales or wheezing if congestive heart failure (CHF) present.

Chest: Note any reproducible pain, although it may be present incidentally with cardiac ischemia.

Cardiac: Note any irregular pulse, murmurs, S3 or S4.

Extremities: Note any pedal edema, seen with CHF.

Rectal exam: Must be performed to rule out occult GI bleeding if you plan to initiate anticoagulation therapy.

Check the ECG

Be sure to compare it to an old ECG. Occasionally, individuals will demonstrate pseudonormalization (e.g., their baseline T-waves are inverted, but now they are upright and normal-appearing on your present ECG) of their ECG, making it difficult to diagnose ischemia changes.

Obtain a CXR

Look for signs of infiltrate, pulmonary edema, pleural effusion, cardiomegaly, or widened mediastinum (suggest aortic dissection).

Check the following labs

Cardiac enzymes

- Myoglobin will show elevations within 2 hours, although it is not specific for cardiac injury.
- Elevation in Trop-I is specific for cardiac muscle injury.

- Elevation in CK can be seen with any muscle injury.
- Individuals with renal failure may have chronically elevated cardiac enzymes.
- NQWMI or non-ST elevation myocardial infarction can only be ruled out by obtaining serial enzymes over a 6- to 12-hr period.

Electrolytes, BUN, creatinine: Rule out electrolyte disturbance or renal failure.

CBC: Ensure that anemia is not the cause of demand ischemia.

A Unstable Angina

Severe paroxysmal pain in the chest associated with an insufficient supply of blood to the heart that is occurring at rest or with increasing frequency. Pain should be relieved with rest or nitroglycerin.

Myocardial infarction

Sudden interruption or insufficiency of the supply of blood to the heart.

Differential diagnosis
    – Chest pain   – Pneumonia   – Pulmonary embolism

P Initiate treatment for ischemia

Institute the following treatment:

- Place the pt on oxygen.
- Give nitroglycerin sublingually or IV if SBP >100.
- Give aspirin 325 mg if not allergic.
- Consider administering β-blocker if heart rate >70 and not hypotensive
- Consider morphine 2–4 mg IV as needed for pain.

If the pt has ECG changes, consider starting heparin therapy.

Titrate medications to provide effective pain relief

Ongoing pain represents continued cardiac muscle injury.

If the pt has ECG changes or has had a recent PCI or CABG, discuss the case with the pt's cardiologist or primary care provider

Discuss initiating glycoprotein IIb/IIIa therapy if the pt has ST depression, positive cardiac enzymes, high risk for ischemia, or if emergency revascularization is planned.

Arrange admission to a monitored nursing floor or coronary care unit

VENOUS THROMBOSIS

S **Does the pt have pain or swelling in one or both legs?**

Deep venous thrombosis (DVT) may involve both legs, but typically is found in only one leg.

Bilateral swelling is more consistent with congestive heart failure (CHF).

Does the pt have any risk factors for a venous thrombosis?

Risk factors include the following:
- Recent surgery or immobilization
- Estrogen or birth control pill use
- Pregnancy
- History of hypercoagulable state
- Tobacco use
- Recent travel
- Cancer
- Prior history of DVT/pulmonary embolism (PE)

Does the pt have any associated symptoms of chest pain or shortness of breath?

May signify a PE and warrants additional evaluation.

Has the pt suffered any trauma to the extremity?

Suggests pain and swelling caused by cellulitis or focal abscess.

Recent fracture or soft tissue injury increases the risk for DVT.

Obtain a thorough past medical history

History of cirrhosis, renal insufficiency, or CHF may explain swelling in lower extremities.

Prior surgery or saphenous vein graft harvest for coronary artery bypass graft is associated with chronic leg swelling postoperatively.

Has the pt been placed on any new medications or have any medications been discontinued?

Any change in CHF or cirrhosis management may lead to increased peripheral edema.

O **Perform a physical exam**

Lungs: Listen for pleural rub, which may be seen with PE.

Cardiac: Listen for new murmurs and palpate for right ventricle heave, which may occur with PE.

Extremities: Measure both calves and compare, palpate for venous cords. Are there any signs of cellulitis (e.g., redness, warmth, swelling, tenderness)?

Check the following labs

CBC, coagulation studies: Baseline studies in case anticoagulation is needed.

Consider checking a D-dimer: ELISA D-dimer is 80% sensitive but nonspecific for DVT.

Consider performing a hypercoagulable evaluation. Important to consider in the ED because testing can be affected by the start of heparin and/or warfarin therapies.

Obtain lower extremity venous duplex

High sensitivity/specificity for proximal veins, but less so for distal calf veins. Test performance is affected by body habitus and tissue edema.

May see Baker (popliteal) cyst as cause of swelling.

Cannot evaluate pelvic veins.

Consider MRI

If there is a strong suspicion for pelvic or inferior vena cava (IVC) thrombosis, which is common after Ob/Gyn surgery.

Consider PE evaluation if the pt has chest pain or shortness of breath

See Pulmonary Embolism, p. 376.

Deep venous thrombosis

A blood clot in the deep veins of the legs. Blood clots above the knee have an increased risk of dislodging and becoming a PE.

Superficial venous thrombosis

A blood clot in the superficial veins of the legs not associated with PE.

Differential diagnosis

- Cellulitis
- Cirrhosis
- CHF
- Nephrotic syndrome
- Lymphedema
- Pregnancy

 Deep venous thrombosis

Begin anticoagulation to prevent clot propagation and PE if no risk factors exist.
- Risk factors include:
  ○ Recent intracranial or subarachnoid hemorrhage
  ○ Active gastrointestinal bleeding
  ○ High risk for falls and subsequent head injury
- Low-molecular-weight heparin or unfractionated heparin can be initiated.
  ○ Can discontinue heparin therapy once warfarin has been therapeutic for 2 days.
- Anticoagulation duration depends on whether the clot is provoked or unprovoked.
  ○ If second DVT/PE or hypercoagulable state is found, the pt will need lifelong warfarin therapy.

Consider IVC filter placement in pts:
- Not suitable for anticoagulation
- Who developed DVT or PE while on anticoagulation
- With tenuous respiratory status where any PE may result in death

Treat pain with NSAIDs.

Superficial venous thrombosis

No indication for anticoagulation therapy unless clot is propagating into deep system.
Initiate conservative therapy.

- Rest
- Warm compresses
- Elevation
- NSAIDs

PULMONARY

PNEUMOTHORAX

S **What are the pt's symptoms?**
Typical symptoms include:
- Sudden onset of pleuritic chest pain on the affected side
- Dyspnea
- Tachypnea
- Cough

Does the pt have any risk factors for a pneumothorax?
- Smoking
- Trauma
- Atmospheric pressure change
- Genetic predisposition (e.g., α-1-antitrypsin deficiency, Marfan syndrome)
- Increased incidence in young, thin, tall men

Has the pt been involved in any trauma?
Penetrating trauma has the highest risk for pneumothorax.

Is there a prior history of pneumothorax?
Recurrent pneumothoraxes may need surgical intervention to prevent future occurrences.

Does the pt have any medical conditions?
Any disease that can affect pulmonary reserve (e.g., chronic obstructive pulmonary disease [COPD], cancer, cystic fibrosis, pulmonary embolus) will make the signs and symptoms of a pneumothorax more severe.

Obtain a social history
Smoking and cocaine inhalation have been associated with pneumothorax.

Perform a review of symptoms
May elicit symptoms consistent with an alternative diagnosis (e.g., pulmonary embolus, pneumonia, bronchitis).

O **Check pt's vital signs**
Ensure that pt is hemodynamically stable.
Hypotension, tachycardia, and tachypnea are seen with tension pneumothorax. Check SpO_2.

Perform a physical exam
General: Is there any respiratory distress?
HEENT: Is there jugular venous distention or tracheal deviation? These are signs of tension pneumothorax.
Lungs: Are breath sounds equal bilaterally? Typically will have diminished breath sounds on the affected side.
Chest: Any signs of trauma? Look for penetrating wounds, crepitus, or signs of blunt injuries.
Cardiac: Are the heart sounds displaced or muffled? Can occur with tension pneumothorax.
Extremities: Any signs of cyanosis?

If there are signs of tension pneumothorax, immediately proceed with needle decompression
Do NOT confirm suspicion with a CXR.

Obtain a CXR
Absence of vascular lung marking peripheral to a **radiolucent line** is diagnostic of a pneumothorax.
Upright expiratory CXR maximizes visualization.
CXR may miss an anterior pneumothorax.
A lateral decubitus CXR may aid in the visualization.

Consider chest CT scan
Highly sensitive and will detect a pneumothorax missed on CXR.

No laboratory studies are needed, although ABG may show hypoxemia and respiratory alkalosis

Pneumothorax
Free air in the pleural space
Four types:
- Primary: No underlying medical condition
- Secondary: Associated with an underlying lung disorder (e.g., COPD)
- Traumatic: Caused by trauma
- Iatrogenic: Result of a medical procedure (e.g., central line placement)

Tension pneumothorax
A true medical emergency
Occurs when air continues to leak from the lung into the pleural space and is unable to escape (one-way valve mechanism), increasing intrathoracic pressure. As the pressure increases, venous blood return is impaired and eventually stops, leading to cardiac arrest.

Differential diagnosis
- Pneumonia
- Pulmonary embolus
- Cardiac tamponade
- Chest wall contusion
- COPD exacerbation
- Asthma exacerbation
- Pleuritis
- Myocardial infarction

Tension pneumothorax
Immediate needle decompression is needed. Insert a 14-gauge needle in the second intercostal space at the midclavicular line. Diagnosis is confirmed when a rush of air is heard on placement and there is immediate improvement in blood pressure and respiratory effort.
Definitive treatment with tube thoracotomy is needed because needle decompression is a temporizing measure.

Pneumothorax
Small primary pneumothoraxes (<15%) in a hemodynamically stable pt can be observed in the ED for 6 hours. If no change is seen on follow-up CXR, the pt can be discharged home with close follow-up.
Pts with a >15% pneumothorax, comorbid conditions, hemodynamic instability, or poor pulmonary reserve should have a pigtail catheter inserted or tube thoracostomy.
Traumatic pneumothoraxes should be treated with the placement of a pigtail catheter or tube thoracostomy. A pigtail catheter is better tolerated, but is not large enough in caliber to evacuate blood, and should be restricted to pure pneumothoraxes.

PULMONARY EDEMA

S **What are the pt's current symptoms?**

Typical symptoms include:
– Dyspnea	– Tachypnea	– Diaphoresis
– Anxiety	– Orthopnea	– Weakness

Determine the type of onset and duration of the pt's symptoms?

Abrupt onset is seen with myocardial infarction, acute mitral regurgitation, hypertensive urgency, or toxic exposure.

Gradual onset is consistent with congestive heart failure (CHF) exacerbation or chronic toxic exposure.

Has the pt been involved in a recent trauma?

Pulmonary edema has been reported with central nervous system (CNS) injuries, trauma, seizures, aspiration, and with re-expansion of the lung after treatment for pneumothorax or effusion (>1 L).

Does the pt have any other medical problems?

Common associated diseases include:
– Aortic stenosis	– Mitral regurgitation	– CHF
– Renal failure	– Liver failure	– Hypertension
– Hyperthyroidism	– Seizures	– CNS injury

Obtain a social history to include occupational exposures

Chemical exposure and inhalation injuries can cause pulmonary edema.

Opioids and cocaine inhalation have been associated with pulmonary edema.

What medication does the pt take?

Will help determine risk factors and medical problems if the pt is unable to communicate.

O **Evaluate the pt's vital signs**

Note SpO_2, respiratory rate, and blood pressure.

Perform a physical exam

General: Respiratory distress? Able to speak in full sentences? Any signs of trauma?

HEENT: Jugular venous distention? Any soot or burns around the nose and mouth? (seen with inhalation injuries)

Lungs: Rales? Wheezing? Decreased breath sounds? Accessory muscle use?

Cardiac: Tachycardia? Murmurs? Gallop? Seen with CHF.

Abdomen: Ascites? Sometimes seen with CHF.

Extremities: Pedal edema, diminished pulses.

Obtain a CXR

Increased vascular markings (cephalization), pleural effusion, alveolar infiltrates, cardiomyopathy, and Kerley B lines (short linear markings in the lung periphery) may all be seen with pulmonary edema.

Obtain an ECG

Exclude myocardial infarction and myocardial ischemia.

Consider obtaining the following labs

CBC to exclude anemia and secondary high-output cardiac failure as cause

BUN, creatinine to evaluate renal function

LFTs to exclude liver failure

Cardiac enzymes to exclude myocardial infarction

BNP to exclude CHF

A **Pulmonary edema**

The leakage of intravascular fluid into the pulmonary interstitium and air spaces

Causes divided into two categories

- *Cardiogenic:* Includes valvular heart disease, cardiomyopathy, pericarditis, myocardial infarction, hypertensive crisis, and volume overload. The pulmonary edema is caused by increased hydrostatic pressure in the pulmonary capillaries, causing intravascular fluid to leak out.
- *Noncardiogenic:* Includes lung re-expansion, occupational or inhalation injuries, drugs (e.g., opioids, cocaine), aspiration, trauma, CNS injury, or sepsis. The pulmonary edema is caused by damage to the pulmonary capillary permeability, which allows fluid to leak out of the intravascular space.

Differential diagnosis

    – COPD   – Pneumonia

    – Adult respiratory distress syndrome   – CHF

 P **Provide supplemental oxygen**

Maintain SpO_2 >92%.

Intubate or place on noninvasive positive pressure ventilation if in severe respiratory distress.

Cardiogenic pulmonary edema

Maximize cardiac function. Goals of therapy are to normalize afterload, preload, and cardiac output.

- If blood pressure is markedly elevated, give vasodilators to decrease afterload.
- Diurese the pt with loop diuretics if volume overload is suspected.
- Treat myocardial ischemia and infarction if present. Emergent reperfusion may be indicated.
- Consider inotropes (e.g., dopamine and/or dobutamine) for pump failure (inadequate cardiac output).

Most pts will require admission. All should be admitted to a monitored bed, and an ICU setting should be considered for any pt who requires mechanical ventilations or is hemodynamically unstable.

Pts with mild symptoms who improve with treatment in the ED, have normal vital signs and diagnostic tests, and have close follow-up can be considered for discharge.

Noncardiogenic pulmonary edema

Generally a self-limited process, and only supportive care is needed.

Treat causative agent and provide respiratory support.

All pts should be admitted and observed closely for progression of the edema.

PULMONARY EMBOLISM

S **What are the pt's current symptoms?**
Common symptoms include:
- Pleuritic chest pain
- Dyspnea
- Cough
- Hemoptysis
- Syncope
- Diaphoresis
- Anxiety
- Restlessness

Does the pt have any risk factors for deep venous thrombosis (DVT)?
See Venous Thrombosis, p. 370

Does the pt have a history of DVT, pulmonary embolus (PE), or hypercoagulable state?
Greater risk for repeat occurrence

Does the pt have any medical problems?
Preexisting pulmonary disorders will decrease pulmonary reserve and increase symptoms.
Cancer, lupus, obesity, and pregnancy are associated with hypercoagulable states and increased PE risk.

Has the pt recently delivered a baby?
Amniotic fluid embolus can occur postdelivery.

Has the pt suffered any long-bone fractures?
Recent long-bone fracture is associated with fat embolus.

Is the pt taking any medication?
May be on warfarin from prior DVT/PE, or estrogen, which increases thrombus risk.
Helps elicit other medical disorders.

Obtain a social history
Smoking increases the risk of thrombus formation.
IV drug abusers can suffer a pulmonary embolus from injected foreign bodies.

O **Check pt's vital signs**
Pay attention to SpO_2 and ensure that the pt is hemodynamically stable. Pts may present in cardiac arrest or shock.
May have a fever.

Perform a physical exam
General: Is the pt in respiratory distress?
Lungs: Wheezing? Rales? May hear diminished breath sounds or pleural rub over the affected area.
Cardiac: Tachycardia? Murmur? Right ventricular (RV) heave?
Extremities: Lower extremity swelling? Homans sign? Calf tenderness?

Obtain CXR
Usually normal. May see a Hampton hump (wedge-shaped infiltrate) or Westermark sign (area of decreased pulmonary vasculature). Pleural effusion may be present.

Obtain the following labs
ABG: May show hypoxemia and respiratory alkalosis.
PT, INR, PTT: Baseline studies before starting any anticoagulation medications.
D-dimer: A degradation product of fibrin, which is elevated in any state that causes a thrombus. Nonspecific but sensitive and can help rule out the diagnosis in low-risk pts (good negative predictive value).
CBC: Baseline study.
UA: Fat molecules in urine help secure diagnosis of fat embolus.
BUN, creatinine: Exclude renal insufficiency if LMWH is to be used.

Obtain a diagnostic study

Individual test will depend on the availability or expertise of your individual institution.

Chest CT scan, helical spiral CT: Very sensitive for proximal PEs but can miss subsegmental/peripheral PE.

Ventilation/perfusion scan: Sensitivity dependent on pretest probability. Underlying lung disease can affect the interpretation of the study.

Pulmonary angiogram: The gold standard, but the most invasive test and requires an angiographer.

Two negative studies are required to exclude the diagnosis if your pretest probability is high.

Obtain an ECG

Most common finding is sinus tachycardia. May show RV strain as evidenced by the classic S1Q3T3 pattern.

Consider lower extremity duplex

DVT does not confirm the diagnosis, but if positive will increase the likelihood of PE and dictate the same treatment be started.

Consider echocardiogram

Look for evidence of RV strain and dysfunction, which are criteria for giving thrombolytics.

 Pulmonary embolus

Virchow triad (i.e., venous stasis, hypercoagulable state, endothelial damage) describes the conditions that increase the risk for PE.

An embolus can be a thrombus, fat particles, or amniotic fluid.

Differential diagnosis

– Congestive heart failure	– Myocardial infarction	– Pneumonia	– Pleurisy
– Pneumothorax	– Asthma	– Chronic obstructive pulmonary disease	

P **Provide supplemental oxygen.**

Maintain SpO_2 >92%

Treat hypotension, if present, with IV fluids

Consider dobutamine if no response to IV fluids.

Start anticoagulation unless contraindicated

Unfractionated heparin versus LMWH (contraindicated in renal failure) at therapeutic doses

Can start warfarin and bridge on day 1 if no invasive procedures are planned

Consider inferior vena cava filter placement. Indicated for

Pts with contraindications for anticoagulation

Recurrent PE despite adequate anticoagulation

Pts with tenuous cardiopulmonary status, where an additional PE can be life ending

Consider systemic thrombolytics or catheter-directed thrombolysis

Indicated in cases where there is documented RV strain and dysfunction by echocardiogram

Consider pulmonary embolectomy in cases of refractory shock

Admit all pts to a monitored bed or ICU depending on status

GASTROINTESTINAL

ABDOMINAL AORTIC ANEURYSM

S **What are the pt's current symptoms?**

Unruptured aneurysms are typically asymptomatic, although pts may experience vague abdominal or back pain.

Ruptured aneurysms typically present with:
- Severe abdominal or back pain
- Weakness/fatigue
- Nausea/vomiting
- Syncope
- Lightheadedness
- Cardiac arrest

Does the pt have hematemesis?
- May signify an aortoenteric fistula. Normally associated with prior abdominal aortic aneurysm (AAA) repair.

Does the pt have a history of AAA?

Useful to know the last known size to make comparisons. Aneurysms typically grow 0.3–0.5 cm per year. Helpful to predict current size.

Does the pt have any risk factors for AAA?

– Atherosclerosis	– Hypertension	– Marfan syndrome
– Male gender	– Tobacco use	– Peripheral vascular disease
– Age >60		

Does the pt have any other medical problems?

Does the pt take any medications? Have any doses been missed?

Uncontrolled hypertension can exacerbate rupture of an aneurysm and is the leading cause of aortic dissection.

Ensure that pt is not on any anticoagulants.

Has the pt had any unexplained weight loss or early satiety?

Superior mesenteric artery syndrome is where the AAA compresses the duodenum, causing nausea, vomiting, and weight loss.

O **Evaluate the pt's vital signs.**

Hypertension will exacerbate ruptures, and hypotension may be seen with severe bleeding.

Perform a physical exam

Abdomen: Rigidity? Guarding? Listen for abdominal bruit. May be able to feel a pulsatile mass. Do not palpate too hard because it may cause rupture.

Skin: Look for signs of retroperitoneal hematoma. Grey-Turner sign is ecchymosis and hemorrhage along the flank. Cullen sign is ecchymosis over the periumbilical region.

Neurologic: May have weakness or numbness in the lower extremities due to spinal cord ischemia.

Obtain the following labs

CBC: May show anemia but is likely to be normal acutely. Establishes baseline.

PT, INR, PTT: Rule out coagulopathy.

Electrolytes, BUN, creatinine: Ensure normal renal function because aneurysm can involve renal arteries and cause renal failure.

Type and cross: Ensure that blood is available if transfusion indicated.

Obtain a diagnostic study

Abdominal ultrasound: Easy bedside test. Can make the diagnosis of aneurysm but insensitive for rupture.

Abdominal CT scan: Highly sensitive for aneurysm and rupture, although can only be done on stable pts. May help establish an alternative diagnosis.

Plain x-rays: Insensitive, but 55%–85% of AAAs (especially if calcified) can be seen on plain films. Classic findings are dilated calcified aortic wall, loss of psoas or renal shadow, or paravertebral soft tissue mass.

A **Abdominal aortic aneurysm**

Most AAAs originate below the renal arteries, and rupture may cause obstruction of renal, mesenteric, or spinal arteries with secondary renal failure, abdominal pain caused by bowel ischemia, and lower extremity paralysis, respectively.

The normal aorta is <2 cm in diameter, and the likelihood of rupture increases with aneurysms >5 cm. Asymptomatic aneurysms >5 cm should be repaired electively.

Differential diagnosis

- Renal colic
- Mesenteric ischemia
- Diverticulitis
- Pancreatitis
- Myocardial infarction
- Aortic dissection
- Peptic ulcer disease
- Biliary colic

P **If asymptomatic**

Elective repair if AAA >5 cm. 5% perioperative mortality with elective surgery.

Serial exams and management of hypertension, atherosclerosis if AAA <5 cm

Discharge pt if AAA is incidental finding, <5 cm, and pt has close follow-up.

If symptomatic

Hypotension: Treat by administering packed red blood cells and IV fluids.

If bedside ultrasound shows AAA and the pt is unstable, the pt should proceed to surgery without any additional diagnostic studies. Approximately 50% perioperative mortality with emergent repair following rupture.

If hemodynamically stable, the pt may undergo additional testing to rule out alternative diagnosis and evaluate extent of involvement of associated vascular structures.

Admit all pts. Most will require ICU admission because they can deteriorate quickly.

APPENDICITIS

S **Does the pt have any abdominal pain? Where is it located?**

Classic abdominal pain starts in the epigastric/periumbilical area and migrates to the right lower quadrant (RLQ) (McBurney point).

Pts at the extremes of age are more likely to have an atypical presentation.

- Pediatric pts may only present with lethargy.
- Elderly pts may present with mental status changes or vague symptoms.

Does the pain radiate anywhere?

Depending on location of the appendix, pain may radiate to the groin or flank.

Does anything exacerbate the pain?

Peritoneal pain is typically worsened by walking, hopping, or hitting bumps on the car ride to the hospital.

Does the pt have any associated symptoms?

    – Anorexia   – Nausea/vomiting   – Fever

Is the pt pregnant?

The pain in pregnancy can be anywhere in the abdomen, and the pt may have an atypical presentation.

When was the pt's last menses?

Ensure that pt is not pregnant and at risk for an ectopic pregnancy. Consider ovarian pathology, dysmenorrhea, or Mittelschmerz.

Does the pt have any other medical problems?

May help elicit an alternative diagnosis (e.g., diverticulitis)

Has the pt been on antibiotics recently?

Pt is more likely to present with an atypical presentation or prolonged, mild symptoms.

O **Evaluate the pt's vital signs**

Is there a fever? Is the pt hemodynamically stable?

Perform a physical exam

General: Does the pt appear toxic?

Abdomen: Point tenderness? Rebound? Guarding? Any pain with heel tap or pelvic shake?

- *Psoas sign:* Increased RLQ pain with extension of the right hip.
- *Obturator sign:* Increased RLQ pain with extension and internal rotation of right hip.
- *Rovsing sign:* RLQ pain with palpation of the left lower quadrant.

Gyn: Adnexal mass or tenderness? Vaginal bleeding? Cervical motion tenderness (CMT)?

- Rule out alternative diagnosis.
- CMT can be seen with any disease process that causes peritoneal signs.

GU: Any testicular masses or tenderness? Penile discharge?

Rectal: Check hemoccult. Rectal pain or tenderness?

Obtain the following labs

CBC: May see a leukocytosis.

UA: Should be normal but may see hematuria and pyuria.

β-hCG: Exclude unknown pregnancy.

Obtain a diagnostic study

Abdominal Ultrasound

Can show dilation of the appendix and abscess. Helpful if positive, but if negative, will often need to evaluate with a CT scan. Consider as a first-line test in very thin individuals or those where there is a suspicion of a pelvic pathology (e.g., ectopic pregnancy, ovarian cyst).

Abdominal CT Scan: With oral contrast can show >90% of appendicitis. Classic findings include appendiceal wall thickening, periappendiceal inflammation, and/or abscess. Very thin individuals make interpretation of CT extremely difficult because there is no separation between the loops of bowel and little adjacent intra-abdominal fat to demonstrate signs of inflammation (stranding).

A Appendicitis

Peak incidence between ages 10 and 30. Results when the appendiceal lumen is obstructed.

Differential diagnosis

- Pancreatitis
- Ectopic pregnancy
- Nephrolithiasis
- Diverticulitis
- Pelvic inflammatory disease
- Gastroenteritis
- Ovarian cyst
- Testicular torsion
- Intestinal obstruction

P Start IV fluids

Administer appropriate pain medication

Small doses of narcotics may help in diagnosis because they can help eliminate guarding and anxiety that confound the exam.

Start antibiotics

Third-generation cephalosporin or penicillin/β-lactamase inhibitor

Add anaerobic coverage with clindamycin or metronidazole if perforation is suspected.

Consult a general surgeon

If the pt is male and has classic findings, a surgeon may proceed to surgery without an imaging study. Appendectomy is treatment of choice.

Admit the pt for serial abdominal exams if diagnosis is not absolute after exam and diagnostic studies are complete.

Consider discharge

If the pt has no peritoneal signs and suspicion approaches zero, is able to tolerate food and liquids, and has close follow-up.

Pts should be observed in the ED for several hours and undergo serial abdominal exams to ensure that symptoms and exam do not worsen before discharging home.

Pts should not be discharged on antibiotics.

BOWEL OBSTRUCTION

S **Does the pt have any abdominal pain?**
Pain may be intermittent and colicky in nature or constant and crampy.
Pain is generally diffuse and difficult to localize.

Does the pt have nausea or vomiting?
May have bilious or fecal vomiting.

Does the pt have a history of abdominal surgery?
Any abdominal surgery increases the risk of adhesion formation and secondary bowel obstruction.
Recent surgery can be associated with an ileus and obstructive symptoms.

Does the pt have any hernias?
Incarceration of the intestine within the hernia can cause strangulation. Internal hernias are also possible, especially in patients with history of gastric bypass.

When was the pt's last bowel movement?
Constipation and lack of flatus are signs of a complete obstruction. A pt may still pass flatus with a partial obstruction.

Does the pt have any other medical problems?
Cancer increases the risk of peritoneal metastasis and adhesion formation.
Ulcerative colitis and Crohn disease can cause bowel inflammation and edema with secondary obstruction.

Is the pt taking any medications?
Obstruction is associated with opiates and anticholinergic medications.

Obtain a social history
Mesenteric ischemia is associated with tobacco use and peripheral vascular disease.

Obtain a review of systems
May help elicit an inciting cause of the obstruction.

O **Evaluate pt's vital signs**
Fever may signify perforation and secondary infection.

Perform a physical exam
General: Is the pt toxic?
Abdomen: Distention? Tenderness? Hyperactive bowel sounds? Seen with obstruction. Rebound tenderness? Suspect perforation.
Rectal: Hemoccult positive? Seen with peptic ulcer disease (PUD), ischemic bowel. Rectal tenderness? Suggests abscess or infection.

Obtain the following labs
CBC: May show leukocytosis.
Electrolytes, BUN, creatinine: Exclude electrolyte disturbance or renal failure.
Lactic acid: Pain out of proportion to exam suggests mesenteric ischemia, often associated with lactic acidosis.

Obtain abdominal x-rays
Classic findings include:
- Dilated loops of bowel
  - Can help localize obstruction by appearance of bowel. Colon has haustra that appear as lines that only partially cross the lumen of the colon. Small bowel has plicae circulares that completely cross the lumen.
- Air-fluid levels
- Lack of air in the rectum and distal bowel
Obtain a decubitus film to demonstrate free air if perforation is suspected.

Consider an abdominal CT scan

Can demonstrate obstruction and transition point (area where obstruction occurred).
   May show an alternative process.
Helps guide operative repair if needed.

A Bowel obstruction

Etiologies include hernia with incarceration, volvulus, intussusception, fecal impaction, adhesions, foreign bodies, bowel ischemia, malignancy, or obstruction caused by medications or electrolyte disturbances.

Differential diagnosis

- Gastroenteritis
- Pancreatitis
- Fecal impaction
- PUD
- Diverticulitis
- Pelvic inflammatory disease
- Appendicitis
- Mesenteric ischemia

P Start IV fluids. Keep pts NPO

Large fluid deficits may be present as a result of prolonged vomiting.

Administer antiemetics for nausea

If nausea is persistent and there is a large amount of abdominal distention, consider placing a nasogastric tube to decompress the stomach.

Consider antibiotics

If perforation is suspected or if there is a possibility of infection as evidenced by elevated WBC or fever
Penicillin/β-lactamase inhibitor or third-generation cephalosporin plus anaerobic coverage with metronidazole or clindamycin

Consult a general surgeon

If mesenteric ischemia, complete bowel obstruction, or strangulated hernia is suspected

Pts with partial obstruction or ileus can be admitted and observed

Treat causative illness if known (e.g., infection, electrolyte disturbance).

In children, colonic intussusception can be diagnosed and treated with a barium or air enema

BILIARY DISEASE

S **Does the pt have risk factors for cholecystitis?**
- Obese
- Female
- Pregnant
- Recent weight loss
- >40 (years old)
- History of gallstones

Does the pt have any pain?
Classic pain is in the right upper quadrant (RUQ) and exacerbated by eating meals with high fat content.
May radiate to the right shoulder.

How long has the pt been having symptoms?
Most pts will complain of intermittent RUQ pain after meals for several weeks or months before they present to the ED with severe pain.

Are there any associated symptoms?
Nausea and vomiting are common.

Does the pt have a fever or chills?
May be seen with cholangitis and acute cholecystitis.

Does the pt have any other medical problems?
Inflammatory bowel disease, cirrhosis, and diabetes increase risk for cholecystitis.
A history of pancreatitis may suggest prior gallstones.

Obtain a social history
Heavy alcohol use can cause cirrhosis, fatty liver, and pancreatitis.

O **Evaluate the pt's vital signs**

Perform a physical exam
HEENT: Scleral icterus or jaundice? Seen with hyperbilirubinemia.
Abdomen: RUQ tenderness? Murphy sign (the pt stops inhaling when the RUQ is being palpated)? Seen with cholecystitis.
Rectal: Should be normal. Positive hemoccult or blood on exam suggests alternative diagnosis. Clay-colored stool suggests biliary obstruction (e.g., pancreatic head mass).

Obtain the following labs
CBC: May see leukocytosis.
LFT: Alkaline phosphatase and bilirubin elevated in choledocholithiasis and may be elevated in cholecystitis.
Amylase/lipase: Elevated in pancreatitis.

Obtain a diagnostic study
RUQ ultrasound:
- May show gallbladder and ductile dilation, gallbladder wall thickening, and pericholecystic fluid.
- "Gold Standard": Visualization of gallbladder can be affected by bowel gas.

Abdominal CT scan:
- Helpful to rule out masses and other pathology. Does not visualize the gallbladder well.

Hepatobiliary iminodiacetic acid scan (HIDA):
- Nuclear medicine study shows uptake of radioactive isotope in the gallbladder from the biliary tree if there is no obstruction. Delayed filling or no filling is diagnostic of cholecystitis.

A **Acute cholecystitis**
Acute inflammation and obstruction of the gallbladder resulting in persistent (>6 hours) pain

Cholelithiasis
Technical term for gallstones

Choledocholithiasis
Obstruction of the hepatic or common bile ducts with stones

Cholangitis
An obstruction and ascending infection of the biliary tree

Biliary colic
Intermittent obstruction of the cystic or common bile ducts results in pain. Often precursor for acute cholecystitis.

Differential diagnosis
- Gallstone pancreatitis
- Abdominal aortic aneurysm/ dissection
- Diverticulitis
- Hepatitis
- Pancreatitis
- Peptic ulcer disease
- Renal colic
- Appendicitis
- Pyelonephritis

P **Start IV fluids and keep pt NPO**

Provide pain relief
NSAIDs are effective in treating biliary colic, but likely contraindicated if the pt requires surgery.
Narcotics may be needed for more severe pain.

Cholelithiasis requires no treatment but increases the risk for acute cholecystitis in the future

Biliary colic can be treated with IV hydration and pain control
Keep pt NPO until symptoms resolve.
Future symptoms may be prevented by avoiding high-fat meals.

Acute cholecystitis
Continue IV fluids, keep NPO, and treat pain.
Consult General Surgery for cholecystectomy.
- May be delayed for several days to allow inflammation to decrease and prevent operative complications.
- May require percutaneous cholecystostomy tube if pt is too unstable for surgery.
Start antibiotics to prevent complications and perforation.

Cholangitis
Requires aggressive treatment to prevent sepsis and hemodynamic collapse.
Start IV fluids, keep NPO, and treat pain.
Start broad-spectrum antibiotics with anaerobic coverage.
Consult General Surgery ASAP and GI for ERCP.
Arrange for biliary decompression via ERCP or percutaneous biliary drainage if ERCP fails.
May require interval cholecystectomy.

DIVERTICULITIS

S **Does the pt have any abdominal pain?**

Commonly complains of left lower quadrant abdominal pain with diverticulitis, although may have pain anywhere.

Typical pain is nonradiating and may be increased by movement, although not positional.

Diverticulosis tends to be asymptomatic, but may cause hematochezia.

Has the pt had any fevers or chills?
Associated with diverticulitis

Does the pt have any associated symptoms?
Common symptoms include:

    – Nausea/vomiting   – Diarrhea/constipation   – Anorexia

Has the pt experienced any rectal bleeding?
Painless rectal bleeding is the hallmark of diverticular bleeds; a common cause of lower GI bleeding in the elderly.

Does pt have a history of diverticulosis or diverticulitis?
Increased risk for diverticulitis in the future

Is the pt pregnant?
May see similar symptoms with an ectopic pregnancy, although diverticulosis is more common in middle-aged pts.

Does the pt have any other medical problems?
History of peripheral vascular disease may suggest alternative diagnosis of mesenteric ischemia and increases sensitivity to anemia with blood loss.

Pts with diabetes tend to have a higher rate of complications.

Obtain a review of symptoms
Vaginal discharge may suggest pelvic inflammatory disease (PID).

Dysuria, polyuria, or hematuria can be seen with urinary tract infection (UTI), pyelonephritis.

O **Evaluate the pt's vital signs**

Is the pt febrile?

Is the pt hemodynamically stable?

Perform a physical exam
Abdomen: Tenderness with or without rebound, guarding, and distention may be seen.

Rectal: Gross blood? Hemoccult positive? May be seen with diverticular bleed. Rectal pain? Suggests colitis or abscess.

Obtain the following labs
CBC: Evaluate for leukocytosis and anemia.

β-hCG: Rule out pregnancy.

UA: Exclude UTI or pyelonephritis.

Type and cross if actively bleeding.

Consider a diagnostic study
Abdominal plain x-rays: Nonspecific, but may demonstrate free air from perforated viscus or signs of obstruction with air-fluid levels.

Abdominal CT scan: In diverticulitis, it will typically show diverticuli, pericolonic inflammation, and bowel wall thickening. May see abscess formation, perforation, or an alternative cause.

    • Should be obtained with oral contrast. IV contrast will enhance the pericolonic inflammation and is necessary to diagnose abscess.

Barium enema: Will show diverticuli but is contraindicated because of the risk of colonic overdistention and perforation.

Sigmoidoscopy/colonoscopy: Can be obtained acutely for lower GI bleeding but are contraindicated in the acute setting for diverticulitis for the same reasons as noted above.

 ### Diverticulosis

Asymptomatic herniation of the colonic mucosa into the muscularis layer. Incidence is increased in the elderly and in societies that eat a low-fiber diet.

Diverticulitis

Acute inflammation and microabscess/perforation of one or more diverticulum, usually caused by an obstruction of the opening. Approximately 50% of pts with diverticulosis will develop diverticulitis over their lifetime.

Diverticular bleed

Acute hemorrhage of a diverticulum. More common in the left colon.

Differential diagnosis

- Appendicitis
- PID
- Inflammatory bowel disease
- Gastroenteritis
- Ectopic pregnancy
- Ischemic colitis
- UTI/pyelonephritis

Initiate IV fluids and keep pt NPO

Diverticulosis

No treatment is needed. Typically an incidental finding found on CT scan or colonoscopy.

Diverticulitis

Start antibiotics. One possible combination is a fluoroquinolone and either clindamycin or metronidazole.

Treat pain with narcotics.

If pt's symptoms are mild, and there is no evidence of systemic disease, gross perforation, or abscess formation, the pt can be discharged home on trial of oral antibiotics.

All pts with severe disease or inability to take oral medications need to be admitted for IV antibiotics and IV hydration.

Diverticular bleed

Take a thorough history to rule out other sources of bleeding and consider gastric lavage via NG tube to rule out upper GI bleed (usually causes melena and not hematochezia).

Admit all pts. Pts who are hemodynamically unstable or at high risk for hemodynamic decompensation should be admitted to the ICU.

Transfuse blood as needed.

Consult Gastroenterology or a general surgeon so that a diagnostic procedure can be performed to localize the source of bleeding.

FOREIGN-BODY INGESTION

S **What did the pt ingest?**

Small button batteries are the most worrisome because they require emergent removal if they become lodged in the esophagus. The battery can cause an alkaline burn and erode through the esophagus in as little as 4 hours.

Does the pt have any difficulty breathing?

Object may cause airway obstruction or press on the trachea, obstructing air flow.

Can the pt swallow?

Obstruction in the esophagus can cause odynophagia or dysphagia.

Does the pt have any chest pain?

May be seen with esophageal perforation or after retching.

Does the pt have any symptoms?

Common symptoms include:
- Coughing/gagging
- Anxiety
- Children may only present with stridor or poor eating
- Nausea/vomiting
- Hoarseness

Does the pt have a history of foreign-body ingestions?

Psychiatric pts, prisoners, and children are more likely to ingest foreign bodies.

Has the pt had any bariatric surgery?

Gastric banding increases the risk of impaction of food boluses.

O **Evaluate pt's vital signs**

Fever and hemodynamic instability may be seen with esophageal rupture.

Perform physical exam

General: Is the pt in distress? Able to swallow own secretions? Drooling? These are signs of severe distress.

HEENT: Perform a thorough inspection of the nose and mouth. Unilateral nasal discharge can be seen with nasal foreign bodies. Listen over trachea for stridor.

Lungs: Listen for wheezing or decreased breath sounds that may be seen with bronchial obstruction.

Abdomen: Generally normal. Note any tenderness, distention, or abnormal bowel sounds.

Obtain a CXR

Will show radio-opaque objects (e.g., button batteries, coins, dense plastic). Coins will often be seen on-end if in trachea or face-on (en face) if in esophagus on frontal (AP or PA) CXR.

Mediastinal and/or subcutaneous air seen with esophageal perforation.

Obtain a lateral neck x-ray if proximal obstruction is suspected

CXR may miss objects in the posterior pharynx.

Consider a Gastrografin swallow

To demonstrate non-radiopaque objects

Consider direct laryngoscopy if the pt feels the object in the upper airway

Allows direct visualization and removal.

Often, foreign-body sensation results from a small laceration or abrasion of the posterior pharynx caused by the foreign body (e.g., chicken bone).

Consider a chest and abdominal CT scan

Very sensitive in localizing foreign objects.

Can evaluate surrounding structures and may show alternative diagnosis.

A   Foreign-body ingestion

Most common objects ingested are coins.

Objects tend to lodge at one of three levels:
- Cricopharyngeal level: Narrowest area in children. Can cause complete airway obstruction.
- T4 level: Aortic arch and carina. Most common in adults.
- Proximal to the gastroesophageal junction.

Differential diagnosis

Croup

Retropharyngeal abscess

Epiglottitis (unvaccinated pts)

P   Most objects that have passed into the stomach and small intestine can be observed and treated expectantly

Arrange for emergent endoscopic removal of any foreign body causing obstruction or airway compromise

All button batteries in the esophagus need to be removed immediately. If the battery has passed into the stomach and intestine, it can be managed expectantly.

Sharp objects (e.g., blades and glass) should be removed as soon as possible.

Schedule elective endoscopy for

Smooth objects in the esophagus that have not passed into the stomach after 24 hours

Button batteries that have remained in the stomach more than 48 hours

Food boluses can be treated with

IV glucagon: Can cause reflex contraction of the esophagus and expel the bolus.

Nitroglycerin/calcium channel blocker: Relax proximal gastroesophageal sphincter.

Endoscopic retrieval (may also push bolus distally).

Do NOT treat with meat tenderizer because it may cause esophageal perforation.

Discharge pts

Who have had objects removed in the ED and have demonstrated that they can tolerate oral intake.

With objects that have passed into the small intestine. Instruct them to monitor their stool.

With button batteries in their stomach, but they will need to return within 48 hours to ensure it has passed into the intestines.

Admit pts with

Esophageal foreign bodies or food boluses that cannot be treated in the ED

GASTROESOPHAGEAL REFLUX DISEASE

S **What are the pt's symptoms?**

Common symptoms include:
- Burning sensation in the chest   – Foul taste or odor in the mouth
- Nausea/vomiting

Atypical symptoms include:
- Hoarseness   – Chronic cough
- Shortness of breath   – Asthma

Do certain foods increase the symptoms?

Foods high in fat content or acidity tend to worsen symptoms.

Are the symptoms increased with certain positions?

Bending over or lying down tend to worsen symptoms.

Determine the pt's use or consumption of alcohol, tobacco, chocolate, or caffeine

All four of these products cause relaxation of the lower esophageal sphincter (LES), increasing gastroesophageal reflux disease (GERD) symptoms.

Has the pt tried any remedies?

Most pts will have already tried over-the-counter antacids, and their response to antacid treatment will help direct your treatment.

Has the pt experienced any dysphagia or odynophagia?

Dysphagia is suggestive of esophageal spasm or stricture.
Odynophagia is suggestive of ulcerative esophagitis.

Does the pt have any other medical problems?

History of coronary atherosclerotic disease (CAD) or risk factors for CAD may warrant cardiac workup because myocardial ischemia can mimic GERD.

What medications is the pt taking?

Opiates, calcium channel blockers, nitrates, theophylline, and anticholinergics can all increase GERD symptoms by relaxing the LES.

O **Perform a physical exam**

Typically normal
Check rectal exam and rule out occult GI blood loss.

Consider obtaining an ECG

Evaluate for myocardial ischemia as cause of symptoms.

Consider obtaining the following labs

CBC: May see chronic anemia caused by esophagitis or peptic ulcer disease (PUD).
Cardiac enzymes: Evaluate for myocardial damage.

Consider obtaining a CXR

May demonstrate a hiatal hernia, although not all hiatal hernias cause symptoms.
Free air or pleural effusion may be seen with an esophageal perforation.
May see an esophageal foreign body.

A **Gastroesophageal reflux disease**

Syndrome caused by the reflux of gastric contents into the esophagus, causing local irritation and inflammation.

Differential diagnosis
- Myocardial ischemia   – PUD
- Cholelithiasis   – Gastritis
- Gastroenteritis   – Esophageal foreign body

P Give a trial of an antacid

A GI cocktail consisting of viscous lidocaine, aluminum hydroxide/magnesium hydroxide, and Donnatal can provide almost immediate pain relief and improvement in symptoms.

Consider starting a proton pump inhibitor or histamine-2 receptor blocker.

Educate the pt on lifestyle modifications

Elevate head of bed 4 inches.

Do not eat within 2 hours of lying down.

Eat small meals and avoid overeating.

Avoid late-night meals or snacks.

Avoid foods that lower the LES tone (e.g., alcohol, caffeine, chocolate, or fatty foods).

Avoid medications that lower the LES tone.

Arrange outpatient evaluation

If diagnosis is unclear or pt has failed antacid treatment, consider:

- Endoscopy: Allows direct visualization of the esophageal and gastric mucosa. Helpful to rule out PUD, hernia, Barrett esophagus, and occult malignancy.
- 24-hour esophageal pH probe: Highly sensitive to secure the diagnosis of chest pain caused by GERD. Not commonly performed, however, because endoscopy can usually make the diagnosis.

Most pts can be discharged home

Consider admission for any pt who has

Severe reactive airway disease

Dehydration

Evidence of esophageal perforation

Evidence of gastrointestinal bleed

GASTROINTESTINAL BLEEDING

 Has the pt noticed any bleeding?

GI bleeding may not be noticed, and the pt may only present with generalized weakness, fatigue, syncope, dyspnea on exertion, or lightheadedness.

Black, tarry stools or melena is commonly seen with upper GI bleeding (proximal to the ligament of Treitz).

Hematochezia (bloody diarrhea) can be seen with a brisk upper GI bleed or more commonly with a lower GI bleed (distal to the ligament of Treitz).

Bright red blood on normal brown stool or on the toilet paper is common with anal fissures or hemorrhoids.

Coffee ground emesis may be seen with an upper GI bleed.

Does the pt have a history of peptic ulcer disease (PUD) or gastritis?
Increases risk for upper gastrointestinal bleeding

Does the pt have a history of diverticulosis?
Common in pts presenting with painless hematochezia, the hallmark of a diverticular bleed

Has the pt been vomiting or retching?
If bleeding follows the vomiting or retching, the cause is likely a Mallory-Weiss tear.

Has the pt been taking any medications?
Heavy NSAID or steroid use increases the risk for PUD and gastritis as the cause of an upper GI bleed.

Iron, bismuth, and charcoal can turn the stool black.

Has the pt recently undergone any endoscopic evaluation?
Ensure that pt is not having any postprocedural bleeding from polypectomy.

Does the pt drink large quantities of alcohol?
Suggests possibility of cirrhosis, portal hypertension, and varices as etiology of blood loss.

What other medical problems does the pt have?
Pt's with coronary atherosclerotic disease (CAD) are at risk for myocardial ischemia with severe anemia.

 Evaluate the pt's vital signs

Ensure that the pt is hemodynamically stable. Look for tachycardia and hypotension.

Perform a physical exam
Chest: Note any stigmata of liver disease (e.g., spider hemangiomas, gynecomastia).
Abdomen: May have tenderness to palpation. Note liver and spleen size (cirrhosis).
Rectal: May note frank blood, hemoccult-positive stool, or melena. Use anoscope to visualize internal hemorrhoids and anal fissures.

Perform a gastric lavage
Place a nasogastric (NG) tube and ensure that there is no blood with aspiration. Need to exclude an upper GI blood source and active bleeding.

Once lavage is performed, NG tube can be removed.

Obtain the following labs
CBC: Evaluate the degree of anemia. In an acute bleed, the hemoglobin may not equilibrate for several hours and is not indicative of actual blood loss. Note platelets and any thrombocytopenia.

PT, INR, PTT: Exclude coagulopathy as a confounding factor in the bleeding.

Type and cross: For blood products as needed.

Electrolytes, BUN, creatinine: Exclude secondary metabolic disturbance or renal insufficiency.

Consider an ECG
Exclude cardiac ischemia with severe anemia.

Gastrointestinal bleeding

Upper sources:

- PUD   - Gastritis
- Esophageal varices   - Mallory-Weiss tear
- Angiodysplasia   - Esophagitis

Lower sources:

- Angiodysplasia   - Diverticular bleed
- Polyp or cancer   - Hemorrhoids
- Anal fissure

In pediatric pts, consider Meckel diverticulum or intussusception.

Differential diagnosis

- Acute abdomen   - Gastroesophageal reflux disease

 Start IV fluids

All pts should have two large-bore (>16-gauge) peripheral IVs established.
Maintain blood pressure with fluid boluses of crystalloid or colloid fluids.

Place on oxygen via nasal cannula

Helps improve oxygen delivery and prevent ischemia.

Transfuse PRBCs

If Hgb <7 and <8 for any patient with cardiac history.

Consult Gastroenterology

Consider emergent endoscopy to localize bleeding site and treat locally.

Consider Surgery consult for severe bleeding that may require surgical intervention

May need tagged RBC scan to localize bleeding.

Consider starting the following medications

Proton pump inhibitor/H_2 blocker: Decreases acid secretion and may prevent rebleeding with PUD and gastritis.

Vasopressin: Potent vasoconstrictor that may help decrease bleeding in variceal or ulcer bleeding.

Octreotide: Decreases splanchnic blood flow (helpful in variceal bleeding).

Follow serial blood counts.

Monitor for ongoing blood loss.

Most pts will be admitted

Admit all pts with ongoing blood loss or borderline vital signs to the ICU.

Discharge home pts who have

Stable vital signs, blood counts, no evidence of active bleeding, and normal coagulation studies

HEPATITIS

S What are the pt's current symptoms?

Common symptoms include:

– Malaise	– Lethargy	– Dark urine or stools
– RUQpain	– Fever	– Jaundice

Has the pt been vaccinated against hepatitis A or B?

Hepatitis B vaccine will protect against hepatitis B and D. A vaccine for hepatitis A has been made available recently and is generally recommended for anyone who is going to travel.

Does the pt have any risk factors for hepatitis?

Viral hepatitis B and C are associated with intravenous drug abuse, unprotected intercourse, tattoos, and blood transfusions.

Hepatitis A is associated with crowded conditions and poor sanitation.

Has the pt been taking any medications?

Acetaminophen, isoniazid, methyldopa, and ketoconazole are just a few of the many medications associated with drug-induced hepatitis.

Review all medications, including chronic medications, because drug-induced hepatitis can occur at anytime.

Does the pt have a history of alcohol use?

Alcohol and viral hepatitis are the two most common causes in the United States.

May need to ask family members about the degree of alcohol use to get an accurate assessment.

Has the pt traveled recently? Does the pt work in a nursing home or day care facility?

Suggests hepatitis A or E because of their spread through the fecal-oral route and association with poor sanitation.

If pt has been camping or hiking recently, ask about ingestion of any wild mushrooms (*Amanita* poisoning).

O Perform a physical exam

HEENT: Scleral icterus? Icterus may be seen under the tongue. Nystagmus and tongue fasciculations may be seen with encephalopathy.

Lungs: Typically normal, but may have dull breath sounds in the bases caused by pleural effusions.

Cardiac: Typically normal, but may have evidence of high-output cardiac failure caused by liver failure.

Chest: Spider angiomas?

Abdomen: Palpate liver; may note knobby texture. Note liver span (decreased in cirrhosis). Fluid wave? Ascites?

Rectal: Hemoccult-positive stool?

Extremities: Asterixis? Palmar erythema?

Neurologic: Stuporous? Lethargic? Comatose? Evaluate mental status.

Check the following labs

CBC: Rule out anemia. May also have an elevated WBC associated with infection.

BUN, creatinine, electrolytes, LFTs: Evaluate renal function. May see electrolyte disturbances, and elevations in LFTs. End-stage hepatitis may have normal LFTs.

- AST/ALT >2 suggests alcohol liver disease.
- Albumin and PT/INR evaluate the synthetic function of the liver.

Ammonia level: Level does not correlate to the degree of encephalopathy present.

Coagulation studies: PT may be elevated when liver synthetic function is impaired.

Acetaminophen level: Exclude acetaminophen toxicity.

Hepatitis serologies:

- HAV: IgM and IgG for HAV. IgM elevation consistent with acute illness.
- HBV: HBs antibody seen with immunization. HBc antibody, HBs antigen, and HBe antigen seen with HBV infection. HBe antigen associated with high infectivity.
- HCV: Check HCV IgG.

A Hepatitis

Etiologies can be from alcohol, viruses (hepatitis A, B, C, D, E, cytomegalovirus, Epstein-Barr virus, herpes simplex virus), toxic exposure (halothane), or drug use.
Chronic hepatitis exists after 6 months of symptoms or persistent lab abnormalities.
Acute hepatitis <6 months.

Differential diagnosis

- Cholecystitis
- Cholangitis
- Biliary cirrhosis
- Steatohepatitis

P Provide supportive care

Consider IV hydration and antiemetics.

Stop any potentially hepatotoxic medications or drugs

Avoid prescribing any hepatotoxic medications (e.g., acetaminophen).

Consider contact prophylaxis for hepatitis A or B

Immune globulin plus vaccination if exposure has been recent.

Treat any coagulopathies with fresh frozen plasma or vitamin K

Start lactulose if hepatic encephalopathy present

Consider paracentesis in any pt with ascites and fever

Exclude spontaneous bacterial peritonitis.

Disposition

Most pts will need to be admitted for IV hydration and further evaluation.
Consider discharge only in those pts with mild symptoms, mild laboratory abnormalities, and who can have close follow-up arranged.
Pts with hepatic encephalopathy, major coagulopathies, or gastrointestinal bleeding will need to be admitted to the ICU.

ISCHEMIC BOWEL

S What are the pt's current symptoms?

The classic description is abdominal pain out of proportion to the exam.
Common symptoms include:

- Abdominal pain   - Nausea/vomiting
- Diarrhea   - GI bleeding

May see:

- Mental status changes   - Fever   - Syncope

Does the pt note anything that exacerbates the pain?

Chronic bowel ischemia typically presents as dull, crampy, postprandial abdominal
pain caused by a narrowing in the visceral (e.g., celiac or superior mesenteric arteries)
from atherosclerosis.

Does the pt have any risk factors for vascular disease?

- Diabetes   - Peripheral vascular disease   - Tobacco use
- Hypercholesterolemia   - Coronary atherosclerotic

What other medical conditions does the pt have?

Helpful to ascertain risk factors and other etiologies for presenting complaints.
Bowel ischemia can be seen post–myocardial infarction (MI) and with congestive heart
failure (CHF), when cardiac output is low enough to cause demand ischemia.

O Evaluate the pt's vital signs

Perform a physical exam

HEENT, lungs, cardiac: Typically normal. May see signs of CHF.
Abdomen: Peritoneal signs? Tenderness? Listen for bruits.
Rectal: Frank blood, hemoccult-positive stool seen with late-stage ischemic bowel.
Neurologic: Note any mental status changes.

Obtain the following labs

CBC: May have elevated WBC. Exclude anemia.
BUN, creatinine, LFT, amylase, lipase, electrolytes: Exclude alternative diagnosis.
  • May see elevations in liver enzymes caused by hepatic ischemia.
  • Typically will have a metabolic acidosis.
Lactic acid level: Sensitive for ischemia, although not specific for bowel ischemia.

Consider obtaining abdominal x-rays

Useful to exclude free air and bowel obstruction. Used less frequently now with CT
scans so readily available.

Consider an abdominal CT scan

May be normal initially. Bowel wall thickening, streaking of mesenteric fat, and lack of
IV contrast filling a visceral artery helps establish diagnosis.

Consider an angiogram

The gold standard in making the diagnosis of arterial insufficiency. May also be therapeutic because an interventional radiologist may open an obstruction with balloon
angioplasty or an injection of papaverine.

Consider colonoscopy or sigmoidoscopy

Allows direct visualization of the colon, which will display ischemic changes.

A Ischemic bowel

Caused by subacute closure or thrombosis of the celiac, superior mesenteric, or inferior
mesenteric arteries (IMA). The IMA supplies the left colon and rectum and has adequate collateral support from the rectal blood supply, so it is not typically associated
with ischemic bowel.

Acute presentations are typically the result of embolic events or as a result of inadequate blood flow caused by CHF, aortic dissection, hypotension, sepsis, or MI.

Chronic presentations (intestinal angina) are caused by atherosclerosis of the blood supply and typically present with postprandial pain and weight loss.

Differential diagnosis

- Intestinal obstruction
- Cholelithiasis
- Volvulus
- Pancreatitis
- Intussusception
- Abdominal aortic aneurysm
- Aortic dissection

P Initiate supportive care

Ensure adequate blood pressure.

- Hydrate with normal saline solution. Pt may require large volumes of fluid replacement.
- Avoid pressors if possible because they may exacerbate the ischemia due to vasoconstriction.

Treat any underlying disorder (e.g., CHF, MI, aortic dissection) that may have incited the ischemia.

Provide adequate pain relief

Pain is typically out of proportion to the exam; however, this should not limit narcotic use except if hypotensive or otherwise contraindicated.

Consider starting IV antibiotics

In order to prevent secondary infection from translocation of bowel flora

Consult a vascular surgeon for possible surgical correction

Interventional radiology consult should also be considered for angiogram and possible balloon angioplasty.

Disposition

All pts should be admitted.

Consider ICU admission for any pt showing any signs of hypotension or hypovolemia.

Mortality rate is 50%–100% without aggressive treatment and repair.

PANCREATITIS

S **What are the pt's symptoms?**
Common symptoms include:
- Midepigastric abdominal pain
- Anorexia
- Nausea/vomiting
- Distention

Has the pt noticed anything that exacerbates the pain?
Pain typically increases several hours after eating and may increase with lying down.

Does anything help alleviate the pain?
Pain typically decreases if the pt avoids eating/drinking.

Does the pt have any risk factors for pancreatitis?
- Alcohol use
- Peptic ulcer disease
- Recent endoscopic retrograde cholangiopancreatography (ERCP)
- Smoking
- Hypertriglyceridemia
- Cholelithiasis
- Scorpion bite (rare)

Does the pt take any medications or herbal supplements?
Oral contraceptives, diuretics, steroids, and aspirin are a few drugs associated with pancreatitis.

Does the pt have any other medical problems?
Pts with a history of pancreatitis may not demonstrate elevations of amylase and lipase. Pancreatitis is associated with cystic fibrosis, lupus, and recent abdominal surgery.
Even after cholecystectomy, patients may develop choledocholithiasis.

Obtain a social history
Alcohol use and cholelithiasis are the two leading causes of pancreatitis in the United States.

O **Perform a physical exam**
HEENT, lungs, cardiac: Typically normal.
Abdomen: Tenderness? Peritoneal signs?
• *Grey-Turner sign:* Ecchymosis along the flank caused by retroperitoneal hemorrhage.
• *Cullen sign:* Ecchymosis around the umbilicus caused by intraperitoneal hemorrhage.
Rectal: Exclude gastrointestinal bleeding.

Obtain the following labs
CBC: Exclude anemia or elevated WBC.
BUN, creatinine, electrolytes: Exclude an underlying renal or electrolyte disturbance.
LFTs, amylase, lipase: Amylase and lipase are typically elevated in acute pancreatitis, although they may be normal in chronic pancreatitis.
• Lipase is more sensitive and specific for pancreatic injury.
• May see elevated alkaline phosphatase, and bilirubin to suggest gallstones.
• Elevations in AST > ALT seen with alcohol abuse.
ESR, CRP: Signs of inflammation and may be elevated in chronic pancreatitis despite having normal amylase and lipase.

Consider abdominal CT scan
Can demonstrate edema and/or necrosis of the pancreas, as well as pseudocyst formation. Calcification and atrophy of the pancreas seen in chronic pancreatitis.

Consider RUQ ultrasound
Poor sensitivity for evaluating the pancreas but useful to rule out cholelithiasis.

Pancreatitis

Inflammation of the pancreas that is associated with edema, autodigestion, necrosis, and
    possible hemorrhage.

Chronic pancreatitis can lead to endocrine dysfunction (diabetes) and exocrine dysfunc-
    tion (malabsorption, fat-soluble vitamin deficiencies).

Ranson criteria can help predict overall mortality.

- Initial criteria include:
    - – Age >55
    - – LDH >350
    - – WBC >16,000
    - – AST >250
    - – Glucose >200

- Criteria after 48 hours:
    - – HCT ↓ by 10%
    - – PaO_2 <60 mm Hg
    - – Mortality nearly 100% if
      >6 criteria are seen
    - – BUN ↑ by 5 mg/dL
    - – Base deficit >4
    - – Calcium <8 mg/dL
    - – Fluid deficit >6 L

Differential diagnosis

- – Peptic ulcer disease
- – Abdominal aortic aneurysm
- – Renal colic
- – Biliary colic
- – Ischemic bowel
- – Intestinal obstruction

P **Provide supportive care**

Pts may require aggressive IV hydration because of fluid sequestration and third spacing.

Keep pt NPO until pain has resolved. May give trial of clear liquids for mild disease.

Provide adequate pain control with narcotics. Treat nausea and vomiting with
    antiemetics.

Treat underlying disorder if possible

Pts with retained gallstones may require surgery or ERCP to decompress the biliary and
    pancreatic system.

Withhold any medications or alcohol that may have caused the pancreatitis.

Consider starting antibiotics

Imipenem has been shown to decrease mortality in necrotizing pancreatitis.

Disposition

Most pts will need to be admitted for IV hydration and pain control.

Consider ICU admission for pts who present with hypotension, have multiple comorbid
    illnesses, or have multiple Ranson criteria because pancreatitis can progress quickly to
    multiorgan system failure and death.

Consider discharging home any pts who are able to tolerate clear liquids in the ED,
    able to adequately hydrate themselves, have mild disease, and have close follow-up
    arranged.

PEPTIC ULCER DISEASE

S **What are the pt's current symptoms?**

Common symptoms include:

- Epigastric abdominal pain   – Heartburn   – Nausea/vomiting
- Melena   – Early satiety   – Bloating

May complain of:

- Hematemesis   – Hematochezia   – Fatigue
- Lethargy

Does the pt have a history of heartburn or peptic ulcer disease (PUD)?

Determine whether the pt's present symptoms are different or whether this is a flare-up.

How are the pt's symptoms related to eating?

Gastric ulcer pain typically occurs immediately after eating.

Duodenal ulcer pain typically occurs 1–3 hours after eating and may actually improve with eating.

What medications is the pt taking?

NSAIDs and steroids increase the risk for PUD.

Medication profile is also helpful to see what medications (e.g., over-the-counter antacids) the pt has tried to alleviate symptoms.

What other medical problems does the pt have?

Helps to exclude other etiologies for the pt's symptoms.

PUD is also associated with renal failure, inflammatory bowel disease (e.g., Crohn disease), and autoimmune disorders that frequently require NSAID or steroid use.

Obtain a social history

Tobacco and alcohol use increase the risk for PUD.

O **Evaluate the pt's vital signs**

Tachycardia and hypotension suggests blood loss or severe dehydration.

Perform a physical exam

HEENT, lungs, cardiac: Typically normal.

Abdomen: Epigastric tenderness may be present. Severe pain suggests perforation.

Rectal: Guaiac positive? Seen with PUD. Frank blood? Suggests a severe bleed.

Obtain the following labs

CBC to exclude anemia.

Electrolytes, LFTs, amylase, lipase to exclude other causes of abdominal pain.

Coagulation studies to exclude a coagulopathy.

Consider sending a type and screen/cross if there are signs/symptoms of recent blood loss

Consider sending *Helicobacter pylori* testing

IgG serology can be sent to see if pt warrants treatment.

Consider obtaining a CXR

Exclude free air secondary to perforation.

Place a nasogastric tube if there has been any hematemesis or hematochezia

Exclude any active upper gastrointestinal bleeding.

Consider emergent endoscopy if active bleeding is noted

Can be diagnostic and therapeutic

Peptic ulcer disease

H. pylori, a urease-producing, gram-negative rod, is the most common cause of PUD.
  • Disrupts the mucosal protective barrier of the stomach and duodenum.
  • Responsible for approximately 95% of gastric ulcers and 85% of duodenal ulcers.
Rare causes include Zollinger-Ellison syndrome and gastrinomas.

Differential diagnosis

- Acute gastritis
- Biliary colic
- Ischemic bowel
- Hepatitis
- Gastroesophageal reflux
- Abdominal obstruction
- Pancreatitis

P **Provide supportive care**

Provide IV hydration and pain control.
Consider a trial of a GI cocktail (i.e., viscous lidocaine, Donnatal, aluminum hydroxide/
  magnesium hydroxide).

Consider obtaining a gastroenterology consult

For emergent endoscopy if there are signs of active blood loss

Educate the pt on lifestyle changes to include

- Bland diet
- Avoid aspirin, NSAIDs
- Small meals
- Alcohol and tobacco avoidance

Start a proton pump inhibitor, H+ blocker, or sucralfate

Decreases acid secretion, allowing the gastric and duodenal mucosa to heal more rapidly

Consider starting treatment for *Helicobacter pylori*

Multiple regimens have been shown to be effective.
Treatment of *H. pylori* has been shown to decrease ulcer recurrence to less than 10%.

Disposition

Most pts can be discharged home with routine follow-up with their primary care
  provider.
Admit any pt with evidence of blood loss, severe symptoms, persistent vomiting, or
  evidence of perforation.

GENITOURINARY

ACUTE RENAL FAILURE

S
What are the pt's current symptoms?
Common symptoms include:
- Nausea/vomiting
- Abdominal pain
- Lethargy
- Oliguria or anuria
- Edema
- Shortness of breath
- Hematuria

Has the pt had decreased oral intake or excess fluid losses?
Dehydration caused by decreased intake, diarrhea/vomiting, or excessive insensible losses can progress to prerenal azotemia and renal failure.

Has the pt had any recent infection or sore throat?
Increases suspicion for poststreptococcal glomerulonephritis.

What medical problems does the pt have?
Diabetes, hypertension, congestive heart failure (CHF), and vasculitis can all contribute to renal failure.
Cirrhosis can lead to renal failure as a result of third spacing and intravascular depletion (prerenal renal failure) or from loss of autoregulation from failure to clear cytokines (hepatorenal syndrome).

What medications does the pt take?
ACE-inhibitor/ARB and NSAID use can inhibit the kidney's autoregulation of blood flow and lead to renal failure.
Diuretic use with excessive fluid loss can cause renal failure.
Recent IV contrast administration and antibiotics (e.g., aminoglycosides) can cause acute tubular necrosis (ATN).

Has the pt had any surgical procedures or interventions done recently?
Vascular surgery, cardiac catheterization, or angiograms can lead to cholesterol embolization and secondary renal failure. Typically occurs 1–2 weeks after the procedure.

Obtain a social history
Intravenous drug abuse increases the risk for embolic disease because of impurities in the drug or endocarditis, both of which can lead to acute renal failure.
Tobacco use increases the risk of atherosclerosis.

O
Evaluate the pt's vital signs
Perform orthostatic vital signs to exclude postural hypotension and dehydration.

Perform a physical exam
Lungs: Rales? Wheezing? Look for signs of volume overload and CHF.
Cardiac: Note any murmurs or gallops. Murmurs may suggest endocarditis; S3/S4 associated with CHF. Note any pedal edema.
Abdomen: Ascites? Costovertebral angle tenderness? Peritoneal signs? May suggest infection.
Neurologic: Mental status changes? Caused by uremia, infection, or dehydration.
Skin: Any rashes to suggest strep infection?

Obtain the following labs
CBC: Evaluate for anemia, which may be the cause of renal failure or a result of it. Increased WBCs can be seen with infection.
BUN/creatinine: Usually elevated. BUN/creatinine ratio >20 suggests prerenal cause.
Electrolytes: Hypo-/hyperkalemia can be seen with renal failure. Ensure that calcium, phosphorus, and magnesium are normal.
LFT: Exclude liver disease.

Urinalysis: May see proteinuria, hematuria. Casts seen with intrinsic renal disease. May see eosinophilia with cholesterol emboli.

FENa: Fractional excretion of urine sodium. If FENa <1, renal failure is typically because of prerenal causes, as the kidneys are retaining sodium and thus water.

Consider serum serologies if vasculitis or rheumatologic cause is suspected.

Obtain blood cultures if postinfectious or if endocarditis is suspected.

Obtain an ECG
Exclude cardiac ischemia and secondary CHF as cause.

Exclude hyperkalemic ECG changes that can quickly progress to cardiac arrest.

Obtain a CXR
Evaluate cardiac silhouette size and whether there is any pulmonary edema to suggest CHF.

Consider renal ultrasound
Evaluate renal parenchyma and exclude postrenal causes (e.g., obstruction).

Evaluate postvoid residual
Useful to exclude an obstructive or postrenal cause of renal failure

A Acute kidney injury

A rapid decline in renal function over hour to days

Causes are divided into prerenal, renal, and postrenal.

Prerenal causes are generally from low intravascular volume or low cardiac output.

Renal causes include ATN, vasculitis, glomerulonephritis, cholesterol emboli, etc.

Postrenal causes are from an obstruction in urine outflow and result in renal damage by increasing tubular pressures.

Differential diagnosis
– CHF   – Anemia   – Cirrhosis

P Treatment is aimed at treating the underlying cause of the acute kidney injury

Consider Foley catheter placement to obtain accurate measurement of urine production.

Consider emergent dialysis in any pt who has
Significant acidosis

Hyperkalemia or electrolyte disturbances that are not responding to conservative treatment or causing ECG changes

Intoxicants such as methylene glycol or aspirin

Fluid overload with blood pressure or respiratory compromise

Symptomatic uremia

Stop any nephrotoxic agent

If prerenal disease is suspected, aggressively hydrate the pt

Disposition
Admit all pts. Morbidity and mortality related to acute kidney injury are significant. Consult Nephrology.

EPIDIDYMITIS

 What are the pt's current symptoms?

Common symptoms include:
- Scrotal pain
- Dysuria
- Fever
- Tenderness to testicle/epididymis

May also complain of:
- Penile discharge
- Scrotal swelling
- Abdominal pain

Was the onset of pain gradual or abrupt?

Pain caused by epididymitis tends to be gradual in onset (>24 hours) and may involve both testicles.

What helps alleviate the pain? What increases the pain?

Epididymal pain typically increases when the pt stands and is relieved with scrotal support or by lying down.

Does the pt have a history of an STD?

Epididymitis in the young (20–30 years old) is most often associated with *Chlamydia* and gonorrhea infections.

Common to have no urethral discharge at the time of presentation.

Has the pt been struck in the groin/testicle?

Exclude trauma from possible etiologies.

Has the pt had a recent viral infection?

Orchitis is commonly associated with viral infections (e.g., mumps, coxsackie A).

Does the pt have any history of urinary retention or recent instrumentation of urinary system?

Epididymitis in older men is associated with *Escherichia coli, Klebsiella,* or *Pseudomonas* and is commonly associated with urinary retention or recent instrumentation.

Obtain a PMH/social history

Include a sexual history and history of STDs.

Inquire specifically about benign prostatic hypertrophy because it increases the risk of urinary retention.

 Evaluate the pt's vital signs

Fever is more commonly associated with a viral syndrome.

Perform a physical exam

Abdomen: Tenderness? Peritoneal signs? Costovertebral angle tenderness? Exclude other pathologies.

GU: Penile discharge? Scrotal swelling? Epididymal tenderness or swelling? Testicle swelling? May all be seen with infection. Inguinal hernia? May suggest incarceration. Cremasteric reflex? If absent, suspect testicular torsion. *Prehn sign:* Decreased pain when testicles and scrotum are lifted; seen with epididymitis, but pain should not change with testicular torsion.

Rectal: Prostate tenderness or fullness? Suggests prostatitis.

Obtain the following labs

Urinalysis: May see WBCs with epididymitis.

Urethral swab for gonorrhea/*Chlamydia*: Exclude STDs.

Consider sending HIV and RPR if suspicion of STD-related epididymitis is high. Increased risk of HIV and syphilis if another STD is found.

If suspicious for testicular torsion, obtain scrotal ultrasound with Doppler flow

If there is any concern about testicular torsion, ultrasound should be obtained as soon as possible.

Epididymitis

Inflammation or infection of the epididymis, generally caused by retrograde spread of
bacteria from the urethra or bladder.

Orchitis

Inflammation or infection of the testicle that can be caused by spread of infection from
the epididymis or from hematogenous spread (e.g., viral).

50% of involved testicles will have residual atrophy.

Differential diagnosis

- Hydrocele
- Testicular trauma
- Varicocele
- Renal colic
- Testicular torsion
- Inguinal hernia

P **Provide effective pain relief**

NSAIDs are generally effective.

Scrotal support with a jock strap.

Limit amount of standing/walking.

Start antibiotics

Sexually active males: Cover gonorrhea/*Chlamydia* with fluoroquinolone (21-day
course) or IM ceftriaxone plus doxycycline (10 days) or single-dose azithromycin.

Older males (>35): Fluoroquinolone (21-day course).

Disposition

Most pts can be discharged home with follow-up with their primary care provider.

Admit pts who are unable to take oral medications or have evidence of an abscess that
may require drainage.

HERNIA

 What are the pt's current symptoms?

Pain or swelling in the area of concern is the most common complaint.
Nausea/vomiting and fever can be seen with incarcerated hernias.

What was the pt doing when the swelling or bulge was first noticed?

An increase in the size of the hernia is normally associated with straining or lifting.

Does the pt have a history of a hernia or hernia repair?

Having a hernia on one side increases the risk of having a contralateral hernia.
Risk of hernia recurrence at the site of a former repair is variable. Rate depends on location, type of repair, and comorbid illnesses that may affect healing.

Is the swelling or bulge related to an area where surgery was performed?

Incision hernias typically appear 18–24 months after the surgery. Typically, pts will
experience some dull pain in the area when they strain, and they will later notice the
bulge.

Is the pt pregnant?

Femoral hernias commonly present in the first trimester of pregnancy.

Obtain a past medical history

Identify comorbid illnesses.

O **Evaluate the pt's vital signs**

Perform a physical exam

Abdomen: While the pt is relaxed and lying supine, palpate the affected area for tender-
ness or mass. Palpate all incisions for defects in the fascia or mass.
GU: Place a finger in the external inguinal ring and have pt perform Valsalva maneuver.
With inguinal hernia, you can feel the hernia sac being pushed out through the ring.
With large inguinal hernias, you may have abdominal contents in the scrotum, allow-
ing one to hear bowel sounds in the scrotum.

Consider obtaining the following labs

Urinalysis: If you suspect urinary tract infection, pyelonephritis, or nephrolithiasis.
CBC: May show leukocytosis with strangulation.
Electrolytes, BUN, creatinine: If pt is vomiting, to exclude electrolyte disturbance.

Consider obtaining a diagnostic study

Typically not necessary because diagnosis can be made with history and physical.
Abdominal x-rays can help screen for obstruction.
Abdominal/pelvic CT with oral contrast can show bowel loops or omentum in an
abdominal wall defect.
Ultrasound/MRI can show abdominal wall defect and bowel.

A **Hernia**

Inguinal hernia: Can be direct (occur through Hasselbach triangle) or indirect (occur
through the internal inguinal ligament). Indirect hernias are the most common and are
congenital, although they may not present until later in life.
Femoral hernia: Herniation into the femoral canal and is more common in women.
Higher risk for incarceration and strangulation.
Incisional hernia: Occur at the site of a surgical incision.
Umbilical hernia: Occur because of a defect in the midline fascia. Higher risk of
incarceration.

Differential diagnosis

– Testicular torsion	– Epididymitis	– Hydrocele/varicocele
– Bowel obstruction	– Lymphadenitis	

Asymptomatic hernias can be observed or repaired electively
Discharge the pt home with instructions to return immediately for pain or if unable to reduce hernia.

Incarcerated hernias need to be reduced ASAP
The longer the hernia is incarcerated, the more edema will form in the bowel wall, making it harder to reduce.
- If the hernia has been incarcerated for more than 4–6 hours, the pt will likely require surgical intervention to reduce the hernia and remove any necrotic bowel. Do not attempt to reduce.

To reduce the hernia, have the pt lie supine and relax.
- Provide analgesia and sedation as needed.
- Place constant, gentle pressure over the mass (herniation) until you are able to push it into the abdominal cavity. Pt should have immediate pain relief.

The definitive treatment for all hernias is surgical correction
Reducible hernias can be repaired electively.

Pts with evidence of bowel obstruction, incarcerated or strangulated hernia, fever, peritonitis, or intractable pain should be admitted for urgent surgical correction.

HYDROCELE/VARICOCELE

 What are the pt's current symptoms?

Most common symptom is painless swelling of the testicle.
  • May have dull ache but typically not painful.
  • Pain typically only seen with large hydrocele/varicocele.
Pt may notice that the size of the testicle changes over time.
Hydroceles can be congenital in approximately 6% of males.
Varicoceles tend to occur in postpubertal males and are more common on the left because of the length of the left gonadal vein (left gonadal vein drains into the left renal vein, right drains into the IVC).

Does anything increase the size or amount of tenderness?

Varicoceles tend to decrease in size when supine and increase in size with standing.
Hydroceles generally do not change with position and increase slowly over time.
  Exception is congenital hydroceles, which are generally communicating from a patent processus vaginalis and have direct flow of peritoneal fluid into the scrotal sac.

Is the swelling/pain unilateral or bilateral?

Bilateral varicoceles can occur in 33% of pts, but underlying testicular pathology needs to be excluded in lone right-sided varicoceles.
Congenital hydroceles are more likely to occur bilaterally.

Has there been any trauma?

Swelling may represent a hematoma.

Does the pt have any other medical problems?

Exclude other disease entities.

What medications has the pt tried?

NSAIDs may help reduce the size of hydroceles by decreasing the amount of fluid produced by the tunica vaginalis.

Obtain a review of symptoms

Systemic and upper respiratory infection symptoms should increase your suspicion for viral orchitis/epididymitis.

 Perform a physical exam

Abdomen: Tenderness? Masses? Peritoneal signs? Costovertebral angle tenderness?
  Exclude infection or alternative diagnosis.
GU: Penile discharge? Epididymal tenderness or mass? Inguinal hernia? Femoral hernia?
  Prehn sign? Cremasteric reflex? Suggests alternative diagnosis. Testicular swelling or mass? Typically seen and tend to be nontender.
  • Does the mass transilluminate? Darken the room and place a light source against the scrotum near the mass. The hemiscrotum should transilluminate if there is a hydrocele.
  • Be sure to thoroughly exclude testicular torsion from your differential.

Obtain the following labs

Urinalysis: Typically normal. Done to exclude any infectious etiology.

Consider obtaining a scrotal ultrasound

If there is any concern at all about testicular torsion, a scrotal ultrasound with Doppler flow should be obtained.
Ultrasound can also help differentiate varicocele from hydrocele and may show any testicular compression with a varicocele.

 Hydrocele

An accumulation of fluid in the tunica vaginalis (a continuation of the peritoneal lining of the abdomen). Fluid can accumulate because of increased production or decreased absorption or can be caused by direct communication between the scrotum and abdominal cavity. The latter is the most common etiology in congenital hydroceles and may require surgical correction.

Acquired hydroceles are normally benign, although they can be a reaction to an underlying testicular pathology (e.g., cancer), which needs to be excluded if the hydrocele persists with conservative treatment.

Varicocele

Caused by dilation of the pampiniform plexus of spermatic veins. Occurs in the left hemiscrotum in most cases because of anatomic differences in venous drainage. It is rare to occur unilaterally on the right, and one-third of cases will be bilateral. Unilateral right varicoceles are rare enough that this finding must increase the concern for inferior vena cava obstruction.

May require surgical repair or endovascular intervention because they can lead to testicular atrophy and infertility.

P Hydrocele

Congenital hydroceles can be treated conservatively with observation, but they have a higher likelihood of needing surgical repair because they are more likely to communicate with the peritoneal cavity.

Supportive care consists of:

- NSAIDs
- Scrotal support
- Pt should follow up with the primary care provider (PCP)/pediatrician/urologist to ensure improvement

Varicocele

Supportive care if there is no evidence of testicular atrophy or if pt is done having children and is not concerned about fertility.

- Scrotal support
- NSAIDs
- Close follow-up with the PCP/pediatrician/urologist to ensure that testicular atrophy does not occur

Consult Urology for possible venous ligation of the gonadal vein if there is evidence of growth restriction of the testis or testicular atrophy in young males.

KIDNEY STONES/NEPHROLITHIASIS

S **What are the pt's current symptoms?**
Common symptoms include:
- Colicky, unilateral flank pain
- Nausea/vomiting
- Hematuria
- Dysuria

Does the pt's pain radiate anywhere?
Typically, the pain will radiate into the groin, penis, or testicles.

Does anything increase or decrease the pain?
Pain from nephrolithiasis tends to be abrupt in onset, colicky, and unchanged by any maneuvers or position changes.

Does the pt have any risk factors for kidney stones?
These include:
- Male gender
- Low water intake
- Immobilization
- High-protein diet (e.g., Atkins)
- Family history
- Spinal cord injury
- Hypertension
- Malignancy
- Gout

Does the pt have a history of kidney stones?
Extremely common to have multiple recurrences of kidney stones.
Document whether the pt has undergone lithotripsy or surgical extraction of a stone in the past.

Has the pt had any fevers?
Not common with kidney stones alone, and a secondary infection will need to be excluded.

Has the pt recently been treated for a urinary tract infection?
Proteus and *Klebsiella* are associated with struvite stone formation because they are urease-positive.

What medical problems does the pt have?
The following medical conditions are associated with increased kidney stone formation:
- HIV
- Cancer
- Gout
- Paralysis
- Primary hyperparathyroidism
- Renal tubular acidosis

Is the pt taking any medications?
Allopurinol and protease inhibitors are associated with kidney stone production.

O **Evaluate the pt's vital signs**
Tachycardia and elevated blood pressure are common because of the associated pain.
Note any fever that may signify an infection.

Perform a physical exam
General: Pts typically are unable to find a comfortable position.
Abdomen: Typically a normal exam. Pain is not reproducible. Note any costovertebral angle tenderness.
Gyn: Exclude pelvic inflammatory disease (PID) and pregnancy.

Obtain the following labs
β-hCG: Necessary before exposing the pt to radiation and to exclude ectopic pregnancy.
BUN/creatinine: Typically normal. May be elevated with complete obstruction.
Urinalysis: Microscopic hematuria seen in >90% cases. Absence of hematuria does not exclude the diagnosis. Note any signs of infection (e.g., leukocyte esterase, WBCs).

Obtain a diagnostic study
Noncontrast helical abdominal CT scan: Gold standard. Will demonstrate stone, hydronephrosis from obstruction, and has the added benefit of being able to differentiate from an alternative diagnosis.

Renal ultrasound: Can exclude hydronephrosis from obstruction, but it is not sensitive enough to see all stones.

Intravenous pyelogram (IVP): Requires an IVP dye load and multiple radiographs. Not done routinely because of the amount of time it takes for the exam and dye load. CT scans are quicker and provide a lot more information.

 ### Nephrolithiasis

There are four types of kidney stones: calcium oxalate/phosphate stones (80%), uric acid stones (10%), struvite stones, and cystine stones.

Knowing the type of stone can help direct treatment in order to prevent recurrences.

Differential diagnosis

- Ectopic pregnancy
- Diverticulitis
- Ovarian torsion
- Pyelonephritis
- Appendicitis
- PID
- Ovarian cyst rupture

 ### Provide effective pain relief

NSAIDs are very effective at alleviating the pain from kidney stones. IV/IM ketorolac can be used in pts with nausea and vomiting.

Narcotic pain medication may be needed initially.

Hydrate the pt with 2 L of normal saline

Treat nausea and vomiting with antiemetics

If stone is less than 5 mm in size

Most of these pts can be treated conservatively because the stone should pass on its own.

Educate the pt on the need to keep adequately hydrated and to drink plenty of liquids in order to flush the stone from the urinary tract. Pts should strain their urine so they will know when the stone is passed and can get it analyzed to see which of the four stone types it is.

Pain control should be provided with NSAIDs and narcotic pain meds.

Stones greater than 5 mm in size

Have a lower likelihood of passing on their own.

Discuss case with the urologist. Pt may require lithotripsy, open pyelolithotomy, or percutaneous nephrolithotomy to remove the stone. Timing of intervention is generally based on the amount of obstruction seen on CT scan.

Antibiotics are generally indicated for any pt with fever or who has evidence of infection on urinalysis

IV ampicillin/gentamicin versus oral fluoroquinolone

PYELONEPHRITIS/UTI

S **What are the pt's current symptoms?**

Common symptoms include:
- Dysuria
- Urgency/frequency
- Suprapubic tenderness/pain

In pyelonephritis, you may also see:
- Fever
- Nausea/vomiting
- Flank pain

Infants and elderly pts may only present with mental status changes, lethargy, or fever.

In males, has there been any penile discharge?

It is rare for males to get urinary tract infections (UTIs); the more common diagnosis is an STD.

In females, has there been any vaginal discharge or odor?

Vaginitis can cause dysuria.

Does the pt have risk factors for a complicated UTI or pyelonephritis?

These include:
- Pregnancy
- Recent antibiotic use
- Diabetes
- Immunosuppressed
- Neurogenic bladder
- History of self-catheterization or indwelling catheter
- Recent hospitalization or residence in nursing home
- Recent instrumentation of urinary system

What medical problems does the pt have?

Multiple comorbid illnesses increase the likelihood of admission versus outpatient treatment.

What medications is the pt taking?

Glucose, nitrite, blood, and bilirubin may be lower or falsely negative on urinalysis in pts who are taking vitamin C.

Obtain a social history

Inquire about sexual history and risk factors for STD/pelvic inflammatory disease (PID).

O **Evaluate the pt's vital signs**

Perform a physical exam

Abdomen: Tenderness? May be seen with PID. Costovertebral angle tenderness? Seen with pyelonephritis.

GU: Inspect penis and testicles for tenderness and signs of STD.

Rectal: Prostate tenderness may be seen with prostatitis.

Gyn: Speculum and bimanual exam to exclude PID/vaginitis.

Obtain the following labs

Urinalysis: Elevated WBCs, positive leukocyte esterase, and nitrite consistent with infection.
- Obtain clean-catch, midstream voiding specimen, or straight cath urinalysis for most accurate results.
- A specimen with large numbers of epithelial cells suggests skin contamination.

Urine culture: Identify organism and antibiotic sensitivities.

CBC: WBCs may be elevated with pyelonephritis.

β-hCG: Exclude pregnancy.

Consider sending blood cultures before starting antibiotics in pts with pyelonephritis who are going to be admitted.

Consider sending gonorrhea/*Chlamydia* cultures in cases where you suspect an STD

Consider noncontract helical abdominal CT or renal ultrasound if concerned about obstruction

Can show renal abscesses, stones, hydronephrosis, and obstruction

Urinary tract infection
Infection of the lower urinary tract (cystitis)

Pyelonephritis
Infection of the upper urinary tract (kidney)

Differential diagnosis
– Urethritis	– Cervicitis	– Prostatitis
– Vulvovaginitis	– PID	– Epididymitis

Consider phenazopyridine to provide some symptomatic relief of the dysuria
Inform the pt that the phenazopyridine will discolor (orange) the urine, tears, and sweat and can permanently stain contact lenses and clothing.

Treat nausea/vomiting with antiemetics and provide IV hydration

Start empiric antibiotics
Uncomplicated UTIs:
- Can be treated with 3–5 days of TMP-SMX, nitrofurantoin, or fosfomycin.
- Other alternatives include cephalosporins and fluoroquinolones.
- Pregnant pts are at high risk of developing pyelonephritis and should be treated with 10 days of cephalexin, nitrofurantoin, or amoxicillin.
- Children and pregnant women should not receive fluoroquinolones.

Complicated UTIs require treatment that will cover resistant organisms (e.g., *Pseudomonas*).
- 10 days of fluoroquinolone, aminoglycoside, or antipseudomonal cephalosporin

Uncomplicated (early) pyelonephritis:
- 5–7 days of fluoroquinolone, oral third- or fourth-generation cephalosporin, 14 days TMP-SMX

Complicated pyelonephritis
- Fluoroquinolone, antipseudomonal penicillin/cephalosporin, and/or aminoglycoside

Discharge the following pts
Uncomplicated UTI

Complicated UTI and uncomplicated pyelonephritis, provided the pt is able to tolerate oral medications and has close follow-up with the primary care provider

Admit pts
Requiring IV medications or who have complicated pyelonephritis.

Consider urology evaluation
For anyone with multiple UTIs/pyelonephritis or any male over the age of 1 with a history of more than one UTI

RHABDOMYOLYSIS

S **What are the pt's current symptoms?**
Common symptoms include:
- – Muscle pain or tenderness   – Low-grade fever
- – Nausea/vomiting   – Dark brown urine

Has the pt done anything that may have caused the rhabdomyolysis?
Associated with overexertion (heavy lifting, exercise, or prolonged seizures), trauma (crush injuries), immobility (e.g., passed out on the floor for hours), and electrical/lightning injuries.

Has the pt recently been bitten by any animal or insect?
Brown recluse spider bites or snake bites can cause necrosis and secondary rhabdomyolysis.

What medical problems does the pt have?
Diabetic ketoacidosis, hyperthyroidism, seizure disorders, polymyositis, and dermatomyositis are all associated with rhabdomyolysis.
Inquire about any psychiatric disorders that may suggest neuroleptic malignant syndrome or serotonin syndrome.

What medications is the pt taking?
HMG-CoA reductase inhibitors, zidovudine, and colchicine have all been associated with rhabdomyolysis or muscle injury.
Antipsychotics can cause neuroleptic malignant syndrome, which is characterized by hyperthermia, mental status changes, and rhabdomyolysis.

Obtain a social history
Cocaine, alcohol, and narcotic use can lead to muscle injury from either overexertion or prolonged immobilization while in a drug-induced coma.

Obtain a family history
Is there a history of any hereditary myopathies?

O **Evaluate the pt's vital signs**
A markedly elevated temperature requires immediate attention and cooling measures to be initiated.

Perform a physical exam
Cardiac: May note tachycardia.
Abdomen: Typically normal but may have some mild tenderness.
Extremities: Note any muscle tenderness, spasticity, or rigidity.
- Ensure that there are strong pulses in all limbs.
- Consider compartment syndrome with any crush injury.
- Note any fractures.
Skin: Note any rash (dermatomyositis), bite marks, or areas of necrosis.

Obtain the following laboratory studies
CBC, coags: Baseline measurements. Exclude anemia, infection, and disseminated intravascular coagulation.
BUN, creatinine, electrolytes: May have elevated BUN/creatinine if there has been renal injury from rhabdomyolysis. Elevated phosphorus and potassium can be seen with cell lysis and decreased renal function.
CK, CKMB: CK will be markedly elevated, but CKMB ratio should remain low. Degree of elevation correlates with degree of muscle injury.
Lactate dehydrogenase and uric acid may be elevated.
Urinalysis: Macroscopic exam will be positive for blood, but microscopic exam will show minimum or no RBCs because of cross-reactivity of the strip reagent with myoglobin.

Obtain an ECG

Baseline and to confirm that there is no cardiac ischemia. Can see arrhythmias and ECG changes with electrolyte disturbances that occur with rhabdomyolysis.

Obtain x-rays of any suspected fracture sites

Check compartmental pressures if compartment syndrome is suspected

A Rhabdomyolysis

Release of muscle's intracellular contents (creatinine kinase, potassium, calcium) from muscle injury and necrosis

It is extremely important to diagnose the inciting cause of the injury so that further injury can be prevented.

Differential diagnosis

- Polymyositis/dermatomyositis
- Acute renal failure
- Vasculitis
- Connective tissue disorders

P Admit all pts

Will need frequent electrolyte monitoring and IV hydration

Start aggressive IV hydration

Mainstay of therapy

Effective in facilitating clearance of myoglobin and preventing renal failure.

Goal for urine output is 200–300 cc/hr.

Loop diuretics may be initiated if there is evidence of volume overload and fluid resuscitation.

Consider alkalinization of urine

Some authorities recommend bicarbonate infusion to help with clearance of myoglobin.

Need to monitor urine pH every 2 hours. Goal for urine pH is >6.5. Adjust bicarbonate infusion as needed to maintain this pH.

Monitor electrolytes every 2–4 hours

Repeat as necessary and be prepared to treat hyperkalemia.

Treat inciting cause

Consider Nephrology consult and dialysis

If pt has inadequate urine output or is developing signs of volume overload.

TESTICULAR TORSION

 What are the pt's current symptoms?
Common symptoms include:
- Abrupt onset of testicular pain
- Nausea/Vomiting

Does anything alleviate the pain?
Typically, the pain is extremely intense and not relieved by any change in position or scrotal support.

How long has the pain been present?
Torsion of the testicular appendage is more common in children and typically presents as scrotal pain that has increased over several days.
Irreversible ischemic damage to the testicle from torsion occurs after 12 hours.

Has there been any trauma or heavy physical exertion?
It is common for a testicular torsion to occur several hours after minor trauma or heavy exertion.
Nocturnal awakening with intense scrotal pain is common in children.

Has the pt ever experienced this pain before?
It is not uncommon for pts to have had intermittent testicular torsion in the past.

Has the pt had any dysuria, penile discharge, or hematuria?
Suggests alternative diagnoses (e.g., STD, renal colic, UTI, epididymitis).

Obtain a medical history
A history of prior testicular torsion increases the risk for torsion on the contralateral side, if patient did not have bilateral surgical fixation or "pexy" of the testes.

Obtain a social history
Include a sexual history to ascertain risk of STDs.

 Perform a physical exam
Abdomen: Tenderness? Masses? Peritoneal signs? Costovertebral angle tenderness? Suggests an alternative diagnosis, although may have tenderness.
GU: Penile discharge? Testicular swelling or mass? Epididymal tenderness or mass? Inguinal hernia? Femoral hernia? Prehn sign? Tenderness and testicular swelling can be seen, but other signs suggest an alternative diagnosis.
- Check the cremasteric reflex. Assessed by stroking or gently pinching the skin of the upper thigh while observing the ipsilateral testis. The testis should elevate toward the perineum. The reflex is usually absent in pts with testicular torsion.
  o In order to get an accurate response, it is important that the pt be relaxed and that the room be warm.
- Testicular manipulation: If torsion is suspected, you can attempt to relieve the torsion by turning the testicle on its long axis away from the midline ("opening the book").
  o Success rate is generally low because testicle can be rotated 180–720 degrees.
  o Alleviation of pain is diagnostic of torsion.

Obtain the following labs
Urinalysis: Typically normal. Done to exclude any infectious etiology if diagnosis is unclear.

Obtain a scrotal ultrasound with Doppler flow
If diagnosis is clear based on history and physical exam, do not delay surgical evaluation and obtain an ultrasound.
Color Doppler ultrasonography is the diagnostic test of choice to differentiate testicular torsion from torsion of the appendix testis or epididymitis. Hyperperfusion of the testis after detorsion can lead to an incorrect diagnosis of epididymitis.

Testicular torsion

Congenitally absent or inadequate attachment of the testicle to the tunica vaginalis, which allows the testicle to twist on the spermatic cord, decreasing arterial blood flow

Peak incidence in neonates and postpubertal boys

Torsion of the testicular appendage

Leading cause of acute scrotal pain in children

The testicular appendage is a small vestigial structure (remnant of the Müllerian duct system) on the anterosuperior aspect of the testis.

Differential diagnosis
- Epididymitis
- Orchitis
- Hydrocele/varicocele
- Renal colic

 Testicular torsion

Obtain a Urology consult ASAP.
- Emergent surgical exploration and repair is needed to prevent testicular necrosis.
- Do NOT delay consultation to obtain laboratory studies or ultrasound.

Intermittent testicular torsion will need surgical repair, although it can be done on a more elective basis.

Provide pain relief with narcotics.

Disposition: Most pts will require admission or transfer for surgical exploration.

Torsion of the testicular appendage

Surgical removal of the appendage is not necessary, although it tends to increase the speed of recovery because pain can remain present with conservative treatment for weeks to months.

Conservative care includes:
- NSAIDs
- Scrotal support
- Ice to scrotum

Disposition: Most pts will be discharged home with follow-up arranged with the primary care provider or urologist.

NEUROLOGY

ALTERED MENTAL STATUS

S **What are the pt's current symptoms?**
Symptoms may range from mild memory loss to comatose state.
Common symptoms include:
- Mood swings   - Delusions   - Hallucinations
- Memory deficits   - Disorientation   - Psychomotor agitation

Was the change in mental status abrupt or gradual?
Abrupt onset can be a result of drugs, poisons, hypoglycemia, seizure, stroke, or trauma.
Gradual onset can be a result of vascular dementia, vitamin deficiencies, infection,
    Alzheimer disease, drugs, or endocrine disorders.

Has the pt had any symptoms consistent with an infection?
In the young and elderly, it is common for the presenting symptom to be mental status
    changes with no other localizing deficits.

Has the pt been involved in any trauma or minor head injury?
Even relatively mild head injuries can result in subdural hematomas and mental status
    changes.

Does the pt have any other medical problems?
Mental status changes can be seen with:
Hepatitis/cirrhosis: Can lead to liver failure and hepatic encephalopathy
Diabetes: Hypo- or hyperglycemia can progress to coma or altered mental status
Chronic obstructive pulmonary disease/asthma: Secondary to hypoxemia or hypercarbia
Hypothyroidism/adrenal insufficiency
Renal insufficiency: Secondary to uremia or decreased clearance of medications
Seizure: Prolonged postictal state or status epilepticus

What medications is the pt taking?
New medications, in particular, narcotics, benzodiazepines, antibiotics, or herbal sup-
    plements, can affect sensorium.
Chronic medications can also be implicated, especially if there has been any change in
    the pt's liver or renal function.

Obtain a social history
Is there any history of alcohol or drug abuse? Think of intoxication or overdose.
Any recent travel? Think about atypical infectious diseases.

Obtain a review of symptoms
Be thorough and obtain collateral information from family or a friend because it may be
    your only clue in determining the etiology of mental status changes.

O **Evaluate pt's vital signs**
Pay particular attention to temperature and SpO_2 to ensure the pt is not hypoxic.

Perform a physical exam
HEENT: Thyromegaly? Meningismus? Dry mucous membranes or signs of head injury?
Lungs: Wheezing? Egophony? Are there any signs of respiratory distress or pneumonia?
Cardiac: Are there any signs of a myocardial infarction or congestive heart failure?
Abdomen: Peritoneal signs? Ascites? Any stigmata of liver disease?
Neurologic: Decorticate or decerebrate posturing? Weakness or numbness? Glasgow
    Coma Scale (GCS) score?

Obtain the following labs
CBC: Leukocytosis supports infection. Exclude anemia.
BUN/creatinine, electrolytes, LFT: Exclude renal, liver, and electrolyte disturbances.
Glucose: Exclude hypoglycemia.

Blood cultures: Exclude bacteremia or occult infection.
Urinalysis, urine culture: Exclude urinary tract infection.
Urine drug screen, EtOH level: Exclude intoxication.

Consider lumbar puncture
If meningitis or encephalitis is suspected or no other cause is apparent

Consider ABG
Exclude hypoxemia, hypercarbia, or carbon monoxide poisoning.

Obtain an ECG
Evaluate for cardiac ischemia or arrhythmia.

Obtain a head CT
Evaluate for intracranial bleed, epidural or subdural hematoma, or mass lesion.

Consider sending RPR, HIV, B$_{12}$, folate, ammonia level, aspirin, and acetaminophen
If history and physical suggests an infectious, metabolic, or toxic cause

 Acute mental status change
Treatment is aimed at correcting the underlying cause. The history and physical is
    essential in narrowing your differential.
Delirium: An acute, transient alteration in cognitive ability secondary to a physiologic
    event
Dementia: Chronic, irreversible change in memory and cognitive function

Differential diagnosis
    – Drug/alcohol intoxication   – Hypoxemia/hypercarbia
    – Poison or toxic ingestion   – Hepatic encephalopathy
    – Uremia   – Anemia

P **Treat the underlying disorder**
Start antibiotics for infections.
Stop offending medications.
Correct hypoxemia/hypercarbia.

Minimize sedation
Should only be used to prevent pts from hurting themselves or others.

Consider Neurology or Psychiatry consults as needed

All pts will need to be admitted
Admission to ICU, monitored bed, or regular bed should be based on pt's ability to
    protect the airway or anticipated progression of the disease process.

HEADACHE

Determine the PQRST of the pain
See Chest Pain, p. 170.
A sudden-onset "thunderclap" headache that is the worst headache of the person's life
is the classic presentation of a spontaneous subarachnoid hemorrhage.

Are there any associated symptoms with the headache?
Common for the pt to suffer from nausea/vomiting, photophobia, and phonophobia.
Sinus pain and pressure suggest a sinus headache.
Neck pain is common with tension or muscular headaches.
Complicated migraines may result in hemiplegia, ataxia, ophthalmoplegia, etc.

Did the pt experience an aura before the headache?
Auras can precede a migraine headache and include visual scotomas, paresthesias,
aphasia, or the perception of a certain fragrance or taste.

Does the pt have a history of headaches?
Determine the frequency of the headaches and the typical severity.
Is this headache like all prior headaches?
Is there anything that causes the headache, or is it associated with menses?
What has worked in the past to relieve the pt's headache?

Has the pt been exposed to any fumes or toxins?
Carbon monoxide poisoning or toxin ingestion can produce headaches.

Has the pt had any upper respiratory infection symptoms, fever, or neck pain?
Will need to exclude encephalitis/meningitis

Does the pt have any other medical conditions?
HIV: Increases suspicion for atypical infection (e.g., toxoplasmosis) or mass lesion from
Kaposi sarcoma.
Cancer: Consider brain metastasis.
Hypertension: Headache may be the first symptom of hypertensive urgency/crisis.

What medications does the pt take?
Ask specifically about over-the-counter pain relievers. Rebound headaches are common
in those who take pain medication regularly.

Obtain a social history
In addition to alcohol, tobacco, and occupational histories, obtain a caffeine history.
Withdrawal from caffeine can result in severe headaches.

Evaluate the pt's vital signs
Note any hypertension or fever.

Perform a physical exam
HEENT: Perform a fundoscopic exam. Sinus tenderness? Neck stiffness? Photophobia?
Phonophobia?
Lungs, cardiac, abdomen: Typically normal.
Neurologic: Complete a full neurologic assessment. Exam is typically normal. May note
paresthesias or other focal neurologic deficits.

Consider the following labs
ABG: Rule out hypoxemia, carbon monoxide poisoning, or hypercarbia.
ESR: May be elevated in temporal arteritis.
CBC: Exclude leukocytosis and anemia.

Consider obtaining a lumbar puncture
Exclude meningitis or encephalitis.
More sensitive than head CT in diagnosing a subarachnoid hemorrhage.

Consider obtaining a head CT

Should be obtained in any individual with neurologic symptoms, atypical headache features, new-onset, severe "worst headache of my life," or HIV with headache to exclude any underlying pathology.

A Headache

Common types of headaches include migraine, trigeminal autonomic cephalgia (e.g., cluster), and tension headaches.

Migraine headaches are subdivided into migraine with or without aura or migraine variant.

- The exact etiology of migraines is unknown, but they are thought to be an imbalance of vascular regulation, resulting in vasoconstriction followed by vasodilation.

Cluster headaches are repetitive headaches that occur for weeks to months at a time, followed by periods of remission. Their exact etiology is unclear.

Tension headaches are the most common headaches and, although they were originally thought to be caused by muscle contractions, recent studies have shown that there is actually more muscle contraction with migraine headaches. The exact etiology of pain remains unclear.

Differential diagnosis

- Stroke
- Meningitis
- Temporomandibular joint syndrome
- Carbon monoxide exposure
- Brain metastasis
- Temporal arteritis
- Sinusitis
- Subarachnoid hemorrhage

P Provide effective pain relief

Supplemental oxygen: Very effective in aborting the pain associated with cluster headaches.

Antiemetics: Prochlorperazine and metoclopramide are very effective in relieving headaches in addition to the nausea associated with them. Low abuse potential. Risk of extrapyramidal side effects.

Analgesics: NSAIDs, acetaminophen, caffeine. Increased risk for withdrawal headaches and dependence on narcotic use.

Ergotamine: Causes vasoconstriction. Risk of coronary ischemia or hypertension.

Triptans: Serotonin agonists that cause vasoconstriction. Same risks as ergotamine.

Consider starting prophylactic treatment if headaches are frequent, debilitating for several days, or extreme in intensity

β-Blockers, SSRIs, calcium channel blockers, valproic acid, and tricyclic antidepressants have all been shown to decrease the frequency and severity of headaches.

Disposition

Most pts can be discharged home.

MENINGITIS

S **What are the pt's current symptoms?**
Common symptoms include:
- – Fever
- – Nausea/vomiting
- – Headache
- – Mental status changes
- – Neck stiffness
- – Photophobia

Does the pt belong to a high-risk group?
- – Elderly
- – HIV-positive
- – College student
- – Neonates
- – Postsplenectomy
- – Recent neurosurgical procedure
- – Alcoholics
- – Immunosuppressed

Has the pt been on antibiotics recently?
Antibiotics will make it more difficult to interpret the results of any cerebrospinal fluid (CSF) studies.

Has the pt been vaccinated against *Neisseria meningitidis, Haemophilus influenzae,* or *Streptococcus pneumoniae?*
Vaccines do not completely prevent infection.
N. meningitidis vaccine only protect against serotypes A, C, Y, or W-135.

Has there been any trauma or recent head injury?
Supportive of an alternative diagnosis (e.g., subarachnoid or intracerebral hemorrhage).

Has the pt been exposed to anyone with meningitis?
Bacterial meningitis is only spread through close personal contact (live in the same household or spend prolonged time in an enclosed space with infected persons).

Has the pt suffered any insect bites recently?
Increased incidence of aseptic (viral) meningitis in the summer, with mosquitoes being a common vector.

What other medical problems does the pt have?
Cancer (metastatic spread of tumor to meninges) and autoimmune disorders are associated with aseptic meningitis.

What medications is the pt taking?
Meningeal symptoms can occur from chemical or drug reactions.

Obtain a social history
Inquire specifically about living situation, close personal contacts, and any recent travel.
Alcohol and drug use increase the risk for meningitis.

O **Evaluate the pt's vital signs**
A fever does not need to be present.

Perform a physical exam
HEENT: Sinus tenderness? (Nasopharyngeal area is the most common source of infections.) Rhinorrhea? Dental abscess? Neck stiffness? Perform a fundoscopic exam to exclude papillary edema (may need to dilate to obtain adequate exam). *Brudzinski sign:* Reflexive hip and knee flexion when the neck of the supine pt is passively flexed.
Lungs, cardiac, abdomen: Typically normal. Note any signs of pneumonia or endocarditis as possible sources of infection.
Extremities: Petechiae may be seen with *N. meningitidis. Kernig sign;* Neck and hamstring pain when the supine pt with hip and knee flexed at 90 degrees as the knee is passively extended.
Neurologic: Mental status changes? Weakness? Numbness?

Obtain the following labs
CBC: May see leukocytosis.
Blood cultures: Isolate causative organism.
Urinalysis, urine culture: Exclude urinary system as source of infection.

Perform a lumbar puncture

Head CT scan is only required before lumbar puncture if there is a risk of a mass lesion or elevated intracranial pressure (risk of herniation).

Send fluid for cell count, glucose, protein, and Gram stain/culture.

Consider sending fungal or tuberculosis cultures, latex agglutination studies, herpes simplex virus (HSV) polymerase chain reaction (PCR).

A Meningitis

Bacterial: S. pneumoniae, N. meningitidis, or H. influenzae are the most common causes. Classic CSF findings are WBC >1,000, decreased CSF-to-serum glucose ratio, increased protein (>150), and elevated opening pressure (classically found in *Cryptococcus*).

Viral: Classic CSF findings are WBC <1,000, normal glucose, protein >200.

Autoimmune, chemical, and carcinomatous tend to have viral CSF picture.

Elderly and newborn pts require a high index of suspicion because they tend to have atypical presentations.

Differential diagnosis

- Migraine   – Stroke   – Brain abscess
- Intracerebral hemorrhage   – Mass lesion

P Start empiric antibiotic treatment ASAP

Do not withhold antibiotics because there will be a delay in obtaining a CT scan or lumbar puncture.

Typical empiric regimen consists of third-generation cephalosporin plus vancomycin (covers cephalosporin-resistant *S. pneumoniae*) ± acyclovir (if HSV is suspected).

Consider adding ampicillin to cover *Listeria* in the elderly, immunosuppressed, or neonatal pt.

Withhold any medications that may be related to a chemical meningitis

NSAIDS, sulfa, OKT3, COX-2 inhibitors, pyridium, and azathioprine

Place the pt in respiratory isolation

Consider starting steroids in children

Decreases risk of residual hearing deficits.

Ideally, the steroids should be given before the antibiotics.

Disposition

Admit all pts to an isolation room.

Contact your health department or infectious disease department if you suspect bacterial meningitis so that close contacts can be evaluated and given prophylaxis with ciprofloxacin or rifampin.

SEIZURES

 Was the seizure witnessed?

Unless tonic-clonic activity was witnessed, the pt may have had a syncopal episode instead of a seizure.

Small muscle twitches (myoclonus) can be seen with syncope.

Does the pt have a history of seizures? If pt has known seizures

Document last known seizure and typical frequency and character of seizures.

Why was the pt transported to the ED for this seizure?

- Bystanders called 911 before the pt being able to inform them that this is their baseline.
    - Atypical seizure?   – Prolonged seizure or postictal state
    - Trauma?
- Has there been any change in the pt's medications?
    - Missed dose   – Increased/decreased dose   – New medication
- Does the pt experience an aura before seizures?
    ○ May experience visual, gustatory, or olfactory changes.
- What type of seizure does the pt typically have?
    ○ *Generalized seizure*—Loss of consciousness with or without tonic-clonic activity
    ○ *Partial (focal) seizure*—Localized seizure usually preceded by aura that does not necessarily result in loss of consciousness, but may evolve (generalize)

Is this a new (first) seizure?

Need to exclude secondary causes of seizure. These include:

- Head injury
- Stroke
- Alcohol or benzodiazepine withdrawal
- Drug reaction
- Intracerebral bleed or mass
- Metabolic disturbances
- Infection
- Drug intoxication (stimulants)

Is the pt pregnant?

May be presenting/defining sign of eclampsia

What medical problems does the pt have?

May suggest secondary causes of new-onset seizure

What medications is the pt taking?

Numerous medications and herbal supplements can lower the seizure threshold and cause iatrogenic seizures.

Obtain a social history

Detailed alcohol and drug abuse history is required. Alcohol or drug intoxication/withdrawal may cause seizures.

Obtain a review of symptoms

Exclude other causes of loss of consciousness (e.g., syncope, hypoglycemia, sleep disorder).

 Perform a physical exam

Postseizure exam is typically normal.

Exclude any injury.

Pt may be postictal as exhibited by confusion, agitation, or a prolonged state of unconsciousness.

If unconscious, ensure that pt is not in status epilepticus.

Obtain the following labs

CBC: Exclude infection, anemia, thrombocytopenia.

Electrolytes, Glucose, BUN/creatinine: Exclude electrolyte disturbances, hypoglycemia, uremia.

Drug levels: Ensure that pt's medications are therapeutic.

Consider sending the following labs:
- Prolactin: Elevated in true seizure, normal in psychogenic nonepileptic seizure (formerly pseudoseizure).
- Urine drug screen/EtOH level: Exclude intoxication.
- Urinalysis, ESR: Exclude infection.

Consider obtaining a head CT

Should be obtained if there is a change in the seizure pattern or characteristic, head injury, fever, or if this is a new-onset seizure.

Consider obtaining an electroencephalogram stat if there is concern about status epilepticus

 Seizure

A change in the pt's baseline behavior caused by brain dysfunction

Status epilepticus: Seizure lasting >30 minutes or recurrent seizure without a return to baseline.

Two classification systems:
- Primary versus secondary (no apparent cause versus known cause)
- Generalized versus partial

Differential diagnosis

– Syncope	– Meningitis	– Hypoglycemia
– Narcolepsy	– Migraines	– Psychogenic nonepileptic seizure

P **Provide supportive care**

Maintain airway.

Provide supplemental oxygen.

Establish IV access.

Treat underlying disorder if resulting from secondary causes

If pt is actively seizing, treat with

Benzodiazepines, phenytoin, or phenobarbital

Goal is to get the pt's seizures under control in <30 minutes to prevent permanent brain injury.

If drug levels are subtherapeutic, consider giving an additional dose

Disposition

Known epileptics can typically be discharged home if their mental status returns to normal and they have appropriate follow-up arranged.

Consult Neurology on all pts with new-onset seizures, persistent mental status changes, or focal neurologic deficits.

Consult local ordinances concerning requirements to report individuals having seizures to the department of motor vehicles.

STROKE

S **What are the pt's symptoms?**
Symptoms are variable. Common symptoms include:
- Expressive or receptive aphasia
- Mental status changes
- Nausea/vomiting
- Weakness/hemiplegia
- Impaired vision
- Ataxia

How long ago did the symptoms start?
If exact onset of symptoms can be determined to be less than 4 hours, the pt may be a candidate for thrombolytics in the ischemic stroke setting. Mechanical thrombectomy may be indicated in pts with last known normal within the past 6–24 hours; however, this is variable depending on the location of the thrombus, presentation, and availability of the resource.
Difficult to ascertain timing when the pt awakens with deficits or is found with them.

Have the symptoms resolved?
Transient ischemic attack (TIA) is defined as a transient neurologic deficit that resolves within 24 hours, although most resolve within 5 minutes.

Has the pt had a stroke before? Are the current symptoms an exacerbation of past deficits?
Sleep deprivation, infections, and electrolyte disturbances can exacerbate prior deficits.

Does the pt have any risk factors for a stroke?
Risk factors include:
- Atherosclerosis
- Atrial fibrillation
- Hypertension
- Diabetes
- Smoking
- Amphetamine/cocaine use

What medical problems does the pt have?
Identify risk factors and comorbid illnesses.

What medications does the pt take?
Warfarin use increases the risk for hemorrhagic stroke.

O **Perform a physical exam**
HEENT: Nystagmus suggests cerebellar infarct. Palpate carotid arteries and listen for carotid bruits (diminished pulse or bruit suggests decreased blood flow).
Lungs, cardiac, abdomen: Typically normal. Irregularly irregular rhythm may be heard with atrial fibrillation. Murmur may suggest endocarditis.
Extremities: Typically normal.
Neurologic: Evaluate mental status, speech, short- and long-term memory. Measure strength in all four extremities. Evaluate cranial nerves. Check deep tendon reflexes, tone of muscles, and Babinski reflex.

Obtain the following labs
CBC, electrolytes, BUN/creatinine, glucose, coagulation studies, urinalysis: Exclude other causes of weakness or mental status changes.
Consider urine drug screen in pts who may have used cocaine/amphetamines.

Obtain a noncontract head CT
Obtained to first exclude hemorrhagic infarct.
Typically normal. May *see* hypodense (dark) area in subacute strokes representing edema or hyperdense (bright) blood.

Consider MRI of brain
More sensitive for ischemia. Can show ischemic infarcts acutely.

Consider lumbar puncture if suspicious of subarachnoid hemorrhage
More sensitive than head CT and brain MRI, which may miss small subarachnoid hemorrhages.

A **Cerebral vascular accident**

Caused by abrupt, focal interruption of blood flow to the brain

May be hemorrhagic (15%) or ischemic.

Ischemic infarcts can occur from embolisms, thrombosis, arterial stenosis, arterial dissection, or venous occlusion.

Differential diagnosis

- Seizure
- Hypertensive encephalopathy
- Hypoglycemia
- Encephalitis
- Meningitis
- Drug effect

P **Provide supportive care**

Maintain airway.

Provide supplemental oxygen.

Obtain IV access.

Consider thrombolytics

In moderate to severe ischemic strokes less than 4.5 hours in duration. Consider mechanical thrombectomy.

Consider transfer to a stroke treatment center.

For ischemic strokes

Start the pt on aspirin.

Monitor blood pressure, but do not treat hypertension unless it exceeds 220/120.

Hypertension may be protective and the brain's attempt to autoregulate blood flow. Decreasing the blood pressure may extend the infarction into watershed areas.

For hemorrhagic strokes

Consult Neurosurgery to consider surgical intervention.

Correct any coagulopathy or thrombocytopenia ASAP.

Disposition

All pts with neurologic deficits need to be admitted to the ICU or Neuro floor, where they can receive frequent neurologic checks.

Pts with TIAs that return to baseline quickly can be discharged home, provided that they are started on antiplatelet therapy and have close follow-up arranged for outpatient evaluation of the TIA.

VERTIGO

 What are the pt's current symptoms?

Common symptoms include:
- Peripheral vertigo
  - Nausea/vomiting
  - Tinnitus
  - Increased symptoms with head movement
  - Fatigable nystagmus
- Central vertigo
  - Intact hearing
  - Vision changes
  - Ataxia
  - No change with head movement
  - Nonfatigable nystagmus

Is the pt complaining of dizziness?

Dizziness is a nonspecific complaint. Have the pt clarify whether the pt means vertiginous dizziness (room spinning) or lightheadedness (near syncope).

Does the pt have or recently had any upper respiratory infection symptoms?

Peripheral vertigo (e.g., labyrinthitis) is associated with viral infections.

Are the symptoms abrupt in onset and intermittent or have they gradually progressed?

Peripheral vertigo is associated with a more acute onset and intermittent symptoms, whereas central vertigo tends to be gradual in onset and more persistent.

Quantify the severity of the duration, and whether any inciting event or activity is associated with the symptoms

What has the pt done to help improve symptoms?

Helpful to narrow differential and determine what an effective treatment might be.

What medical problems does the pt have?

Central vertigo can be associated with mass lesions, migraines, strokes, multiple sclerosis, peripheral vascular disease, and intracerebral hemorrhages.

Peripheral vertigo can be seen with acoustic neuromas, meningiomas, and posttrauma.

What medication is or has the pt been on recently?

Numerous medications have ototoxicity (e.g., aminoglycosides, loop diuretics, chemotherapeutic agents). Take a thorough medication history.

Obtain a social history

Exclude drug or alcohol abuse as etiology.

O **Perform a physical exam**

HEENT: Note any nystagmus (vertical, horizontal, or rotary) and whether it is fatigable. Evaluate tympanic membranes to exclude otitis media.
- Perform Dix-Hallpike maneuver: Have the pt sit on the bed, turn head to one side, and then lay supine quickly so the head can hang off the end of the bed. Note any nystagmus (type and duration), raise the pt to a seated position rapidly and note any nystagmus. Repeat with the head turned to the opposite side.
- In peripheral vertigo, this maneuver should exacerbate symptoms and show nystagmus that is short in duration (<1 minute), fatigable, and starts after a short latency period.
- Central vertigo will last >1 minute, has no latency period, and will not be fatigable. Symptoms are generally mild.

Lungs, cardiac, abdomen: Typically normal.

Neurologic: Complete a full neurologic exam to exclude any deficits that would suggest a central cause.

Labs are generally not helpful
Obtain to exclude secondary causes if suspected.

Obtain a noncontract head CT
If the pt has central vertigo, focal neurologic deficits, or any evidence of trauma or stroke

Consider obtaining an MRI
Increased sensitivity for cerebellar disease and early cerebrovascular accident (CVA)

A   Vertigo
Central vertigo: Caused by brainstem or cerebellar disease. Common etiologies include
   CVA, intracerebral hemorrhage, cancer (metastatic or primary central nervous system),
   multiple sclerosis, or migraines.
Peripheral vertigo: Most common is benign positional vertigo, which occurs from crystal
   forming in the semicircular canals. Dix-Hallpike maneuver may be diagnostic and
   therapeutic.
Other causes include labyrinthitis, acoustic neuroma, meningioma, and drug ototoxicity.

Differential diagnosis
– CVA	– Seizure	– Migraine
– Syncope	– Hypoxia	– Drug intoxication
– Ménière disease		

P   Pt with central vertigo should be admitted for a complete evaluation
Although symptoms may be mild, the causes are more ominous.

Peripheral vertigo care is supportive
Antiemetics for nausea and vomiting.
Antihistamines, scopolamine, and benzodiazepines have all been used as vestibular
   suppressants.

Perform brandt-daroff, semont, or epley maneuvers for benign positional vertigo
A series of head and neck movements that has approximately 60% success rate in alleviating symptoms. Goal is to move the canoliths or debris in the semicircular canals into
   the utricle, where they cannot interfere with the function of the endolymph.
A modified Epley maneuver can be taught for self-treatment at home.

Disposition
Admit all pts with central vertigo, intractable vomiting, or if diagnosis is unclear.
Discharge pts with peripheral vertigo who are able to tolerate oral intake, have a steady
   gait, and have close follow-up.
Consider ENT consult for pts with persistent or severe symptoms.

WEAKNESS

S **Has the weakness been gradual in onset or abrupt?**
Abrupt onset is more typical of cerebrovascular accident (CVA).
Gradual onset seen with multiple sclerosis (MS), amyotrophic lateral sclerosis
(ALS), myasthenia gravis (MG), Lambert-Eaton myasthenic syndrome (LEMS), and
myopathies.

Does the pt have true muscle weakness?
Functional weakness (pt feels weak but there is no loss of muscle strength) can be
caused by medical conditions such as exercise intolerance, joint pain, anemia, congestive heart failure, or depression.

Does the weakness improve with exertion?
LEMS tends to improve with exertion, whereas MG gets worse.

Does the pt have any visual complaints (e.g., diplopia, blurred vision)?
MS, LEMS, and MG typically have visual complaints. Pts with ALS have normal vision
and sensation.

Does the pt have any muscle pain or tenderness?
Suggests dermatomyositis or (less likely) polymyositis

Does the pt complain of any alteration in sensation (e.g., paresthesias)?
ALS and MG do not affect sensory functions.

What activities is the pt having difficulty doing?
Proximal muscle weakness is characterized by an inability to rise from a seated position
associated with deltoid, quadriceps, and axial muscle group weakness.
Distal muscle weakness is characterized by decreased grip strength, foot drop, and wrist
flexion/extension. Pt may have difficultly opening jars and standing on tips of toes.

What medical problems does the pt have?
MG is associated with autoimmune disorders (e.g., autoimmune hypothyroidism, rheumatoid arthritis, systemic lupus erythematosus) and thymoma.
70% of LEMS pts will have a cancer (commonly small cell lung cancer), but the neurologic symptoms often develop before the cancer is diagnosed.
Dermatomyositis and polymyositis also have an increased association with cancer.

What medications is the pt taking?
Chronic steroids, antimalarial agents (e.g., chloroquine), penicillamine, and colchicine
have all been attributed to muscle weakness.

Obtain a social history and a review of symptoms
Living in the northern latitudes before puberty increases the risk for MS.

O **Perform a physical exam**
HEENT: Perform a fundoscopic exam to look for optic neuritis. Note nystagmus, weak-
ness of extraocular movement, ability to swallow.
Lungs, cardiac, abdomen: Ensure adequate respiratory effort and strength.
Extremities: Check for muscle atrophy, tenderness, or rash.
Neurologic: Perform a complete exam to include functional testing (e.g., open a jar,
stand from seated position). Rate strength of all major muscle groups. Check reflexes
in all limbs and Babinski reflex.

Obtain the following labs
CBC: Exclude anemia.
Electrolytes: Exclude hypo-/hyperkalemia, hypo-/hypercalcemia, and hypomagnesemia.
CK: Elevated in myositis and myopathies.
Blood cultures, urinalysis, and urine culture: Exclude occult infection.
TSH: Exclude hypothyroidism.

Consider obtaining a head CT
Exclude intracranial hemorrhage and CVA.

Consider obtaining a chest CT
Evaluate for thymoma (MG) and lung cancer (LEMS).

A   Weakness
Multiple sclerosis: Most common autoimmune inflammatory demyelinating disease of the central nervous system. Onset is 20–40 years of age.

Amyotrophic lateral sclerosis: Most common motor neuron disease characterized by upper and lower motor neuron degeneration.

Myasthenia gravis: Autoimmune disease characterized by the development of acetylcholine receptor antibodies.

Lambert-Eaton myasthenic syndrome: Paraneoplastic autoimmune disease similar to MG with a high association with small cell lung cancer.

Differential diagnosis
- Botulism
- Tick paralysis
- Guillain-Barré syndrome
- Stroke
- CNS tumor
- Hypothyroidism

P   Consider a Neurology consultation

Provide supportive care: IV hydration, supplemental oxygen

Disposition
Admit all pts with new onset of symptoms who do not have a diagnosis.

Monitor respiratory status closely because progressive respiratory muscle weakness may require intubation. Follow forced vital capacity and negative inspiratory pressure.

Pts with known disease, mild symptoms, and no signs of respiratory compromise can be discharged home if close neurologic (same or next-day) follow-up is arranged.

Treat any underlying electrolyte disturbance or infection

Inpatient testing to be considered
MRI of brain: More sensitive for demyelination and inflammation associated with MS.

Lumbar puncture: Exclude occult infection. Oligoclonal bands and elevated IgG seen in MS.

Muscle biopsy: Denervation seen with ALS. Inflammation seen with myositis.

Electromyogram: To differentiate muscle from nerve abnormalities.

Acetylcholine receptor antibody: Positive in 85% of MG pts.

Tensilon test: Edrophonium challenge will temporarily reverse symptoms in MG pts.

TRAUMA

ANIMAL BITE

S **When, where, and how did the bite occur?**
Document the time, place, and events leading up to the bite.
Document the areas of injury and whether any self-treatment has occurred.

What animal was involved in the bite? Was the bite provoked?
Dog bites are usually associated with a crush or tearing injury.
Cat bites are typically puncture wounds and have a higher associated risk of soft-
tissue infection and osteomyelitis with the introduction of bacteria directly into the
periosteum.
Wild animal bites (bats, coyotes, foxes, raccoons) increase the risk of rabies exposure.
Rodents (e.g., mice, rats, squirrels) except for the ground hog are considered a low risk
for rabies transmission. There is no transplacental transmission of the virus, and most
rodents are killed in the attack that would transmit the virus.
Unprovoked attacks or animals that are acting bizarrely are more likely to be infected
with rabies.

Can the animal be observed or is the animal known to the pt?
If the animal cannot be observed for 10 days for signs of rabies and its rabies vaccination
status is not known, the pt should start the rabies vaccine series.

Is the pt's tetanus immunization up-to-date?
Tetanus should be updated if the last booster was more than 5 years ago and the wound
is high risk for tetanus.

Has the local animal control service been notified?
Most jurisdictions require that all bites be reported to the local animal control warden.
Check with your ED on reporting requirements.

Does the pt have any medical problems?
Pts with diabetes or peripheral vascular disease are at increased risk for infectious
complications.

O **Perform a physical exam**
Note location, size, number, and shape of all bites. Consider drawing a diagram.
Explore all wounds carefully to exclude foreign bodies, joint space involvement, or any
bone/tendon injury.
Consider anesthetizing the area to ensure an adequate exam.
A complete skin exam is warranted, especially in children, to document any other
injuries.

Consider obtaining an x-ray of the involved area
Use x-rays judiciously to exclude fractures and foreign bodies. Most foreign bodies can
be seen on plain films.
Ultrasound, fluoroscopy, CT scan, or MRI can also be useful in localizing foreign bodies.

Consider obtaining wound cultures
If the area appears infected or purulent, wound culture can help direct antibiotic
therapy.

Consider blood cultures in those pts who are systemically ill

A **Animal bite**
Wound infections are common, involving 80% of cat bites and 5% of dog bites.
Bacteria associated with infection include:
- Skin flora: *Staphylococcus* or *Streptococcus*
- Cats: *Pasteurella, Moraxella, Neisseria*
- Dogs: *Pasteurella, Capnocytophaga cynodegmi*

Wash wounds thoroughly and debride as needed

Most wounds should be allowed to heal by secondary intention to minimize the risk of infection and abscess formation.

Consider primary closure of wounds on the scalp and face that can be disfiguring.

Ensure that tetanus immunization is current

Administer tetanus-diphtheria vaccine if not current and the pt has been immunized in the past.

If wound is tetanus-prone and pt has not been immunized in the past, administer tetanus immune globulin and tetanus vaccine.

Consider antibiotic therapy

Antibiotics should be prescribed for all distal extremity wounds and moderate- to high-risk wounds because of the high rate of infection.

Amoxicillin/clavulanic acid is the antibiotic of choice. Clindamycin plus a fluoroquinolone or TMP-SMX is an alternative in penicillin-allergic pts.

Consult Orthopedics for any injuries that involve fractures, tendon involvement, or compromise the joint space

These wounds require extensive irrigation and debridement that is more suitable for the OR.

Consider rabies immunoprophylaxis

In high-risk wounds, the pt should receive the rabies vaccine and rabies immune globulin.

Treatment can be delayed if the animal can be observed and is healthy-appearing.

Disposition

Most pts can be discharged home on oral antibiotics, if indicated.

Admit pts with systemic symptoms or joint infections, who fail to respond to outpatient therapy, or who have significant comorbidities requiring IV antibiotics.

ANKLE SPRAIN

S **How did the pt injure the ankle?**

Document whether the pt inverted or everted the ankle.

Inversion injuries are associated with injury to the lateral malleolus and associated ligamentous structures (commonly anterior talofibular ligament).

Eversion injuries are associated with injury to the medial malleolus (commonly deltoid ligament).

Has the pt been able to bear weight and walk since the injury?

Ask the pt how he or she got to the ED. Often, the triage nurse will place the pt in a wheelchair, but he or she was able to walk to the triage desk.

Inability to walk four steps is an indication to obtain x-rays.

Where does the pt localize the pain?

Localizes the area of injury and helps exclude foot injuries with referred pain.

What self-treatment has the pt done to date?

Pain medications and ice may alter your physical exam.

Document past medical history, medications, allergies, and social history

Exclude comorbid illnesses, possible medication interactions with your prescribed treatment, and allergies.

Complete documentation is needed in order to bill.

O **Perform a physical exam**

Note any tenderness, ecchymosis, or swelling.

- Specifically check for tenderness over:
  - Fifth metatarsal head: Exclude a Jones or dancer's fracture.
  - Navicular: Exclude fracture/dislocation.
  - Fibula head: Exclude a Maisonneuve fracture (proximal fibula fracture, disruption of the interosseous membrane, and medial malleolus fracture or deltoid tendon rupture).

Document normal sensation and pulses.

Perform the thompson test

Ensure that the Achilles tendon is intact. With the foot in a neutral position, squeeze the calf muscles. The foot should plantar flex. Lack of movement suggests complete rupture of the Achilles tendon. Movement will be normal with partial ruptures.

Test the stability of the ankle joint

Anterior draw: Test the anterior talofibular ligament (ATFL). Push the tibia posterior while pulling the heel forward. Increased laxity or movement when compared with the unaffected side suggests injury.

Talar tilt: Tests the ATFL and calcaneofibular ligament. Plantar flex the foot and test for laxity with inversion and eversion. Compare with the unaffected side.

Consider obtaining radiographs

According to the Ottawa ankle rules, an ankle series is indicated for:

- Inability to bear weight immediately after injury and walk four steps
- Bony tenderness on posterior edge or tip of either malleolus
- Bony tenderness over the fifth metatarsal head or navicular (include foot series)

Obtain a full tibia/fibula series if pt has pain over the proximal fibula.

A **Ankle sprain**

Ligamentous sprain that is graded 1, 2, or 3:

- Type 1: mild stretch of the ligament with fibers remaining intact
- Type 2: partial disruption of ligament fibers
- Type 3: complete disruption; ATFL is the most common tendon injured

Achilles rupture

Risk of rupture increased with use of prednisone, fluoroquinolones, and age older than 60.

Ankle fracture

Foot fractures

Jones fracture: Fracture of the proximal fifth metatarsal.

Dancer's fracture: Avulsion fracture of the base of the fifth metatarsal.

P Provide supportive care

All injuries should be treated with rest, ice, compression, and elevation (RICE).

NSAIDs may be needed for pain relief. Narcotics should be used sparingly.

Ankle sprains

Pt should bear weight as tolerated.

Severe (type 3) sprains should be treated with posterior splint, non–weight-bearing
status, and referral to Orthopedics.

Air or gel stirrup braces can help prevent recurrent sprains while allowing plantar and
dorsiflexion.

Pts with persistent pain after 2 weeks of conservative therapy should be referred to
Orthopedics.

Achilles rupture

Orthopedics consultation

Treatment is controversial. Options include operative repair or conservative therapy
with casting and non–weight-bearing status.

Ankle fractures

Orthopedics consultation for any open fracture or unstable fracture.

Open fractures also require antibiotic treatment (i.e., cefazolin) and ensuring tetanus
immunization is up-to-date.

Stable fractures can be managed with splint (posterior stirrup), non–weight-bearing
status, and orthopedic referral.

Foot fracture

Posterior splint

Orthopedics referral

Disposition

Most pts will be discharged home, with follow-up arranged with orthopedics or primary
care provider.

Admit all pts with open or unstable fractures that will require operative repair.

BURNS

S **When, where, and how was the pt burned?**

Document time and place of burn.

Document type of burn (e.g., electrical, thermal, or chemical).

- If chemical, attempt to identify the exact chemical involved, and at a minimum, if it is an acid or alkali.
- Acids cause coagulation necrosis, which limits depth of injury.
- Alkalis cause liquefaction necrosis, resulting in deep penetration.

Systemic effects are possible.

Ask specifically what burned because toxic vapors can be released from the burning process.

What self-treatment has the pt tried?

Inquire about any ointments or creams that may have been applied because they can alter the burn's appearance, and depending on the cream/ointment, may increase the risk of infection.

Does the pt have any difficulty speaking or breathing?

Thermal burns of the airway and nasopharynx can result in dysphonia, and respiratory compromise from edema.

Bronchospasm, pneumonitis, and adult respiratory distress syndrome (ARDS) can all result from inhalation injuries.

Is the pt's tetanus immunization current?

All burns that involve the dermis are tetanus-prone. Update if the last booster was >5 years.

Is the pt's or parent's story consistent with the injuries seen?

Consider child abuse in any child presenting with burns where the story does not match the pattern of injury seen.

Obtain a past medical history, medication list, allergy list, and social history

Sulfa allergies are common. Do not apply silver sulfadiazine without taking a thorough history.

O **Evaluate the pt's vital signs**

Monitor SpO_2 and ensure that oxygenation is adequate.

Perform a physical exam

Document location and thickness of burns.

First-degree burn: superficial erythema (e.g., sunburn).

Second-degree burn (partial-thickness): dermis involved; erythema, pain, and blistering present.

Third-degree burn (full-thickness): painless; visible thrombosed vessels are pathognomonic.

Fourth-degree burn: full-thickness burn that includes muscle and bone

Body surface area of burns can be estimated by the rule of nines in adults.

- 9% of body surface area is given to each arm and head/neck
- 18% for each leg, anterior torso, and posterior torso
- 1% perineum

Consult a Lund and Browder chart for estimating body surface area of burns in children.

HEENT: Note any soot or burns around nares and mouth. Note any singed nose or facial hair. Predicts upper airway injury and risk of respiratory compromise.

Lungs: Note any wheezing, signs of consolidation, respiratory distress.

Cardiac, abdomen: Typically normal. Tachycardia may be present.

Extremities: Ensure adequate range of motion if burns involve hands or cross joints.

Consider obtaining the following labs

CBC, electrolytes, BUN, creatinine, ABG, carboxyhemoglobin: Exclude carbon monoxide poisoning, ensure proper oxygenation, and exclude electrolyte disturbance.

Obtain an ECG with any electrical injury

Exclude cardiac injury and arrhythmia.

Obtain a CXR if evidence of inhalation injury is present

Exclude pneumonitis, ARDS, underlying pulmonary disease.

A Burn

Minor burn: Involves <15% of body (<10% in elderly/children)

Moderate burn: 15%–25% of body (10%–20% in elderly/children)

Severe burn: >25% (>20% in elderly/children) or burns that may cause cosmetic or functional deficits (e.g., face, perineum, hands) or burns that compromise respiratory function

P Ensure that pt has an intact airway

Intubate for respiratory distress or if there are severe facial/neck burns. Early intubation is recommended because airway edema may preclude intubation later.

Provide IV hydration for moderate and severe burns

Burns require large-volume fluid resuscitation because of insensible losses and fluid shifting. Use the Parkland formula to estimate fluid needs.

Ensure that pt's tetanus Immunization is up-to-date

Booster required if the last injection was >5 years.

Oral and IV antibiotic prophylaxis are not needed for minor burns and are controversial in severe burns

Follow your local treatment protocols.

Local burn management

Dress minor burns with nonadherent dry gauze after applying topical antibacterial cream (e.g., silver sulfadiazine, mupirocin). Avoid using sulfadiazine on the face.

Provide effective pain relief

NSAIDs and/or narcotics for pain

Disposition

Follow local reporting guidelines if child abuse is suspected.

Consider transferring all severe burn pts to a local burn treatment center.

Minor burn pts can be discharged home with close follow-up.

Circumferential, electrical, moderate, and severe burn pts should be admitted.

Second-, third-, and fourth-degree burns may require skin and muscle grafts.

FRACTURE

 How, when, and where did the injury occur?

Attempt to identify the exact mechanism of injury. Helps predict the type of fracture.
Prolonged time to presentation for care increases risk of compartment syndrome and
    rhabdomyolysis. Determine time of injury.
What treatment has the pt received before arrival in the ED?

Document the pt's dominant hand

Plays an important role in deciding promptness of surgical repair versus conservative
    management of fractures

Is it an open fracture?

Any fracture associated with an overlying laceration. An orthopedic emergency because
    of the increased risk of osteomyelitis if not cleaned, debrided early, and antibiotics are
    given (e.g., cefazolin).
Document last tetanus immunization and update as needed.

Does the pt have any weakness or numbness?

Exclude associated nerve injury.
Often the pt will not want to move limb, but you must test strength and sensation distal
    to the fracture.

Does the pt have any other medical conditions?

Peripheral vascular disease, diabetes, and osteoporosis all may attribute to delayed bone
    healing and/or increased fracture risk.

 Evaluate the pt's vital signs

Tachycardia can be from pain but may also be the first sign of significant internal blood
    loss. A femur fracture, for example, may result in large-volume blood loss.

Perform a physical exam

Fully expose any area of concern.
Document the pt's ability to ambulate and any abnormality to the gait.
Note any tenderness, erythema, ecchymosis, deformity, crepitus, or decreased range of
    motion.
For hip pain, document any leg-length discrepancy and position of leg when in position
    of comfort (e.g., internally or externally rotated).
Evaluate for ligamentous or tendon instability or tenderness.
Fully evaluate the joints above and below the area of concern.
Document sensation and strength before and after any movement or splinting of affected
    area.
Document pulse strength and quality along with capillary refill.
Complete a full exam to exclude any occult injuries.

Obtain x-rays of the concerned area

Ensure that x-ray includes the joint above and below the area of concern.
Need a minimum of two views (e.g., posteroanterior and lateral) to exclude fracture.
Describe the fracture:
  • State whether it is open (associated with laceration) or closed.
  • State the area of the fracture (e.g., epiphysis, metaphysis, diaphysis).
  • State the type of fracture (e.g., transverse, oblique, spiral, greenstick, comminuted).
  • State angulation, rotation, or displacement using the proximal fragment as your
    reference point.
  • State any associated dislocation or joint involvement.

Consider obtaining the following labs if presentation is delayed

CBC, electrolytes, BUN, creatinine, creatinine kinase: Exclude rhabdomyolysis, second-
    ary renal failure, and anemia.

A **Fracture**

Can be caused by trauma, pathology (e.g., metastatic bone lesions), or stress.

Open fractures require emergent orthopedic evaluation for aggressive irrigation and
  debridement in order to prevent osteomyelitis.

Differential Diagnosis

- Sprain   – Contusion   – Dislocation
- Arthritis   – Tendon/ligament tear

P **Provide effective pain relief**

NSAIDs and/or narcotics are effective.

Rest, ice, compression, elevation (RICE).

Open fractures

Irrigate with copious amounts of sterile normal saline.

Ensure that bone fragments remain covered with moist gauze soaked in normal saline.

Provide tetanus immunization if not current.

Administer IV antibiotics (e.g., cefazolin) as soon as possible.

Splint the affected area

Document neurovascular status pre- and postsplinting.

The splint should immobilize the joint above and below the fracture.

Disposition

Open fractures/dislocations that cannot be adequately reduced and fractures associated
  with neurologic deficits require immediate orthopedic referral.

Most hip or femur fractures are admitted for operative repair the following day.

All other pts can be discharged home after the fracture is splinted with orthopedic
  surgery follow-up.

HEAD INJURY

S **How, when, and where did the pt get injured?**

If pt was assaulted, check to see what your local reporting requirements are.

Was the event witnessed? Attempt to get a first-hand account of the event.

Did the pt ever lose consciousness?

Document the time of unconsciousness and how the pt was after consciousness was regained.

- Was the pt confused? Can be seen with a postictal state resulting from a seizure or closed head injury.
- Consider a syncopal episode if the pt had loss of consciousness (LOC) for a few seconds and immediately awoke once he or she was lying down.

Pts who have an LOC, awaken, and have a *lucid interval*, and then develop a change in mental status or LOC may have suffered an epidural hematoma (EDH).

Was any seizure activity noted?

Ask bystanders specifically what they saw because the layperson's idea of seizure activity varies.

Does the pt have a history of falls or head injuries?

Repeated falls or head injuries increase the risk of subdural hematomas (SDHs), especially in the elderly.

Does the pt have any neck pain?

Consider spinal injury in any pt who has a significant head injury or mechanism of injury.

Does the pt have any weakness, numbness, or paralysis now?

Indicates a more severe head injury with either a severe contusion or intracerebral bleed.

Does the pt have any other medical problems?

Document any prior head injuries or neurologic disease or surgery.

Cardiac history may suggest arrhythmia and secondary syncope.

What medications is the pt taking?

Inquire specifically about warfarin, aspirin, clopidogrel, direct oral anticoagulants (DOACs), and other blood thinners that can increase the risk of intracranial bleeding.

Obtain a social history

Document any recent alcohol or drug use. Both can obscure your evaluation of the pt's mental status.

O **Evaluate the pt's vital signs**

Glasgow Coma Score should be included as a vital sign.

Perform a physical exam

HEENT: Note any ecchymosis, lacerations, or abrasions.

- Inspect skull for any depressions or step-offs consistent with fracture.
- Note any hematotympanum or blood/cerebrospinal fluid (CSF) draining from ear, which may suggest basilar skull fracture.
- Inspect nares: Note bleeding or CSF drainage.
- Inspect mouth: Note any loose teeth, fractured teeth, or lacerations.
- Inspect neck: Note any vertebral tenderness or step-offs. Pt should be placed in a c-collar until x-rays are obtained, if there is any significant head injury.

Neurologic: Perform mental status exam. Test all cranial nerves. Note any focal weakness, numbness, Babinski sign, hypo- or hyperreflexia.

Obtain a C-spine series

Exclude vertebral injury.

Obtain a head CT scan

Without contrast and with bone windows. Exclude skull fracture, intracerebral bleed, EDH, or SDH.
- Classic EDH appears as a convex (lens-shaped) hyperdensity with shift of midline structures, compression of ipsilateral lateral ventricle, and can lead to herniation.
- Classic SDH appears as a crescent-shaped concave hyperdensity. Large SDH can also cause herniation and compression of the ventricles.

Consider obtaining the following labs

CBC, coags, bleeding time: Exclude thrombocytopenia, hypocoagulable state, or platelet dysfunction if the pt has significant bleeding or intracerebral bleeding.

Type and screen: If blood products (fresh frozen plasma or platelets) are needed to correct bleeding state.

EtOH level, urine drug screen: Exclude intoxication or drug effect as cause of mental status changes.

 ### Head injury

EDH usually caused by a temporal-parietal skull fracture with laceration of the medial meningeal artery is the classic description. Death can result quickly from uncal herniation.

SDH usually caused by the tearing or laceration of bridging veins that transverse the subdural space. Associated with cerebral contusions, cerebral edema, and diffuse axonal injury.

Mild traumatic brain injury (concussion): Diffuse reversible brain injury that occurs at the time of trauma. Characterized by a change in mental status with or without LOC (may last up to 6 hours).

Differential Diagnosis

   – Seizure   – Syncope   – Cerebrovascular accident

 ### Supportive care

Ensure that pt is able to maintain airway and intubate if needed.

Treat hypotension with IV fluids. Hypertension should be treated very cautiously and typically does not require treatment.

Seizure prophylaxis with an antiepileptic is generally recommended.

Perform frequent neurologic checks.

Consult Neurosurgery for any epidural or subdural hematoma or intracerebral bleed

An EDH with impending herniation requires immediate surgical decompression. A burr hole may need to be placed in the pt's head in the ED as a temporizing measure.

Disposition

Pts with mild head injuries who have no neurologic deficits, have a normal head CT scan, and have family/friends who can watch them closely can be discharged home.

Admit all pts with intracerebral bleeds, SDH, EDH, or neurologic deficits to the ICU for close monitoring and frequent neurologic checks.

LACERATION

S **How, when, and where did the pt obtain the laceration?**

Primary wound closure (closure at time of initial evaluation) is generally not recommended if the laceration is more than 8 hours old because of an increased risk of infection. Facial lacerations may be closed up to 24 hours later in order to get a better cosmetic outcome.

Lacerations caused by glass, wood, and other organic material have an increased risk for retained foreign bodies.

Abide by local regulations requiring reporting any child abuse or assault.

If wounds are suspicious for an assault, be sure to ask the pt how the lacerations were obtained in private because the companion may be the perpetrator.

Did the pt sustain a puncture wound to the foot?

Plantar puncture wounds have an increased risk of infection because of *Pseudomonas* and a retained foreign body if the pt was wearing shoes at the time.

When was the pt's last tetanus immunization?

If the last immunization was >5 years ago, pt will require a booster dose.

What other medical problems does the pt have?

Diabetes and peripheral vascular disease increase the risk for wound infections and delayed wound healing.

What medications is the pt taking?

Chronic steroid use or other immune suppressing medications will delay wound healing.

Document any medication allergies, social history, and review of symptoms

O **Evaluate the pt's vital signs**

Tachycardia is the first sign of significant blood loss. Hypotension is a late sign.

Perform a physical exam

Document the length, depth, shape, and location of all lacerations. Consider drawing a diagram.

Thoroughly irrigate and explore the wound(s) to exclude underlying tendon, blood vessel, joint or muscular injury, and foreign bodies.

Document pt's handedness on all lacerations involving the arms or hands.

Evaluate the capillary refill, distal pulses, distal sensation, and the function of any underlying joints.

Complete a full physical exam to exclude any other injuries.

Consider obtaining an x-ray of the area involved

Plain radiographs can be useful for demonstrating foreign bodies. Glass (down to 2 mm in size with or without lead), gravel, and metallic bodies can easily be seen, as they are radiopaque. Organic material (e.g., wood) and plastic are often missed.

Fluoroscopy, CT scan, or ultrasound can also be useful in localization of organic or plastic foreign bodies.

A **Laceration**

Differential diagnosis

| – Bite | – Crush injury | – Open fracture |

P **Control bleeding**

Apply direct pressure on the wound or just proximal to the wound.

A blood pressure cuff applied to the limb can be inflated to slow blood flow.

A local tourniquet can be applied to aid in controlling blood flow while the wound is being closed. Tourniquet time should be limited.

Provide pain relief

NSAIDs, narcotics, or local anesthetics can all be effective.

Update tetanus immunization

If the wound is tetanus-prone and the pt has never received tetanus immunization, the
pt should receive tetanus immune globulin and a tetanus-diphtheria vaccination.

Anesthetize the wound

Local or topical anesthetics can be used. Anesthetic with epinephrine can reduce
the amount of anesthetic required and aid in controlling bleeding by causing
vasoconstriction.

Consider a regional nerve block if local infiltration of anesthetic will alter wound edges
and prevent a good cosmetic closure.

Irrigate the wound

The wound should be irrigated with a minimum of 500 cc normal saline (use more if
heavily contaminated). A 30-cc syringe with an 18-gauge angiocatheter provides an
ideal pressure stream to flush bacteria and debris without causing tissue damage.

Remove any foreign bodies that are visualized.

Debride the wound

Remove any devitalized tissue and revise the wound edges as needed to obtain a clean
edge that will prompt wound healing.

Close the wound

Closure can be done with sutures, staples, topical skin glue, or skin-closure tape as
indicated

Ensuring that the wound edges are everted, there is minimum tension across the suture
line, and the wound edges are lined up will provide for excellent cosmetic closure and
prevent wound dehiscence.

Wound should be dressed with antibiotic ointment and dry sterile dressing.
Consider splinting a finger or limb if the laceration crosses a joint

Disposition

Most pts will be discharged home to have their sutures or staples removed by their
primary care provider.

General guidelines for suture/staple removal:

- Face: 3–5 d
- Upper extremity: 7–10 d
- Over joints: 14 d
- Scalp: 10–14 d
- Lower extremity: 10–14 d

Admit pts with severe wound infections, joint involvement, or repairs that will require
surgery.

Antibiotics are generally not indicated but should be given for bites, plantar puncture wounds, or heavily contaminated wounds

V
PSYCHIATRY

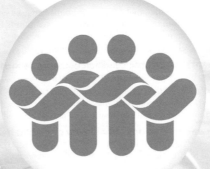

GUIDELINES FOR CONDUCTING A PSYCHIATRIC INTERVIEW

The Psychiatry SOAP notes will guide you through the thought process for making specific psychiatric diagnoses. However, the following questions should be addressed for each patient, regardless of diagnosis.

1. Is the patient's psychiatric condition caused/exacerbated by a substance or medication?

A complete inventory of ALL the substances that a patient takes should be reviewed. This includes prescription medications, OTC drugs, health food supplements, herbal preparations, alcohol, and illicit substances. Ask the patient the following:
- The amount or dosage that is being taken
- The duration of usage for each substance
- Any temporal relationship between the usage or withdrawal of the substance and the onset of their current symptoms
- Does using the substance make their symptoms better or worse?
- Does abstaining from the substance make their symptoms better or worse?

Addressing any substance or medication that might cause or contribute to the patient's presentation will always be a part of the treatment plan.

2. Is the patient's psychiatric condition caused or exacerbated by a medical condition?

A complete inventory of the patient's medical history should be taken.

A variety of medical conditions can present with psychiatric manifestations, and managing comorbid medical conditions would be a part of the treatment plan.

3. Does the patient have any prior history of mental health treatment?

Patients should be asked the following:
- Prior mental health diagnoses? What were the symptoms that the patient displayed that lead to the diagnosis?
- Prior medication trials? Identify the med, the dosage, the duration of treatment, whether the med was effective, and the reason for discontinuation.
- Prior psychotherapy? Identify the duration of treatment, the style of psychotherapy employed, and the reason for discontinuation.
- Prior hospitalizations? Ask about the circumstances surrounding the admission and the duration of the hospital stay.

4. Is this patient currently undergoing any mental health treatment?

Ask the patient to detail his or her current medication and/or psychotherapy regimen.

5. Is there a family history of psychiatric conditions?

This would include a family history of substance use disorders, suicidal ideation (SI), or suicide attempts.

6. Consider any pertinent social history

Information that can be addressed in this section: childhood/upbringing; marital status/relationship history/whether they have children; current living situation; educational pursuits and employment history; legal history; trauma history; and religious affiliation.

7. All patients should be assessed for the presence of SI

SI with a plan and intent is most concerning and will usually warrant a referral to higher level of care, such as an inpatient admission. Ask about parasuicidal behaviors, which are self-inflicted injuries that are intended to cause harm, but not to inflict an injury severe enough to result in death (e.g., superficial cutting, hitting oneself). Does the patient have access to firearms?

8. All patients should be assessed for the presence of HI

HI with intent and an identifiable target warrants further intervention, which can involve an inpatient admission or notifying the authorities. The clinician should know their state's laws regarding their duty to warn or their duty to protect a potential victim.

9. Perform a mental status exam

Document these findings: appearance, attitude, speech, motor, mood, affect, thought process, thought content (includes SI/HI), cognition (orientation, attention, memory), insight, and judgment.

PERSONALITY DISORDERS

S **Assess the patient's personality traits**

Interview the patient and collateral informants. Continue to evaluate the patient's personality traits over the course of your professional relationship.

When did the traits first become apparent?

Personality traits are evident in youth to early adulthood.

Are the traits constant or intermittent?

Personality traits are stable over time and should be consistent as the patient interacts with others and their environment.

Are the patient's personality traits induced/exacerbated by a substance or a medication?

See Guideline #1 on p. 446.

Are the patient's personality traits induced/exacerbated by a medical condition?

See Guideline #2 on p. 446. TBI, epilepsy, and dementia are medical conditions that can be associated with personality changes.

O **Assess the patient's vital signs and perform a physical exam as part of the assessment for medical causes of personality disorders, if applicable**

Pertinent labs and other diagnostic tests

There are no specific labs tests for the diagnosis of personality disorders; correlate the medical necessity for further studies with the clinical presentation and physical exam findings.

A **Personality disorders**

Personality disorders involve a maladaptive pattern of thinking about oneself, interacting with the environment, or relating to others. By definition, personality disorders are constant and evident across a range of scenarios.

Cluster A personality disorders

Paranoid: suspicious and distrustful of others, holds grudges, quick to take offense

Schizotypal: "magical thinking"; odd behaviors or affect, can be paranoid

Schizoid: no interest in interacting with others, prefers to be alone

Cluster B personality disorders

Histrionic: desires to be the center of attention

Narcissistic: inflated sense of self; primarily interested in others as a source of affirmation

Antisocial: lack of regards for others; violates rules, laws, or societal norms

Borderline: tumultuous relationships; SI or self-harm with real or imagined abandonment, emotional lability, fragile self-image

Cluster C personality disorders

Dependent: requires constant affirmation; fears being alone

Obsessive compulsive personality disorder: rigid, rule oriented, perfectionistic

Avoidant: sensitive to rejection; tends to be self-conscious

P **Psychotherapy is the primary therapeutic intervention for personality disorders**

Dialectical behavior therapy, in particular, is helpful with borderline personality disorder. CBT can address personality disorders by teaching patients to develop more adaptive ways of perceiving themselves, others, and their environment.

Medication management that is targeted toward certain personality traits can be beneficial

There are no medications that directly affect personality disorders, but medications can be used to target specific symptoms that are associated with these conditions. Antipsychotic medications can be beneficial in treating the paranoid ideation associated with Cluster A personality disorders.

Mood stabilizers and atypical antipsychotics show efficacy in treating the mood lability associated with borderline personality disorder. It is always appropriate to initiate medication management to treat any comorbid mental health conditions.

PSYCHOTIC DISORDERS

 What are the patient's current symptoms?

Hallucinations?*: perceptions in the absence of an actual stimulus
Delusions?*: e.g., false, fixed beliefs
Disorganized speech?*: e.g., verbigeration (repetition of words or phrases)
Disorganized behavior?*: e.g., echopraxia (imitating others' behavior)
(* = the positive symptoms of psychosis)
Negative symptoms: e.g., lack of motivation and lack of spontaneous speech

What is the duration of the patient's symptoms?

Brief psychotic disorder (1): at least 1 day—resolution of symptoms by 1 month
Schizophreniform disorder (2): 1 month—less than 6 months
Schizophrenia (2): greater than 6 month
(#) = the minimum number of symptoms present; at least one symptom must be a hallucination, delusion, or disordered speech

Are the patient's symptoms induced/exacerbated by any substance or medication?

See Guideline #1 on p. 446. Cocaine, cannabis, amphetamines, steroids, Parkinson meds, and antibiotics can be associated with psychosis.

Are the patient's symptoms induced/exacerbated by a medical condition?

See Guideline #2 on p. 446. Delirium, TBI, brain tumors, epilepsy, or dementia can be associated with psychosis.

Does the patient have any comorbid mood symptoms?

If so, then consider schizoaffective disorder, MDD w/ psychotic features, or BAD w/ psychotic features.

Does the patient have a personality disorder?

Cluster A personality disorders can be associated with psychotic features; see Personality Disorders, p. 448.

Patients with psychosis need a detailed assessment for safety concerns.

See Guidelines #7 and 8 on pp. 446 and 447.

 Assess the patient's vital signs and perform a physical exam as part of the assessment for medical causes of psychosis

Pertinent labs and other diagnostic tests

B12/folate, CMP, HIV, RPR, EEG, neuroimaging, UPT, UDS/BAL, toxin screen, ESR/ANA, drug levels, U/A, CBC w/ diff

A **Differential diagnosis**

Brief psychotic disorder, schizophreniform disorder, MDD with psychotic features, schizophrenia, cluster A PD, delusional disorder, schizoaffective disorder, medication/substance-induced psychotic disorder, psychotic disorder due to another medical condition.

P **Determine the appropriate setting for treatment**

An inpatient stay is warranted if there are concerns for severe agitation, SI, or HI, or if the patient's symptoms are severe enough to warrant daily monitoring and intervention.

Start an antipsychotic medication.

An atypical antipsychotic (e.g., aripiprazole, quetiapine) is the first-line medication. Typical antipsychotics (e.g., haloperidol, fluphenazine) are also effective but can be associated with a higher risk of abnormal movements and less efficacy in treating negative symptoms. If compliance is a concern, then a number of these medications can be administered as a long-acting injection. Clozapine or ECT is a treatment recommendation for refractory symptoms. Patients taking antipsychotic medications should be monitored for weight gain, sedation, abnormal movements, and metabolic side effects. If there are comorbid mood symptoms, then an antidepressant or mood stabilizer would be warranted.

Address any contributing medical conditions, medications, or substances

Perform a thorough medical evaluation for the patient who presents with their first episode of psychosis.

Therapy can be useful

Therapy centered around family support, psychoeducation, and vocational rehabilitation can be beneficial. CBT can be useful in addressing specific psychotic features, such as delusions.

ANXIETY DISORDERS

S **What are the patient's symptoms?**

Fear of public speaking or interactions with others? Fear of leaving one's home? Fear of a clearly identified object or situation? Worry about a variety of things? Intrusive, repetitive thoughts? Repetitive behaviors to alleviate anxiety? Physical symptoms associated with anxiety?

Ask the patient to elaborate on why he or she feels worried or afraid

The patient's response can alert you to the potential for comorbid mental health conditions. For example, fear in the context of a prior history of trauma suggests the possibility of PTSD should be considered. However, fear as part of a persecutory delusion, suggests the possibility of a psychotic disorder.

Are the symptoms induced/exacerbated by a substance or medication?

See Guideline #1 on p. 446. Substances that can be associated with anxiety are cocaine, amphetamines, albuterol, steroids, and caffeine.

Are the symptoms induced/exacerbated by a medical condition?

See Guideline #2 on p. 446. Medical conditions that can be associated with anxiety are hyperthyroidism, COPD, asthma, heart disease, and pain.

O **Assess the patient's vital signs and perform a physical exam as part of the assessment for medical causes of anxiety**

Pertinent labs

TFTs, UDS, drug levels

A **Anxiety disorders**

Anxiety disorders are characterized by the presence of fear (apprehension about a clearly defined object or situation) or anxiety (apprehension without a clearly defined cause) that is typically out of proportion to the actual situation.

Differential diagnosis

Anxiety disorder due to another medical condition, GAD, OCD*, panic disorder and panic attacks, PTSD*, separation anxiety disorder, specific phobia, substance/medication-induced anxiety disorder

*OCD and PTSD aren't anxiety disorders, but anxiety is frequently a part of their presentation.

P **Cognitive behavioral therapy (CBT) is the psychotherapy of choice to address anxiety disorders.**

CBT targets anxiety by challenging patients to critically evaluate their worries and to replace worry with more constructive and realistic thoughts. ERP is a variant of CBT that targets specific phobias and fears by encouraging the patient to confront the object or situation that prompts fear, while simultaneously resisting their usual fear response. Take the example of a boy who runs away whenever he sees a dog. With ERP, the boy would be encouraged to have progressive contact with a dog. Rather than run away, the boy would be taught alternate methods to deal with his fear, such as engaging in deep breathing exercises. The ultimate result is that the boy would learn to tolerate being around dogs and his original fear response would be extinguished.

There are also medication options to treat anxiety

Anxiety medications can be scheduled or given PRN. The first-line choice for a scheduled medication would be an SSRI (e.g., fluoxetine, sertraline), an SNRI (e.g., duloxetine, venlafaxine), or buspirone. TCAs and MAOIs are also effective for anxiety, but these medications are used less frequently because of their side effect profiles.

PRN medications such as hydroxyzine and benzodiazepines (e.g., alprazolam, lorazepam) are effective options for panic and anxiety.

Propranolol is a PRN option that can be effective for performance issues within the context of social anxiety disorder. Patients should be cautioned that these PRN medications carry risk for sedation, and caution should be used when the patient drives or performs other tasks that require alertness. Propranolol can also be associated with hypotension, and benzodiazepine usage should be time-limited as long-term use can lead to dependence.

MOOD DISORDERS

S **Is the patient depressed?**

Depressed mood*, loss of interest*, decreased energy, changes in sleep, changes in appetite, suicidal ideation, decreased concentration, feelings of guilt or worthlessness, psychomotor retardation.

*One of these symptoms must be present + four additional symptoms for at least 2 weeks to diagnose a major depressive episode.

Is there a history of mania?

Excessively elevated, euphoric, or irritable mood**; increased energy**; distractibility; decreased need for sleep; flight of ideas; grandiosity; increase in goal-directed behaviors; indiscriminate behaviors; or talkativeness.

**These symptoms must be present + ≥ three additional symptoms (≥four symptoms if mood is irritable) for at least 1 week to diagnose a manic episode.

Is there a history of hypomania?

Symptoms are the same as mania, but the severity is more attenuated.

Did any stressors cause or contribute to the onset of the depressed mood?

If so, then consider other diagnoses on the differential. For example, mood symptoms associated with a traumatic event could indicate the presence of PTSD.

Are the patient's mood symptoms induced/exacerbated by substance use?

See Guideline #1 on p. 446. Substances that can be associated with depression are cannabis, NSAIDs, antihypertensives, or oral contraceptives. Substances that can be associated with mania are steroids, cocaine, and PCP.

Are the patient's mood symptoms induced/exacerbated by a medical condition?

See Guideline # 2 on p. 446. Medical conditions that can be associated with depressive or manic symptoms are lupus, MS, malignances, or diabetes.

The patient's risk for suicide requires special consideration

See Guideline #7 on p. 446.

O **Assess the patient's vital signs and perform a physical exam as part of the assessment for medical causes of psychosis**

Pertinent labs and other diagnostic tests

B12/folate, electrolytes, LFTs, UDS, neuroimaging, UPT, BAL, TFTs, drug levels, CBC w/ diff

A **Differential diagnoses for MDD**

Dysthymia, MDD with psychotic features, seasonal affective disorder, premenstrual dysphoric syndrome, substance/medication-induced depressive disorder, depressive disorder due to another medical condition

Differential diagnoses for bipolar

BAD I (at least one episode of mania; periods of hypomania or depressive episodes are optional), BAD II (periods of hypomania + periods of MDD), cyclothymia (periods of hypomanic and depressive symptoms; criteria for mania, hypomania, or MDD are never met), BAD with psychotic features, substance/medication-induced bipolar disorder, bipolar disorder due to another medical condition.

P **MDD**

SSRIs are the first line of choice; however, other antidepressant choices are also reasonable. MAOIs and TCAs are effective in treating depression, but these medications are used less frequently because of their side effect profiles. All patients should be assessed for a history of mania prior to initiating an antidepressant because this class of medications can unmask manic symptoms.

Bipolar I and II

Initiate a mood stabilizer to address manic or hypomanic symptoms. Mood stabilizers are atypical antipsychotics, some anticonvulsants, and lithium, and the choice of medication should to be tailored to the patient's individual needs.

Treatment recommendations for MDD, BAD I, and BAD II

Monitor for safety concerns. Inpatient treatment is warranted for the patient who is at acute risk for SI or HI and is also appropriate for the patient whose symptoms are severe enough to warrant daily intervention. Finally, psychotherapy can be beneficial to treat mood disorders and should be offered to patients in addition to medication management.

DISSOCIATIVE DISORDERS

S **What are the patient's symptoms?**

Lapses in memory? Inability to recall details of their past? Periods of time that the patient can't account for? Is the ability to form new memories disturbed? Sensation that their environment is distorted or unreal? Sensation their body are thoughts are distorted or unreal? The presence of more than one personality? If so, then what is observed (e.g., changes in voice, changes in demeanor or behavior)?

Was the onset gradual or abrupt? Are the symptoms persistent or intermittent?

Memory disruption with dissociative episodes is typically abrupt in onset and the symptoms can be intermittent. Dementia would typically be associated with memory deficits that are gradual in onset and persistent.

Are the patient's symptoms induced/exacerbated by a substance or medication?

See Guideline #1 on p. 446. Hallucinogens and PCP can be associated with dissociative symptoms.

Are the patient's symptoms induced/exacerbated by a medical condition?

See Guideline #2 on p. 446. In particular, is there any history of head trauma, seizures, dementia, or delirium?

Does the pt have any history of trauma or PTSD? Were the symptoms precipitated by some distressing event?

Dissociation can be seen in patients with a history of trauma. Dissociative identity disorder (DID) is common in patients with a history of childhood trauma.

Are there other co-occurring mental health conditions?

Dissociative symptoms can be associated with personality disorders, namely borderline personality disorder, anxiety disorders, and depressive disorders. Dissociative symptoms should be distinguished from an underlying psychotic disorder. Affect fluctuations that can occur with DID should be differentiated from the mood fluctuations associated with bipolar disorder.

Any suspicion that the pt is intentionally manufacturing their symptoms?

See the discussion on Malingering and Factitious Disorder under the SOAP for Somatic Disorders, p. 462.

O **Assess the patient's vital signs and perform a physical exam as part of the assessment for medical causes of dissociation**

Pertinent labs and other diagnostic tests

BAL, EEG, drug levels, neuroimaging, UDS

A **Dissociative disorders**

Dissociative disorders involve lapses in or distortion of patients' memories, sense of self, or their perception of their environment. Dissociative disorders are often associated with a history of trauma. Dissociation is a defense mechanism that allows the individual to avoid memories or situations that are traumatic or have some other negative connotation associated with them.

Differential diagnosis

Depersonalization/derealization, DID, dissociative amnesia, dissociative fugue, factitious disorder, malingering, personality disorders, substance/medication-induced dissociative disorder.

P Address PTSD or any trauma history, as applicable. Treat other comorbid mental health conditions

Patients with a history of dissociative symptoms need a thorough evaluation for a history of trauma. Although there are no medications that directly affect dissociative symptoms, patients can be offered medication management to treat any comorbid anxiety, depressive or PTSD symptoms. Address any substances or medications that could contribute.

Make a psychotherapy referral to target the dissociative disorder and any associated psychiatric conditions

CBT is useful in addressing anxiety and PTSD symptoms. DBT is useful in addressing the emotional dysregulation associated with borderline personality disorder.

IMPULSE CONTROL DISORDERS

S **Does the patient have an urge to engage in a behavior that is hard to resist?**
Ask the pt to describe the behavior(s). Does the patient experience anxiety when they attempt to resist these urges? Is the anxiety relieved if the patient engages in the behavior? Does the patient enjoy engaging in the behavior?

Any co-occurring mental health conditions?
Impulsive behaviors need to be distinguished from:
- Indiscriminate behaviors that can occur during a manic episode
- Indiscriminate behaviors that can occur during substance intoxication
- Disorganized thought pattern or behaviors associated with psychosis
- Obsessive and compulsive behaviors associated with OCD
- Acts that show a willful disregard for others; typically associated with
- Conduct disorder or antisocial personality disorder
- Conditions associated with impaired judgment, such as dementia

O **There are no specific physical exam findings, labs, or other diagnostic tests suggested**

A **Impulse control disorders**
Impulse control disorders involve the urge to engage in maladaptive behaviors. The patient typically finds the urge to be gratifying and difficult to resist.

Differential diagnoses
There a number of conditions that are in this category. Some of the more commonly encountered are pathological gambling, sexual compulsions, compulsive shopping, kleptomania (stealing), pyromania (fire setting), intermittent explosive disorder (aggressive impulses), trichotillomania (hair pulling), and skin picking.

P **Medication management might be beneficial**
SSRIs, naltrexone, and clomipramine have shown efficacy in treating impulsive behaviors.

Psychotherapy interventions are also beneficial for impulse control disorders
Participation in self-help groups can help to lessen the impact of these disorders. In particular, self-help groups and motivational interviewing have been shown to benefit pathological gambling. Habit reversal training is a form of CBT in which the patient is taught to perform an alternate, more adaptive behavior in lieu of the original, maladaptive behavior. Take the example of a patient who picks his or her skin. Rather than give in to this urge, the patient is taught another behavior, such as taking deep breaths.

NEUROCOGNITIVE DISORDERS

S **Is there a change in the patient's cognitive status from his or her baseline? What are the patient's current symptoms?**
- Memory deficits? Is long-term versus short-term memory involved?
- Language difficulties, any aphasias?
- Personality changes (e.g., irritability, apathy, tearfulness, inappropriate behavior)?
- Difficulties w/ ADLs (e.g., ability to feed and dress themselves)
- Hallucinations or perceptual disturbances? Any changes in sleep?
- Any decline in executive functioning (e.g., ability to plan, to multitask)?
- Age at the time of onset?
- Any sundowning (symptoms worse in the evening)?

Is the patient delirious?
Dementia is typically associated with a gradual onset, intact attention, and a relative stability in the symptoms over time. However, delirium would be associated with an acute onset, inability to sustain attention, and a waxing and waning course. The cognitive changes associated with delirium typically improve when the underlying cause of the delirium is addressed. If a patient with dementia has an abrupt onset of AMS, then a delirium superimposed on the baseline dementia should be considered.

Are the cognitive issues induced/exacerbated by a medical condition?
See Guideline #2 on p. 446. Conditions that can be associated with a cognitive decline are CVAs, Parkinson diseaese, TBI, HIV, or Wernicke encephalopathy.

Are the cognitive issues caused/exacerbated by a substance or medication?
See Guideline #1 on p. 446.

Does the pt have comorbid mental health conditions?
Depression, ADHD, and anxiety can be associated with poor concentration and focus. Severe depression, in particular, can be associated with "pseudodementia," which is transient memory deficit. There is typically a temporal relationship between the onset of the cognitive deficits and the worsening mood. The clinician should also see an improvement in cognition with treatment of the depression.

O **Assess the patient's vital signs**
Perform a physical exam.
Neuro: assess for abnormal movements, motor or sensory deficits, aphasia.

Pertinent labs and other diagnostic tests
Neuroimaging, neuropsychological testing, CBC w/ diff, electrolytes, blood glucose, LFTs, EEG, HIV, UDS/BAL, LP w/ CSF study, toxin screen, vitamin levels, TFTs, PET scan

A **Neurocognitive disorders**
Neurocognitive disorders are associated with a cognitive decline that affects the patient's daily functioning. They can be classified by the underlying etiology, if known.

P **Address all medical comorbidities and any contributing substances**
Maximize the medical treatment for etiology of the dementia, if known, and for other comorbid medical conditions. Taper or discontinue any offending substances or medications. Have any vision or hearing deficits been addressed?

Try environmental modifications
Patients should have access to a calendar and clock for orientation. Maintain a calm environment; use lighting to clearly distinguish between day and nighttime.

Medication management slows down the progression of disease, but doesn't provide a cure

Cholinesterase inhibitors (e.g., donepezil, rivastigmine) are usually given in combination with memantine, an NMDA receptor antagonist. Provide med management to treat other comorbid mental health symptoms, such as depression, anxiety, agitation, or insomnia.

Therapy can be beneficial

Offer cognitive rehabilitation and skills training for the patient; family support groups for their loved ones.

SOMATIC SYMPTOMS

S **What are the patient's current symptoms?**
  • Preoccupation with having physical or neurological symptoms?
  • Preoccupation with having or acquiring a specific disease or medical condition?
  • Do the health concerns cause distress?

Has a thorough medical evaluation been conducted?
Only consider a somatic disorder after the patient has had the appropriate evaluation to address his or her concern. Patients with this disorder may not be reassured by normal diagnostic study results.

How does the patient address concerns about his or her health?
  • Avoids seeking medical attention out of fear that an illness will be diagnosed
  • Excessive checking for signs of illness or disease
  • Excessive amount of time spent thinking about or researching the illness
  • Overutilization of medical services (e.g., frequent doctor's visits, requests unnecessary tests)

Any suspicion the symptoms are being intentionally produced? If so, then what is the patient's motivation to do so?

Factitious disorder
Factitious disorder is the intentional production or exaggeration of physical symptoms or a disease state for primary gain, which is a motivation that is internally driven. An example of primary gain is a desire for attention by assuming the sick role. A factitious disorder can also be imposed upon another person.

Malingering
Malingering is an intentional production or exaggeration of physical symptoms or a disease state for secondary gain, which is a motivation that is externally driven. An example of secondary gain is a person pretends to be injured in order to win a lawsuit.

O **Assess the patient's vital signs, perform a physical exam, and conduct pertinent lab work and diagnostic studies, as applicable**
The clinician should carefully review the patient's treatment history, including previous medical records and prior results of any labs and diagnostic studies to determine the best course of action. The goal is to validate the patient's concerns; however, the clinician should avoid pursuing unnecessary or redundant medical evaluations.

A **Somatic disorders**
The cardinal feature in this category of diagnoses is the patient's level of distress regarding his or her physical state is deemed to be disproportionate to his or her actual health status.

Differential diagnoses
Conversion disorder, factitious disorder, illness anxiety disorder, malingering, somatic symptom disorder

P **These treatment recommendations should be implemented in tandem with the primary care provider's management of the patient's health concerns**

Offer CBT
Somatization can involve increased sensitivity to physical sensations and a vulnerability to interpret these sensations as negative. CBT can reduce somatic preoccupation by addressing the negative thought process that causes the patient to misinterpret his or her physical sensations as being indicative of illness.

Initiate medication management to treat any comorbid psychiatric conditions

Comorbid depression and anxiety can be common, and an SSRI (e.g., fluoxetine, paroxetine) is typically the first line of treatment. Consider a TCA (e.g., amitriptyline, nortriptyline) or an SNRI (e.g., duloxetine, venlafaxine) if the patient has pain in addition to mood or anxiety symptoms.

A factitious disorder imposed on another requires that care be taken to ensure the safety of the injured person

The case would need to be referred to the appropriate agency (e.g., Social Services, Child Protective Services).

SLEEP DISORDERS

S **How much sleep does the patient get?**

Does the patient feel well rested when he or she wakes up? Trouble falling or staying asleep? What does the patient do when he or she can't sleep? Early morning awakening? Poor concentration during the day? Excessive sleepiness during the day? Napping during the day? If so, then how long? Nightmares or vivid dreams? Sleep paralysis? Hypnagogic or hypnopompic hallucinations? Constant leg movement or aches?

Does the patient's bedtime ritual allow him or her to relax before bed?

Any habits that interfere with sleep (e.g., using electronic devices too close to bedtime)?

Does the patient's sleep environment that negatively affect sleep?

E.g., excessive light, temperature issues, an uncomfortable sleeping arrangement

Are the patient's sleep issues induced/exacerbated by a substance or medication?

See Guideline #1 on p. 446. Avoid stimulants, such as caffeine, prior to bedtime. If possible, avoid sedating substances during the day.

Does the patient have signs of sleep apnea or other medical conditions that could affect his or her sleep?

See Guideline #2 on p. 446. Sleep apnea can be associated with snoring or periods of interrupted breathing. Other medical conditions that can be associated with poor sleep are pulmonary disease, RLS, gastric reflux, or pain.

Does the patient have any comorbid mental health conditions?

Anxiety, depression, or PTSD can be associated with alterations in sleep.

O **Assess the patient's vital signs**

HTN can be associated with sleep apnea.

Select physical exam findings associated with disordered sleep:

Appearance: large neck circumference, obesity, appears somnolent during the exam

Oropharynx: narrow airway, large tonsils, or uvula

Cardiac: signs of heart failure

Pulmonary: signs of pulmonary hypertension

Neuro: confusion, memory deficits

Pertinent labs and other diagnostic tests: drug levels, MSLT, sleep study, UDS

A **Sleep disorders**

Sleep disorders are disturbances that affect the quality and/or quantity of sleep.

Differential diagnoses

Central or obstructive sleep apnea, hypersomnia, medical conditions that can affect sleep, narcolepsy, RLS, sleep disturbances associated with the REM phase, sleep disturbances related to alterations in circadian rhythm, substance/medication-induced sleep disorder.

P **Encourage the patient to improve his or her sleep hygiene**

Maintain set times to go to bed and to wake up and to avoid activities that can be stimulating prior to bedtime, such as exercising or using electronic devices. Use the sleep environment for sleep and sexual activity only, and sleep in a comfortable temperature and on a comfortable mattress and bed linens. Items that can deter sleep, such as a TV, should be removed. Develop a bedtime ritual that fosters relaxation. Limit daytime napping <30 minutes.

Address any medical conditions or substances that contribute to the presentation

Consider a sleep study for the patient who has chronic sleep disturbance.

There are a variety of sleep aids that can be offered to address insomnia

Ideally, sleep aids should be for short-term usage. Dependence can develop with long-term usage of some classes of sleep aids. Counsel patients on the risk for falls, sedation, and the need to use caution when performing other tasks that require alertness. Sleep aids can be associated with having behaviors during sleep that the person doesn't recall, such as eating or having conversations.

Stimulants, such as modafinil or methylphenidate, are used to treat hypersomnia or narcolepsy

ChCBT and mindfulness training can incorporate relaxation training to facilitate sleep

EATING DISORDERS

S **What strategies does the patient use to lose/maintain weight?**

Behaviors that restrict weight gain

Excessive dieting or fasting; excessive exercise; strategies that alter metabolism or suppress appetite (e.g., using stimulants, diet pills, insulin or thyroid medication to lose weight).

Behaviors that disrupt nutrient/fluid absorption ("purging")

Laxative, enema, or diuretic abuse; induced vomiting

What is the motivation to engage in these behaviors?

Anorexia nervosa (AN) and bulimia nervosa (BN) are often driven by a desire to lose weight or to avoid gaining additional weight.

Does the patient have comorbid mental health conditions?

MDD can be associated with poor appetite and subsequent weight loss. Psychosis, OCD, and BDD can be associated with disordered thinking regarding food or body image.

O **Assess the patient's vital signs**

AN can be associated with hypothermia, bradycardia, or hypotension with orthostasis.

Select physical exam findings for AN

Appearance: low body mass index (BMI)
Derm: hair is brittle and/or thinning; formation of lanugo hair; dry skin
Cardiac: abnormal heart rhythm
Hematologic: bruising
Renal: signs of dehydration
Endocrine: cold intolerance, menstrual abnormalities
Musculoskeletal: pathological fractures, muscle wasting

Select physical exam findings for BN

Appearance: normal to high BMI
Derm: Russell sign—calluses on the back of hand from induced vomiting
HEENT: parotid gland swelling; bad breath, dental caries, enamel erosion
Cardiac: abnormal heart rhythm
GI: abdominal pain or tenderness, bloating, constipation
Endocrine: menstrual irregularities

Pertinent labs and diagnostic tests

CBC w/ diff, bone density studies, electrolytes, ECG, LFTs, TFTs, UPT, vitamin levels, bone density studies

A **Eating disorders**

Eating disorders involve maladaptive eating habits that can lead to extreme weight loss, malnutrition, or other medical complications. **AN** is primarily associated with behaviors that seek to control weight through restrictive measures. However, purging can also occur as part of AN. **BN** is associated with episodes of binge eating, followed by episodes of restricting or purging behaviors to counteract weight gain.

Differential diagnoses

Avoidant/restrictive food intake behavior; binge eating disorder (BED); medical conditions associated with weight loss; weight loss secondary to other psychiatric conditions that are associated with obsessions, delusions or other distortions regarding food, eating, or body image

Medical stabilization is a priority

Vital sign instability, electrolyte abnormalities, or nutritional deficits require medical attention. Cardiac arrhythmias and re-feeding syndrome are the major sources of mortality associated with eating disorders.

Psychotherapy is effective for eating disorders

CBT targets the maladaptive thoughts about eating that are associated with BN and BED. Family therapy addresses the family dynamic's effect on the patient's eating patterns in AN.

Medication management is also be beneficial

Offer an antidepressant for comorbid depression, anxiety, or OCD symptoms that affect the patient's symptoms. Bupropion should be avoided as it can decrease the seizure threshold in patients with eating disorders. Topiramate, fluoxetine, lisdexamfetamine, and phentermine show benefit in treating binge eating. Olanzapine can be used to maintain weight gain in AN.

SEXUAL DYSFUNCTION

S **What are the patient's current symptoms?**

For Men	For Women
– A decline in desire?	– A decline in desire?
– Inability to achieve or maintain an erection?	– Insufficient lubrication?
– Premature ejaculation or inability to ejaculate?	– Difficulty having an orgasm?
– Genital pain? penile deformity?	– Vaginal pain w/ intercourse?

Are the symptoms new in onset or were they always present?

Are the symptoms situational or likely to occur during most sexual encounters?

Are the patient's symptoms induced/exacerbated by a substance or medication?

See Guideline #1 on p. 446. Substances that can be associated with sexual dysfunction are antidepressants, antihypertensives, alcohol, and opiates.

Are the patient's psychosis symptoms induced/exacerbated by a medical condition?

See Guideline #2 on p. 446. Conditions that can be associated with male sexual dysfunction are heart disease, diabetes, atherosclerosis, and prostate disease.

Conditions that can be associated with female sexual dysfunction are menopause and vaginal prolapse.

Has there been any trauma to the genital area?

Peyronie disease is a curvature of the penis that can occur as a result of trauma. Falls, blunt trauma to the genitals, urethral injury from catheterization, or vigorous sexual activity can be sources of trauma with subsequent sexual dysfunction.

Any comorbid mental health conditions?

MDD could be associated with a loss of interest in sexual activity; somatic disorders and BDD can be associated with somatic preoccupations that affect desire or performance; PTSD associated with sexual trauma can be associated with avoidance of sexual activity.

Assess the patient's attitudes about his or her sexuality and current sexual relationship

Are there cultural or religious beliefs that adversely affect the patient's sexuality? Is relationship conflict a contributing factor?

O **Assess the patient's vital signs**

HTN can be associated with sexual dysfunction.

Perform a physical exam

Female: external genital exam (prolapses, lesions, tears, Pap smear)
Male: external genital exam (lesions, Peyronie disease, prostate exam

Pertinent labs and other diagnostic tests

For men: PSA, A1C, NPT testing, penile U/S or angiogram
For both genders—U/A, hormone levels

A **Sexual disorders**

Sexual disorders affect sexual performance in the areas of desire, arousal or orgasm.

Differential diagnoses

Delayed or premature ejaculation, dyspareunia, ED, anorgasmia in women, vaginismus, disorders that affect desire or arousal.

Treat any medical comorbidities

This includes maximizing treatment for any contributing medical conditions, making lifestyle changes such as weight optimization, and addressing any offending substances, including nicotine.

Treatments for erectile dysfunction

PDE-5 inhibitors (e.g., sildenafil, tadalafil), penile pump or implant, alprostadil injections, testosterone

Treatments for premature ejaculation

PDE-5 inhibitors, SSRIs, tramadol (avoid SSRIs + tramadol due to the risk for serotonin syndrome)

Treatments for delayed ejaculation

Amantadine, buspirone, cyproheptadine

Treatments for low female desire

Estrogen or androgen therapy, flibanserin

Treatments for low female arousal

Vaginal lubricants, vaginal estrogen

Treatments for vaginal pain

Address medical or structural issues (e.g., prolapse, infections); topical analgesics; sexual positions that allow the patient to control the depth of penetration

Psychotherapy can also be beneficial

Therapy can address attitudes about sexuality and relationship dynamics. CBT can target anticipatory anxiety regarding penetration that is often associated with vaginal pain syndromes.

SUBSTANCE USE DISORDERS

S **Is there a current or past history of alcohol, illicit substance, OTC medication, or prescription medication abuse? Also, ask about tobacco and caffeine usage**

What is the amount or dosage that is being used? What is the route of ingestion? Any IVDA? If so, then assess for infections, such as cellulitis, hepatitis C, and HIV. Does the patient ever appear intoxicated? Can you smell substances when you interact with the patient (e.g., alcohol on their breath)? Any drug-seeking behaviors, such as asking for early refills? Do collateral informants raise concerns for substance abuse?

When was the patient's last usage of the substance? Any withdrawal symptoms when they stop using the substance?

Timely detoxification for alcohol, benzodiazepines, and barbiturates can prevent life-threatening withdrawal.

Prior treatment for substance abuse? What's the longest period of sobriety?

Inpatient or outpatient rehabilitation programs? Any medications to curb substance usage? How successful were the interventions? Patients with substance abuse often struggle in their efforts to achieve sobriety.

Has the patient suffered any negative consequences as a result of the substance use?

Legal issues or health complications? Social, professional, or financial impact?

O **Assess the vital signs**

Substance intoxication or withdrawal can be associated with abnormalities in HR, respirations, BP, or temperature.

Select physical exam findings that can be associated with substance abuse

Appearance: needle marks from IVDA, sweating, shaking, yawning
HEENT: fixed or dilated pupils, nystagmus, eyes tearing, runny nose
Cardiac: Abnormal heart rhythm, enlarged heart, endocarditis
GI: jaundice, enlarged liver, ascites, vomiting, diarrhea
MS: cramping, myalgias, muscle rigidity
Neuro: seizures, confusion, ataxia, unsteady gait, slurred speech, agitation

Pertinent labs and diagnostic tests

BAL, CBC w/ diff, drug levels, drug screen (urine, blood, breath, saliva), electrolytes, ECG, hepatitis panel, HIV, LFTs, UPT, neuroimaging

A **Substance use disorders**

Substance use disorders involve a maladaptive usage of a substance. Associated conditions include acute intoxication and withdrawal.

P **Treat alcohol, benzodiazepines, and barbiturates with an appropriate detoxification protocol to prevent life-threatening withdrawal**

Symptomatic relief can be offered for substances without life-threatening withdrawal, such as cocaine, opioid, or cannabis. For example, patients with opioid withdrawal can be offered NSAIDs to treat myalgias; loperamide for diarrhea; clonidine, methadone, or buprenorphine for withdrawal symptoms; or melatonin for insomnia.

Consider medications that promote abstinence

Opiates

Methadone and buprenorphine can be provided long term to deter illicit opiate usage. Buprenorphine + naloxone is another long-term medication option with a formulation that deters abuse of the drug. Naltrexone promotes abstinence by blocking the effects of opiates. Because of their mechanism of action, both buprenorphine and naltrexone can precipitate withdrawal if they are taken while the patient still has opiates in their system.

Alcohol

Naltrexone and acamprosate curb cravings; disulfiram deters abuse by adversely affecting alcohol's metabolism

Nicotine

Nicotine replacement therapy, bupropion, and varenicline can curb cravings

Therapy, such as 12-step programs or other peer support groups, can help patients to maintain their sobriety

Family-focused groups, such as Al-anon, can provide support to the loved ones of people struggling with addiction. Motivational interviewing is a technique that allows patients to explore their readiness to make the changes necessary to achieve sobriety.

POSTTRAUMATIC STRESS DISORDER

S **Did the patient experience a trauma?**

Trauma is a circumstance that caused or could have caused death or serious injury. Trauma can be personally experienced, witnessed, or experienced by learning the details of an acquaintance's trauma.

When did the patient's symptoms start in relation to the trauma?

For PTSD: the symptoms can start at any time after the trauma, but the duration of symptoms must be at least 1 month before the diagnosis of PTSD is made. For acute stress disorder: the symptoms start by the third day and must be resolved by 1 month after the trauma occurred.

What symptoms does the patient experience?

- Re-experiencing (e.g., nightmares, flashbacks)
- Changes in thought process or mood (e.g., person believes that they are to blame for trauma; inability to remember details about the trauma)
- Increased arousal (e.g., anger, insomnia)
- Avoidance (e.g., avoids "triggers," which are reminders of the trauma)

Any concern for substance abuse or other comorbid mental health conditions?

See Guideline #1 on p. 446. Substance abuse, BPD, MDD, and anxiety are common comorbidities with PTSD. Comprehensive treatment for PTSD would involve addressing substance abuse and other comorbid mental health conditions.

Was the trauma associated with a TBI?

A TBI can be associated with symptoms such as insomnia, poor recall of the trauma, or irritability that can overlap with PTSD.

The patient's risk for suicide requires special consideration

See Guideline #7 on p. 446. Increased rates of SI and suicide attempts are associated with PTSD.

O **Assess the patient's vital signs, perform a physical exam, and conduct pertinent lab work and diagnostic studies**

A **PTSD**

PTSD can encompass a wide constellation of symptoms after suffering a trauma. There can be vivid recollections of the trauma, a conscious effort to avoid recalling the trauma, or little to no recall of the trauma as part of a dissociative process. There can be a higher level of arousal, which can manifest as insomnia, hypervigilance, or irritability. Finally, PTSD can lead to negative self-appraisal (e.g., guilt, blame), which can foster depressive and anxiety symptoms.

Differential diagnoses: acute stress disorder, adjustment disorder

P **Consider medication management**

An SSRI is typically offered as a first line of treatment because of its tolerable side effect profile and its usefulness in addressing other comorbid mental health conditions, such as depression or anxiety. In particular, paroxetine and sertraline are the SSRIs with the FDA indication to treat PTSD. Venlafaxine, an SNRI, is another antidepressant that has been shown benefit for treating PTSD. Prazosin, an α1 receptor agonist, can be useful in targeting trauma-related nightmares. Benzodiazepines (e.g., clonazepam, alprazolam) are contraindicated because of their risk for dependence and their ability to interfere with the trauma processing that occurs in therapy.

Therapy is also beneficial

CBT is highly effective in treating PTSD by targeting negative self-appraisal. Within CBT, ERP can be used to target avoidance and hyperarousal symptoms when the patient is confronted by a trigger. EMDR is another type of therapy that is useful in treating PTSD. During EMDR, the patient recounts aspect of the trauma while tracking the lateral movements of the therapist's finger or another object. Mindfulness training can be helpful in targeting symptoms associated with PTSD, such as anxiety and insomnia.

Size	Description	Etiology
Anisocytosis	Abnormal size variation	Any severe anemia
Macrocytes	Large cells (MCV > 100)	Megaloblastic anemia, liver disease, hemolysis, liver disease, hypothyroid
Microcytes	Small cells (MCV < 80)	Iron deficiency, sideroblastic anemia, thalassemia, lead poisoning

Shape	Description	Etiology
Acanthocytes	Small cells with thorn-like projections	Hereditary or postsplenectomy
Burr cells	Indented, shriveled cells	Hemolysis, uremia, DIC
Ovalocytes	Oval-shaped cells	Hereditary, iron deficiency
Poikilocytosis	Abnormal shape variation	Any severe anemia
Schistocytes	Fragmented cells	Intravascular hemolysis, postsplenectomy
Sickle cells	Twisted crescent shape	Sickle cell
Spherocytes	Sphere-shaped cells	Hereditary, extravascular hemolysis, transfusion
Stomatocytes	Slit-like center (vs normally round center)	Hemolysis, thalassemia, burns, SLE, lead poisoning, liver disease
Target cells	Dark center in the middle of the normally clear center of the cell	Liver disease, thalassemia, hemoglobinopathy
Teardrop cells	Teardrop-shaped cells	Myeloproliferative disease, thalassemia

Inclusions	Description	Etiology
Basophilic stippling	Small, dark dots (lead, iron)	Hemolysis, lead poisoning, thalassemia
Heinz bodies	Dark inclusions (denatured hemoglobin)	G6PD with hemolysis, some hemoglobinopathies
Howell-Jolly bodies	Purple spheres (nuclear debris)	Hyposplenism, pernicious anemia, thalassemia
Nucleated RBC	Nuclei still present (young RBC)	Hemolysis, myeloproliferative disease–like leukemia, polycythemia vera, marrow infiltration, multiple myeloma, any severe anemia
Pappenheimer bodies	Blue granules (iron)	Sideroblastic (iron-loading) anemia, postsplenectomy

INDEX

Note: Page numbers followed by "t" indicate tables.